W9-AWP-533

Face to Face

A Guide to AIDS Counseling

Updated Version

About the Editors

James W. Dilley, MD is Associate Clinical Professor of Psychiatry at the University of California San Francisco and has been the Director of the UCSF AIDS Health Project (AHP) since 1984. Since that time, he has lectured and published widely on the psychiatric and neuropsychological aspects of HIV disease. He is the Executive Editor of *FOCUS: A Guide to AIDS Research and Counseling,* AHP's well-respected monthly review and co-author of *AIDS Law for Mental Health Professionals,* and is working on a companion anthology to *Face to Face* that will be published by AHP in the spring of 1994.

Cheri Pies, MSW, DrPH is a private consultant with an emphasis in reproductive ethics, public health, and health education practice. She has worked extensively in the past as an AIDS prevention trainer and educator and as a consultant to a variety of AIDS agencies, media projects, and research studies. She is the author of *Considering Parenthood* (Spinster's Inc., 1985), a workbook for lesbians and gay men seeking to make parenting decisions.

Michael Helquist is Director of AIDSCOM, an international HIV prevention project managed by the Academy for Educational Development in Washington, DC. He has been a consultant to the World Health Organization, the Centers for Disease Control, and various AIDS organizations. He is editor of *AIDS, Social Marketing, and Communication* (1993), Founding Editor and Editorial Consultant to *FOCUS: A Guide to AIDS Research and Counseling,* editor of *Working with AIDS: A Resource Guide for Mental Health Professionals* (AIDS Health Project, 1987), and co-editor of *AIDS: A Self Care Manual* (AIDS Project Los Angeles, 1987). He produced "The Helquist Report," a health promotion and AIDS research column in *The Advocate,* and, since 1982, has published more than 500 HIV-related articles.

Face to Face

A Guide to AIDS Counseling

Updated Version

Editors

James W. Dilley
Cheri Pies
Michael Helquist

Published by the AIDS Health Project
University of California San Francisco

Distributed to the Trade by
Celestial Arts
Berkeley, California

Copyright © 1993   AIDS Health Project   All rights reserved.

For information and comments:
AIDS Health Project
Box 0884
San Francisco, California 94143-0884

For trade discounts and returns:
Celestial Arts
P.O. Box 7327
Berkeley, CA 94707

No part of this book may be reproduced by any mechanical, photographic, or electronic process, or in the form of a phono-graphic recording, nor may it be stored in a retrieval system, transmitted, or otherwise be copied for public or private use without the written permission of the publisher.

First Printing, September 1989
Second Printing, February 1990
Updated Version, April 1993
Second Printing, September 1995

Made in the United States

Front cover painting by Daniel Phill, Copyright © 1987
"Cubis 7" oil on canvas 48" x 62"
Courtesy of Daniel Phill and the John Pence Gallery, San Francisco

Index: Sayre Van Young

Library of Congress Cataloging-in-Publication Data

Face to face.

        1. AIDS (Disease)—Patients—Counseling of.
I. Dilley, James W., 1951 -   . II. Pies, Cheri, 1949 -   . III. Helquist,
Michael, 1949 -   .   IV. AIDS Health Project.   [DNLM: 1. Acquired
Immunodeficiency Syndrome-psychology.   2. Counseling.   WD 308 F138]
RC607.A26F33   1989   362.1'969792   89-20217
ISBN 0-89087-583-9

Face to Face: A Guide to AIDS Counseling is published by the AIDS Health Project, an affiliated unit of the Langley Porter Psychiatric Institute, School of Medicine, University of California San Francisco, and was supported in part by a grant from the California State Department of Mental Health.

To all those living, working, and dying with AIDS and
to all past and present employees
of the AIDS Health Project

Acknowledgements

Many significant contributions to the overall effort of publishing this book have been made, small and large alike. To chronicle each would be impossible. Yet there are those individuals who stand out, those who saw the project through from beginning to end and those who brought special skills or knowledge to the task and without whose stamina and expertise the project would not have been completed. Special acknowledgement goes to:

Dorothy Stinnett, whose patience, keen sense of organization and unflagging attention to detail kept the editors going as she typed her way through multiple drafts.

Joseph Wilson and Leslie Samuels, whose knowledge and skill with desktop publishing allowed us to publish the book "in house."

Ron Moskowitz, who gave freely of his time and expertise, finding a publisher and distributor, and negotiating contracts with them.

Paul Quin, who helped us pay attention to the multiple design and format issues required of any book.

Daniel Phill, who spontaneously and generously offered us the use of his paintings for the cover art.

Sayre Van Young, who indexed the book during her vacation.

Glenda Rhea, Anne Pollack, and Kathy Barr whose sharp eyes and red pens kept us honest and out of trouble.

Our thanks also go to the California State Department of Mental Health, Apple Computer, Inc., and David Hinds and Paul Reed of Celestial Arts Publishing, and the many individuals who guided our thinking, including Renetia Martin, Francie Kendall, Sally Jue, Leon McKusick, Paul Ahmed, and the AIDS Health Project staff.

Finally, for all their patience and understanding, special thanks to Jorge Morales, the life partner of Jim Dilley, to Marcy Fraser, cherished companion of Cheri Pies, and to Ray Faure, Jack Stein, and Bill Woods, valued friends of Michael Helquist.

Foreword to the Updated Version

Face to Face: A Guide to AIDS Counseling was published in September 1989—the first book specifically written for mental health professionals and AIDS counselors who work on the "front lines" of the epidemic. Based largely on the experiences of University of California San Francisco AIDS Health Project (AHP) staff, *Face to Face* offers a comprehensive review of the psychosocial challenges faced by people at risk for HIV disease and provides sixteen case histories to help mental health providers develop treatment plans with HIV-related concerns in mind.

Since its first printing, *Face to Face* has enjoyed significant success and has earned a well-deserved place in the history of works dedicated to AIDS counseling. Reader feedback has been consistently positive, and AIDS educators have described the book as a "standard in the field." A third printing has become necessary to meet the increasing number of requests for information about HIV-related psychosocial concerns from Europe, Asia, and Oceania as well as the United States.

Early Intervention
Today, the landscape surrounding HIV disease and AIDS has changed. While *Face to Face* still provides a comprehensive and accurate overview of the field, we believe it is important to address in this printing some of the most significant of these changes. We have highlighted these changes by adding editor's notes and updated references to several chapters and including two articles on issues that have become increasingly important (see Appendix D, "Updates: New Issues," page 376).

The single most important change in HIV-related care has been the evolution and general acceptance of early medical intervention (see updated Appendix A: "Natural History of HIV Disease," page 358). Early intervention has shifted the attitude of the medical community and, in large measure, the communities of those historically at risk of infection, to favor antibody testing. While in the early years of the epidemic antibody testing was seen by community activists as invasive and of little use, today a consensus exists among AIDS organizations and AIDS professionals alike, that antibody testing should be promoted among those at greatest risk.

This increase in testing also brings additional challenges. Among these is the likelihood that people learn of their infection earlier in the course of the disease, they live with the information for longer periods of time, and thus further stress their capacities to cope. Despite the change in attitude toward treatment and testing, however, the issues outlined in "The Decision to Test: A Personal Choice," page 49, remain accurate.

The reason attitudes towards testing have changed, of course, is simple: knowledge of infection can lead to the use of antiviral treatment, prophylactic treatment of common opportunistic diseases, medical monitoring, alternative treatments, and ultimately increased life-span. Knowledge of serostatus has come to mean power: the power to take control and fight back. Also significant, the participation in early intervention activities has added to the psychological and social challenges outlined in "The HIV-Positive Client," page 15.

The Changing Epidemic

A second change that has occurred over the past few years is a shift in the demographics of the disease in the United States. While still primarily a disease of gay and bisexual men in their thirties and forties, HIV infection has emerged increasingly among people of color, women, and younger gay men in their teens and twenties (see "Ethnic Minorities, HIV Disease, and the Growing Underclass," page 230; "The Epidemiology of HIV among Intravenous Drug Users," page 108; and "Youth and HIV: No Immunity," page 249). This shift in the demographics means that mental health professionals will be asked more and more to provide services to an increasingly diverse group of individuals.

Third, as the number of people affected by HIV infection grows, so do the number of deaths. Because AIDS continues to be largely a disease of communities, these deaths mean that HIV-infected people have often lost significant others to the epidemic. As a result, they face the grief of multiple loss along with the other burdens of HIV disease. Furthermore, they must face this grief without the strength of support systems that were comprised of friends who have now died. This situation has mushroomed since *Face to Face* was written, and we have addressed it by including an article on multiple loss in Appendix D. Readers should also note that while this article highlights this issue among gay men, it is also a factor for intravenous drug users, women who have lost children and perhaps partners, and people of color.

Fourth, "relapse," or the strain of maintaining behavior change over time, has surfaced particularly in gay male communities where prevention efforts have spanned more than a decade. Mental health professionals working with those at risk of infection need to be aware of this phenomenon and help their clients maintain safer behaviors. Material in Appendix D also addresses this issue.

Finally, the statistics cited in *Face to Face* have been updated where possible.

The Universality of the Challenge

Reviewing the book today, we were struck not so much by what was missing from or obsolete in the book, but rather, by the degree to which the book still meets its original mission. Taken in its entirety, *Face to Face* and its clinical approaches continue to be as relevant today as they were in 1989. This speaks as much to the universality of the challenges posed by HIV disease as to the success of our efforts; responding to the epidemic remains a function of living with a life-threatening illness, making behavioral changes, coping with stigma, sickness, and disability, managing grief, and focusing on the challenges of finding meaning, value, and quality of life in the face of this illness.

We are pleased to offer this third printing of *Face to Face* in the spirit of its main theme: living with HIV disease should not be something a person faces alone. HIV-related counseling ensures that it is addressed instead face to face.

For the Editors,
James W. Dilley, MD

Foreword to the Original Version

From the very beginning, the AIDS epidemic has placed multiple demands on virtually every sector of the the health care system. Among these has been the need for health care workers in general, and mental health providers in particular, to develop expertise in the area of AIDS counseling. The AIDS Health Project (AHP) began in 1984 with the intention of providing psychological support services to those affected by the epidemic and to bring the understanding of the behavioral sciences to the task of helping people learn to cope with the threat of this disease. The Project was among the first AIDS prevention counseling programs to be developed in response to the epidemic and has been a leader in developing mental health programs for people with AIDS and those at risk ever since. In addition, the Project has championed the cause of educating the professional community about the psychosocial consequences of the epidemic.

Face to Face represents an extension of an earlier work published by the Project, *Working with AIDS: A Resource Guide for Mental Health Professionals* (UCSF AIDS Health Project, 1985). Both books reflect the experience and commitment of many dedicated individuals—mental health professionals who saw firsthand the psychological devastation of the epidemic and wanted to apply their skills and training to reduce the distress of those affected. These books were designed to convey the experience of the Project staff in providing services to those affected by a spectrum of HIV-related disorders. These two volumes, along with AHP's highly regarded monthly newsletter, *FOCUS: A Guide to AIDS Research and Counseling*, help inform and educate health care workers about the mental health and psychosocial implications of the AIDS epidemic. The need to do so only keeps growing.

The role of AIDS prevention counseling has grown exponentially over the years. The first test of the importance of counseling came with the licensing of the HIV antibody test in 1985 and the establishment of the federally funded Anonymous Testing Program. Initially conceptualized as a program wherein individuals wishing to be tested would call a telephone operator to learn their results, the AHP and others argued forcefully for the establishment of a face to face procedure of counseling that was both humane and ensured that individuals would learn how to protect themselves and others from infection. As a result, the AHP was asked to develop a model program that included a protocol for pre- and post-test counseling. The model was developed and placed in operation in June 1985 and has become the prototype used throughout California as well as the United States and abroad. The AIDS Health Project has counseled over 50,000 individuals through this program in San Francisco since that time.

Over the years, AIDS prevention counseling has been identified as an essential standard of care. Providing these services raises many difficult issues, including dealing with sexual functioning and orientation, having to face death and dying issues, confronting racism and the lack of resources available to minority communities, and accepting substance abuse as a larger part of our social fabric than anyone would like to believe. Being an AIDS counselor means struggling with these issues. It asks a great deal of those who are willing to accept its challenges.

In this book, we provide thoughtful information for counselors and mental health professionals confronted with the task of serving those coping with the threat of HIV. While it was not possible to address every issue raised in counseling those with HIV concerns, we hope the approaches described here and the discussion of the issues presented will be useful in a variety of settings. We have also tried to be supportive of those doing the work. For those interested in a more detailed analysis of the "how-to" of AIDS counseling, the reader might consider *AIDS: A Guide to Clinical Counselling* by Riva Miller and Robert Bor of the Royal Free Hospital in London (available from Science Press, 20 Chancellor's St., Hammersmith Riverside, London W6 9RL, UK). This book provides an excellent primer for someone starting out in the field who would like to read verbatim examples of how AIDS prevention counseling is performed and would serve as an excellent companion volume to *Face to Face*.

Nearly a decade has passed since HIV was identified. Thousands of health and human service workers have graduated from training programs and have gone on to provide service to their clients—many of whom have been at high risk for HIV infection or have actually been infected. The presence of this virus in our midst is disruptive and disturbing. Yet it is a fact of modern life that must be confronted. While remarkable advances have been made in understanding the basics of the disease and in treating its complications, the challenges of AIDS prevention counseling remain. We hope this book will be helpful to all those learning to confront AIDS face to face.

James W. Dilley, MD
Cheri Pies
Michael Helquist
August 10, 1989

An Introduction and Personal Perspective from a Counselor with AIDS

I welcome the publication of a quality book on AIDS counseling from two perspectives. First, as a psychologist and a Certified Rehabilitation Counselor, I know that the need to increase skills in this area continues to grow. Second, as a person with AIDS, I know firsthand how much mental health care workers must be sensitive to the many issues and feelings related to counseling people with HIV disease.

The media and epidemiologic reports about AIDS so often focus our attention on the prevention of HIV infection and the treatment of the illnesses that occur. Usually ignored or minimized are the significant emotional needs of people diagnosed to be somewhere along the continuum of HIV disease. These needs include counseling for those who are considering taking the HIV antibody test, those who have received their results, those struggling with loss of physical and mental abilities, and those individuals overcome by the recurring loss of friends and family members. *Face to Face* addresses these counseling issues with valuable information and with the solid perspective of people experienced in AIDS work.

As a therapist before the AIDS crisis began I worked extensively with hearing-impaired clients and those with various physical, emotional, and mental impairments. Many felt isolated and ostracized from the "general public." They also experienced a loss of belonging due to the many barriers that kept them from full participation in society. Many of these clients found that counseling offered them an opportunity to turn their anger and rage into empowerment—by acknowledging and respecting their own feelings and by using social and political strategies to assert their own important roles in society.

When I left my work in December 1986 due to HIV disease, I had many of the same experiences my clients often told me about.

I learned what it meant to be a disabled person, struggling with a physical condition that limited my abilities and facing a range of societal attitudes about me because I was HIV antibody positive. Not only did I face a life-threatening disease, but also a fear that certain people and groups (e.g., family, colleagues, insurance companies) would learn of my health status, reject me and possibly discriminate against me.

My therapist became the focal point through which I channeled all my conflicts, fears, and hopes. In the midst of my shock and despair, I relied on him to be nonjudgmental, informed, and forthright. He helped me recognize my special inner strength with which to face my life circumstances and to make constructive, though difficult, decisions. I cannot imagine speaking with a counselor who was not sensitive to issues related to HIV disease.

Later, as I began to adjust to living with AIDS, I reached out by giving support to others. I became involved with the organization People with AIDS, San Francisco, and with the effort to make HIV treatments more quickly available to the people who need them. As a result of my speaking engagements, the AIDS Health Project invited me to join its training program for volunteer therapists. For two years I have been a panel member, speaking about my experiences with AIDS, and I feel great satisfaction with the opportunity to help other counselors understand the diverse issues that come with doing AIDS work.

I am excited that *Face to Face* will become an integral part of this educational process and that mental health workers will have it as a resource. Whether readers have had previous experience with AIDS counseling or not, this book will enhance their ability to work with people with HIV disease. Counseling people affected by HIV can be challenging and not without its stressors. Yet in the counseling session, the trained counselors may experience from their clients the strength of the human soul in the form of courage, faith, and inner wisdom. In turn, people with HIV disease may benefit from an emotional and mental healing that cannot be measured by their physical health or appearance.

David Glassberg, MA, CRC, CIRS
San Francisco

Contents

Appendices

I
Counseling People With HIV Disease

- **The Psychological Needs of People With AIDS**
  Judy Macks, MSW, LCSW

- **The HIV-Positive Client**
  David Silven, PhD and
  Thomas J. Caldarola, MA, MFCC

- **Cross-Cultural Counseling:**
  The Extra Dimension
  Bart K. Aoki, PhD

The Psychological Needs of People With AIDS

Judy Macks, MSW, LCSW

People with AIDS (PWAs) face a complex set of psychosocial concerns and issues as they confront the reality of an AIDS diagnosis (1,2,3). Various models of psychological responses to an AIDS diagnosis, such as the situational distress model of crisis (4) and adaptive responses by stage and task (5), have been described in the literature. Interestingly, many of the psychological responses and coping mechanisms utilized by people with AIDS are similar to those used by people with illnesses such as cancer and heart disease. However, the complex sociocultural nature of AIDS and the ways in which it is transmitted set it apart from other diseases. The fact that AIDS invokes cultural taboos concerning homosexuality, sex, death, and drugs attaches a particular stigma to this illness. This stigma can play a significant role in the individual's adaptation and response to an AIDS diagnosis. Therefore, in program planning and implèmentation, attention must be paid to both the psychological as well as the sociocultural impact of AIDS on those affected by the disease.

Psychosocial Concerns

Ten psychosocial dimensions which highlight the most profound areas of concern for people with AIDS will be described in this chapter. The first six dimensions include 1) need for information, 2) need for services, 3) substance abuse, 4) neuropsychiatric complications, 5) diverse concerns of at-risk populations, and 6) search for hope. Each of these will be considered in terms of key concerns and specific interventions designed to address those concerns. The remaining four dimensions include 7) distressing feelings, 8) periods of crisis, 9) social support, and 10) medical treatment experiences.

Need for Information

People with AIDS often feel they must sort through rapidly changing medical and epidemiological information in order to make informed choices about their health care. This can be an overwhelming task given the amount of information regularly reported in the media and medical journals. Additionally, many important medical questions regarding treatment, prognosis, and the course of illness remain unanswered, often engendering confusion and anxiety. Many PWAs feel frustrated with the lack of consistent answers and the degree of uncertainty which they face. Accurate information is needed whenever possible to maximize a sense of control over their lives.

Educational interventions, whether individual or group, can be crucial for the person with AIDS. Education must be provided not only by medical professionals but also by mental health and social service professionals. In particular, information about the medical aspects of AIDS, treatment options and side effects, course of illness, transmission of HIV, infection control, and risk reduction guidelines for sexual activities and needle sharing is essential.

PWAs need access to a wide range of resources, including medical, mental health, social services, and alternative therapies. Since information and referral services are utilized frequently, printed lists of available resources can be extremely useful.

Finally, many PWAs need education about adaptive emotional responses and what they may experience emotionally throughout the course of the illness. Knowing what to expect in advance—and being reassured that certain responses are normal and extremely common—can allay fears and anxieties about becoming emotionally overwhelmed and losing control.

Need for Services

A person with AIDS may also need financial benefits, housing, transportation, legal services, and attendant care. Obtaining financial benefits quickly is essential given the sometimes rapid progression of the disease, the continued need for medical services in both inpatient and outpatient settings, and the life-threatening nature of the illness. Housing concerns may be critical for a person with AIDS who suddenly cannot meet rent or mortgage payments, who has been evicted from a living situation because of the diagnosis, who has moved to a new area seeking better medical attention, or who has had a history of unstable living arrangements. In particular, women with AIDS who also have children frequently face difficulty in securing housing.

Important and complex legal issues may confront the person with AIDS. Wills, power of attorney, custody decisions, and wishes regarding life support and funeral arrangements need to be discussed and documented legally. Legal documentation becomes particularly significant for the gay client who wishes his partner to retain power of attorney and assume other primary decision-making roles. Without this safeguard, biological families can intervene, and the PWA's wishes may not be respected.

At some point during their illness, most people with AIDS require home care services. These services can include nursing care, attendant care, practical support such as cleaning, cooking, and laundry, public health nursing, psychological intervention, and hospice care. The need for outpatient and home care services varies according to the physical state of the person with AIDS. For example, the individual discharged from the hospital may need assistance in the home only for a short period of time. However, toward the end of the illness, those wishing to remain in their homes can require 24-hour attendant care. Although the cost effectiveness of providing outpatient and home care services has been documented, these services are rarely or inadequately funded.

Substance Abuse

Issues related to AIDS and substance use raise complex challenges for the PWA and the provider alike. People with AIDS may display a wide range of substance-using behaviors. For some, substance-using behavior, including the use of alcohol, may affect health status, high-risk behaviors related to HIV transmission, psychological adaptation to the diagnosis, social support and quality of life. For others, the AIDS diagnosis is secondary to IV drug use. Health care providers can play a crucial role by accurately assessing a client's substance-using behaviors. It is only by ascertaining the degree to which an individual's alcohol or drug use currently interferes with his or her social, occupational, psychological and physical functioning that effective interventions can be initiated.

Those individuals considered to be substance abusers present additional psychosocial concerns. Because of the nature of substance abuse and the life-threatening risks associated with it, substance abusers commonly deny the threat or reality of AIDS. The stigma associated with IV drug use coupled with the alienation and exclusion from systems of health care and AIDS services increase the difficulty of coping with an AIDS diagnosis for these individuals. In addition, it is not uncommon for substance abusers to experience guilt and internal conflict regarding their substance-abusing behaviors. For those who are recovering addicts or alcoholics, the stress of dealing with a life-threatening illness and the recovery process simultaneously can be profound and requires additional support.

Substance abuse treatment programs, both residential and outpatient, must be accessible and sensitive to people with AIDS. This will require, in many communities, advocating for additional services in order to meet the needs of those individuals seeking treatment, including women with children.

Neuropsychiatric Complications in AIDS

Increasing documentation details the prevalence of neurologic complications in AIDS (6,7,8,9). Researchers estimate that 66%-90% of those diagnosed with AIDS will experience some degree of cognitive impairment (10,11,12,13). This can be caused by an opportu-nistic infection, such as toxoplasmosis or cryptococcal meningitis, or from HIV infection in the brain. PWAs experiencing organically based symptoms, such as short-term memory loss, confusion, disorientation, depressive symptoms, or behavioral changes, require a thorough assessment and recommendations for management.

Those experiencing these symptoms frequently feel terrified and extremely frustrated. For many individuals, the changes in cognition, affect and behavior wax and wane throughout the course of the illness. It is during periods of lucidity or awareness of the symptoms that people with AIDS feel the most anguish. Others may not be aware of their own difficulties with memory or concentration. However, loved ones may be acutely aware of these changes and begin to respond differently to the person with AIDS. When this happens, the person with AIDS may feel angry, frustrated or confused about the new responses received from loved ones.

The onset of organically based symptoms marks yet another point of deterioration and loss in the disease process. It is not uncommon for the person with AIDS to feel distressed and hopeless or to appear depressed at these times. PWAs need support and reassurance from providers and family members that they "are not going crazy" and that there are ways to manage and cope with these deficits.

Diverse Concerns of Populations At Risk

All people with AIDS share the common experience of profound distress associated with learning they have a life-threatening illness. In addition, the stigma of AIDS affects all diagnosed individuals. Each unique group of people with AIDS, however, has special concerns.

Services for gay and bisexual men, for example, should be sensitive to the cultural, economic, ethnic, political, and social diversity of gay communities. Intravenous drug users need the coordination of several systems including health care, substance abuse treatment, mental health and AIDS service delivery systems. For women, special needs arise, including concerns about perinatal transmission, pediatric AIDS and civil liberties issues related to reproductive freedom. People with hemophilia who also have AIDS confront the double burden of having two medical illnesses, each of which often results in discrimination. Many are angry about their exposure to HIV, feeling that it should have been prevented.

Special needs of these and other populations must be recognized and clarified. Such identification can then lead to implementation of services which are both sensitive and accessible.

Search for Hope

Maintaining hope is a primary task for every person with AIDS, and it is one of the most difficult. Feelings of hope fluctuate daily, and sources of hope differ from person to person. Maintaining hope is a daily process, not a state that is ultimately attained. The degree of hope people feel can be affected drastically by how well they feel physically, emotionally or spiritually that day. Hope is fostered when individuals feel powerful and in control of their lives to as great a degree as possible.

Hope is frequently associated with developing or maintaining spiritual and religious practices, finding new meaning in experiences, becoming politically active, altering one's attitude and way of thinking, maintaining significant social and familial ties, and being able to help others. For many individuals, hope is also tied to medical treatments or alternative healing options.

Maintaining hope often requires reframing and redefining what feels hopeful. If hope is associated with more global or long-term achievements, a person with AIDS may become frustrated and lose hope. However, if hope becomes associated with day-to-day accomplishments and events, the possibilities for feeling hopeful are greatly increased.

Denial, an important and protective defense mechanism, is integrally intertwined with maintaining hope. People with AIDS need to find ways to live on a daily basis without the constant preoccupation of threat. Constructive denial allows for much needed cognitive and emotional breaks from AIDS, and it cushions the impact and intensity of emotional reactions. When denial helps a person with AIDS attend to daily living in the fullest way possible, it contributes greatly to feelings of hope.

The most important factor in maintaining hope is active participation in decision making, health care and life activities. Ultimately, any intervention that enables a person with AIDS to feel in control serves to strengthen feelings of hope.

Distressing Feelings

Stages of grief identified by Kübler-Ross—including denial, anger, bargaining, depression and acceptance—can all be experienced by the person with AIDS. Most clients describe their feelings as a roller coaster of emotions. Mood fluctuations, compounded by a profound sense of helplessness and hopelessness, can impair social and occupational functioning.

Many people with AIDS face multiple losses throughout their illness including the loss of previous sexual behaviors and intimate relationships, disfigurement and damaged self-image, changes in employment patterns, loss of self-esteem and, possibly, the death of loved ones to AIDS. It is not uncommon, for example, for a person diagnosed with AIDS to have been deeply affected by multiple losses in the past several years.

Sociocultural factors and societal responses to AIDS seem to intensify distressing reactions of guilt, self-blame, and lowered self-esteem. These feelings may stem from unresolved conflicts about one's sexual orientation or internalized manifestations of homophobia, racism, or sexism. For example, messages in the media blaming homosexuals or prostitutes for AIDS can influence significantly an individual's feelings about the disease. Rather than identifying the virus as the cause of the illness, many feel they have caused the disease because of who they are or because of their lifestyle choices.

Some individuals feel contaminated, particularly in association with sexuality and physical and affectional closeness. While not uncommon for persons with a life-threatening illness, these feelings are complicated by the sexual transmissibility of HIV. They can be further intensified by the unnecessary and irrational procedures adopted by some providers and institutions, such as the excessive use of masks, gowns, gloves, and goggles.

People with AIDS may need assistance in adapting to the varied physiologic and psychosocial changes that occur throughout the disease and that result in a perceived loss of status. Close to 70% of those diagnosed with AIDS are 20-39 years of age; many are at the beginning or the peak of their careers. Some may be forced to abandon their source of income and social support, leading to a loss of self-esteem. Others may feel they have failed and experience disappointment that dreams, plans for the future, and intentions of creating a more stable life will not be realized. The drastic change in lifestyle faced by a young person experiencing chronic fatigue, debilitation, loss of mobility, and loss of bodily functions can result in isolation, boredom, increased substance use, inability to care for children, and depression. As the individual increasingly relies on friends, family and support systems for basic care, a loss of independent functioning contributes dramatically to the perceived loss of status.

Finally, profound fear of rejection contributes to high levels of distress for people with AIDS. Many are rejected by their biological families, by their partners, their social support systems, employers, and roommates. Whether real or anticipated, rejection and loss can affect profoundly the client's psychosocial functioning.

Periods of Crisis

Many people with AIDS need assistance at particular points of crisis that can occur throughout the progression of this disease. Such times include the initial diagnosis, the onset or recurrence of a particular symptom or infection, a sudden or profound loss of mobility, treatment failure, rejection by a family member, or the terminal stage of the illness. At these times, PWAs may be prone to psychological decompensation. People with AIDS commonly express suicidal ideation, particularly in times of crisis. Most frequently, suicidal ideation reflects an attempt to manage feelings of despair, loss of control, helplessness, and fear of future events. Previous functioning and coping skills prior to diagnosis may be the best indicators of the PWA's ability to manage periods of crisis.

Social Support

Social support is important for its ameliorative effect on depression and coping with medical illness (14,15,16). People with AIDS are better able to live with their disease when they maintain or develop ties with supportive family, friends and community members as well as with others who are living with the disease. Adequate social support systems help people with AIDS maintain feelings of hopefulness and interconnectedness with others while providing practical support and consistency in managing daily activities of living.

Because of the stigma and secrecy associated with the AIDS epidemic, maintaining or strengthening one's support system can be complex and difficult. Some people have been rejected by family members, partners, friends and co-workers. Others anticipate rejection and isolate themselves. The disclosure of an AIDS diagnosis to family or friends can precipitate a crisis which can have a positive or negative effect on the support system. Although people with AIDS and their families who reach out for support risk being rejected, most have found that many people respond with attentive caring, love, and courage.

Medical Treatments

People with AIDS face complicated decisions and barriers when they begin to consider treatment options. First, most treatment options are not readily available. Medical treatments are costly and may be financially inaccessible. Most treatment options are experimental and limited to small numbers of subjects who are able to qualify for investigational treatment protocols. A number of experimental drugs have not been tested for their efficacy but are, nevertheless, being used "underground" by people with AIDS.

The decision to embark on a particular treatment requires consideration of a number of factors. Is a particular treatment available, accessible and financially possible? Does the individual have the desire and ability to maintain a strict regimen which may be required for alternative or traditional treatment? What are the side effects? How ill is the person willing to feel from the side effects of a particular treatment?

Specific Interventions

Biopsychosocial Assessment

With a life-threatening disease involving progressive physiologic and often cognitive deterioration, a biopsychosocial assessment provides particularly useful information if gathered as baseline data. The biopsychosocial assessment provides for simultaneous attention to the relationship of the physiological, psychological and sociocultural aspects of AIDS for each individual. It is particularly important to gather data regarding pre-morbid personality, coping skills, strengths and weaknesses, risk for psychological decompensation as evidenced by psychiatric history, occupational and social functioning, family history, substance use, self-esteem, feelings about AIDS and the individual's risk factor. Attention to cultural, religious, and spiritual values and attitudes is critical, especially as they affect communication styles and contribute to feelings about homosexuality, drug use, death, dying and grief.

Crisis Intervention

Many PWAs require intervention at times of acute crisis. Interventions should be designed to enhance adaptive and integrative functioning through past and newly acquired coping skills. Whenever possible, having crisis services available in medical or community settings can provide early intervention and possibly prevent further crises.

Individual Therapy

A wide range of individual therapies can be helpful for the person with AIDS including supportive, cognitive-behavioral, and insight-oriented approaches. Individual therapy can be particularly useful in addressing the PWA's ability to manage distress and crises, deal with the ramifications of perceived loss of status, enhance support systems, maintain hopefulness, and maximize decision-making skills. Often, individual therapy offers a structure in which to recognize and resolve grief. Many clients identify individual therapy as their intervention of choice. Furthermore, for the chronically mentally disabled, individual therapy may be the primary modality in which education and support can be provided effectively.

Family Interventions

In most instances, an individual's AIDS diagnosis affects family members. This group may include a spouse or partner, children, extended family and support network, and family of origin. Family systems, despite their configuration, risk fracture as they attempt to manage the enormous impact of AIDS on their lives. Lack of social and financial support, as well as the possible presence of substance-abusing adults in the family, increases this risk of family disruption. The overall goals of family intervention include enhancing the family's ability to support each other, to focus on the immediate crisis and environmental situation, to provide substance use treatment when appropriate, to assist the grieving process, to encourage resolution of long-standing conflicts, and to decrease each member's isolation by facilitating social support outside of the family system. Practitioners may utilize case management, couples counseling, family therapy, home visits and group interventions to address these goals.

Support Groups

Group interventions have been found useful for people facing life-threatening illnesses (17,18,19). In particular, groups allow for the enhancement of social support. They provide clients with the opportunity to discuss issues and problems related to the illness with others experiencing similar problems. A range of group modalities may be useful, including cognitive behavioral groups, therapy groups, and self-help groups for clients and family members.

Group interventions alone are sufficient for many; however, others find a group setting in conjunction with individual treatment more beneficial. In some settings clients are encouraged or sometimes required to be in individual therapy while participating in a group if they are assessed to be at high risk for psychological decompensation, have characterological disorders, or are actively suicidal. Some clients may not be appropriate for group participation if it seems at the time of assessment that they would be too disruptive to the group process or would be unable to gain from the group experience.

For individuals facing life-threatening illnesses, a short-term closed-group model can provide predictable consistency, thereby enhancing the development of social support. The structure offers a contained environment which provides models for managing overwhelming feelings and provides ongoing support which can often lead to feelings of empowerment and hopefulness. The short-term nature of this model also provides the best opportunity for maintaining the integrity of a group, given the fluctuation in physical status and the high mortality rate for people with AIDS.

Long-term groups can offer increased opportunities for in-depth therapeutic intervention, but there may be difficulty in maintaining consistent group attendance due to physical illness and death of group members. Drop-in groups can be especially useful for persons requiring immediate support or for those individuals whose emotional and physical state may prevent them from making a commitment to a time-limited or ongoing closed group.

Conclusion

The care of people with AIDS requires a multi-disciplinary approach including the collaboration of medical, mental health, social service, substance abuse, and community organization professionals as well as community activists. Certainly no single service or intervention can meet the complex physiological, psychological, and sociocultural needs of the various groups of individuals with AIDS. During the early years of the AIDS epidemic, services were designed and implemented in reaction to the immediate crisis. With the recognition that this epidemic will be present for years to come, assessing community needs and program evaluation have become more important. Lessons learned from these reviews must be incorporated into a long-range plan for comprehensive service delivery systems on local, regional, and federal levels.

The psychosocial impact of this epidemic is most intensely experienced by the individual with AIDS. How well their needs are met will ultimately determine and reflect how well communities and societies cope with AIDS.

■

References

1. Tross S, Hirsch DA: Psychological distress and neuropsychological complications of HIV infection and AIDS. Am Psychologist 1988; 43(11):929-934
2. Morin SF, Malyon AK, Epstein D, et al: Meeting psychological needs in the AIDS crisis, in AIDS: A Self Care Manual. Edited by Moffatt BC, Speigel J, Parrish S, et al. The AIDS Project Los Angeles, Santa Monica, CA, IBS Press, June 1987
3. Faulstich, ME: Psychiatric aspects of AIDS. Am J Psychiatry 1987; 144:551-556
4. Nichols SE: Psychosocial reactions of persons with acquired immunodeficiency syndrome. Ann Intern Med 1985; 103:765-769
5. Dilley JW: Treatment interventions and approaches to care of patients with Acquired Immune Deficiency Syndrome, in Psychiatric Implications of Acquired Immune Deficiency Syndrome. Edited by Nichols SE and Ostrow D. Washington, D.C., American Psychiatric Press, Inc., 1984
6. Buckingham SL, Van Gorp WG: AIDS dementia complex. J Contemporary Social Work 1988; 69(6):371-375
7. Wolcott DL, Fawzy FI, Pasnau RO: Acquired Immune Deficiency Syndrome (AIDS) and Consultation-Liaison Psychiatry. Gen Hosp Psychiatry 1985; 7:280-292
8. Loewenstein RJ, Shartstein SS: Neuropsychiatric aspects of acquired immune deficiency syndrome. International J Psychiatry in Med 1983-1984; 13:255-260
9. Holland J, Tross S: The psychosocial and neuropsychiatric sequelae of the acquired immunodeficiency syndrome and related disorders. Ann Intern Med 1985; 103:760-764
10. Snider WD, Simpson DM, Nielsen S, et al: Neurological complications of acquired immune deficiency syndrome: analysis of 50 patients. Ann Neurology 1983; 14:403-418

11. Perry S, Tross S: Psychiatric problems of AIDS inpatients at the New York Hospital: preliminary report. Public Health Reports 1984; 99:200-205

12. Navia BA, Jordan BD, Price RW: The AIDS dementia complex: clinical features. Ann Neurology June 19, 1986; 517-524

13. Buckingham SL, Van Gorp WG: Essential knowledge about AIDS dementia. Social Work 1988; 33(2):112-115

14. Cavanaugh S, Clark D, Gibbons R: Diagnosing depression in the hospitalized medically ill. Psychosomatics 1983; 24:809-815

15. Moos R: Coping With Physical Illness. Edited by Moos R. New York, Plenum Medical Book Co., 1977

16. Cobb S: Social support as a moderator of life stress. Psychosomatic Med 1976; 38:300-314

17. Rahe RH, Ward HW, Hayes V: Brief group therapy in myocardial infarction rehabilitation: three to four year follow-up of a controlled trial. Psychosomatic Med 1979; 41:229-242

18. Hacket TP: The use of groups in the rehabilitation of the post-coronary patient. Advances in Cardiology 1978; 24:127-135

19. Spiegel D, Yalom ID: A support group for dying patients. International Journal of Group Psychotherapy 1978; 28:233-235

■

Judy Macks, MSW, LCSW works as an independent consultant specializing in AIDS and organization development. Formerly the Director of Training for the UCSF AIDS Health Project, she has published extensively on the psychosocial aspects of AIDS and the impact of AIDS on providers.

The HIV-Positive Client

David Silven, PhD and
Thomas J. Caldarola, MA, MFCC

The prospect of counseling clients who are HIV antibody positive understandably raises serious concerns for counselors. For some, misplaced fear of contagion from casual contact, a reluctance to talk about sexual matters, or concern about having to confront illness and potentially progressive disability in their clients are primary considerations. For others, deciding to work with this population involves, at least in part, a desire to confront directly one's own discomfort and anxiety about AIDS. For most, there is confusion stemming from the lack of clear professional guidelines or precedents about how to work with this client population.

Fears of inadequacy and of becoming overwhelmed or "burned out" are also common sources of hesitation. Anticipating the client's high level of need and urgent wish for change can add to the anxiety of counselors who may already question their capacity to be helpful. In this chapter, common themes raised by those who are seropositive will be discussed, and practical suggestions for ways to intervene will be offered.

Common Themes

Clients who seek counseling after receiving an antibody positive test result often do so with acute subjective distress, including anxiety, depression, and feeling "out of control." They may also complain of a general lack of feeling, or a sense of being "numb." More commonly, clients report some combination of these feelings and describe feeling emotionally overwhelmed on the one hand, and emotionally numbed on the other. In essence, they report their experience as that of being on an emotional "roller coaster." They speak freely of a sense of imminent doom and describe the terror of sickness and dying, of becoming physically disabled and unable to care for themselves, and of ending their lives by suicide. Clients often question whether they can continue with their day-to-day routines and responsibilities, including jobs and social relationships. Hopelessness is a prominent theme; and a fundamental question, often not stated explicitly, is whether to prepare to die or to continue directing one's focus toward living.

Uncertainty is another recurring theme for seropositive individuals and is seen in virtually all areas of their lives. Uncertainty about the future is prominent as individuals ask themselves about their ability to cope with the knowledge of their antibody status and wonder about the future state of their health. They are beset by a host of questions about how to handle this new information; they may question plans for the future, current life situations, and personal relationships. Additionally, there is often uncertainty about how to avoid infecting others, how best to take care of their own health, whether to continue in a job or relationship which is stressful or displeasing, and whether to disclose their antibody status and to whom. These many levels of uncertainty often leave seropositive clients feeling they have lost control of their lives, a source of anxiety in itself.

Managing Stress

Seropositive individuals frequently experience a range of stressful physical and psychological symptoms. Depression and anxiety are common and can result in sleep and appetite disturbances, fatigue, loss or a lessening of sexual desire and sexual impotence. Panic attacks, phobic reactions, impaired concentration, and ruminative thinking which involves a repeated and frequent focus on the hopelessness of the situation or about the unfairness of an "early death," are also common and can complicate the client's ability to cope. The stress experienced is often intensified by the perception that stress must be lowered to protect an immune system already compromised by HIV.

Self-Esteem and Social Isolation

Lowered self-esteem and a sense of social isolation are frequent reactions of those who learn they are infected with HIV. The seropositive client's self-esteem is challenged on several fronts. First, self-image as an essentially healthy being is challenged and may be temporarily or permanently lost. Seropositive individuals often describe feeling contaminated or dirty. These feelings parallel negative societal messages about HIV. Secondly, because most individuals became infected through sexual contact, many feel they have done something wrong or have been a "bad" person who has gotten what was "deserved."

For the gay man who is seropositive, learning his antibody status may trigger internalized homophobia as he "blames" his being infected on his homosexuality. The gay man who has chosen to remain largely "in the closet" often struggles with his own homophobia when he contemplates disclosing his antibody status to others. Alternatively, the gay man who is comfortable being open about his sexual preference may be distressed at the prospect of his HIV disclosure as he remembers painful coming-out experiences from the past.

Heterosexuals may feel they are now unable or unwilling to take the risk of parenting since they may infect their unborn child or their sexual partner or may not live to see their children grow to adulthood. This potential loss of the ability to have children can have profound effects on feelings of self-worth.

Isolation is another significant issue for seropositive clients. Most seropositive people encounter social isolation to some degree as they experience or fear rejection from large segments of society, including friends, family, and co-workers. Urban areas with large visible gay populations offer readily available opportunities for peer support to gay seropositive men, yet these services are often missing for heterosexuals. It is very common for women or heterosexual men who are seropositive to be entirely alone with the information. They are likely to know few if any heterosexuals with HIV. Smaller communities may offer no support services to either gay or heterosexual seropositives. Consequently, both groups typically feel a mixture of sadness and disappointment as well as anger at the lack of responsiveness of others in the community.

Gay men who live in high AIDS incidence areas often experience an additional source of isolation due to the loss of significant others in their lives who have died of AIDS. They mourn both the loss of companionship as well as the support of now-deceased friends. In areas with large gay populations, clients often describe their environment as a "war zone" because so many have died and because their community has been so hard hit by illness and death.

Decision-Making Dilemmas

Seropositive individuals confront a host of decisions that need to be made, and frequently there is a feeling that these decisions need to be made immediately. For example, seropositives often question how deeply to immerse themselves in thinking and learning about HIV. Many worry that they will miss something important to their health if they don't stay current about ongoing developments with treatments for HIV. On the other hand, many feel overwhelmed by trying to keep up with the ever-increasing volume of AIDS information and tend to avoid reading about HIV or attending informational meetings.

The progressively grim statistics concerning the course of HIV infection leaves many seropositives caught between their desire to know as much as possible about HIV and their fear of becoming immobilized by bad news. Those who are monitored closely by their physicians (See Appendix A: "Natural History of HIV Disease") are frequently buffeted by changes in their laboratory values which are an ever-present reminder of the slow deterioration of their immune systems.

A related issue is whether to pursue medical treatments. This decision frequently touches on the issues of denial versus confrontation. Deciding to pursue treatment is tantamount to acknowledging directly that a serious situation exists. Yet some seropositive individuals come to view the decision to pursue treatment as a means of regaining a sense of control and mastery in their situation. (See Editor's Notes, page 25.)

Another important decision often faced is whether to remain in a job or other life pursuit that is less than satisfying. The question is often related to the ambiguity about medical prognosis ("How much longer will I be healthy enough to remain active?"). Some clients worry that they may not live much longer and that they cannot afford to waste time unhappily. Or, they worry that remaining in a stressful situation will only hasten the progression of illness because of the suspected negative effects of stress. Others may feel trapped in their present work situation because of the real fear of the loss of health insurance were they to leave their job, or they fear being rejected for new jobs because of their antibody status.

Disclosure

Most seropositive clients question whether to tell others about their status. At a time when they are already feeling emotionally fragile and isolated because of their antibody status, they fear further alienation from those who they imagine might reject or abandon them. Fears of discrimination at one's job as well as in other areas of life, including housing, health insurance and medical care, are reinforced by the abundance of anecdotes concerning mistreatment of seropositive individuals in the general community. The client may have already experienced adverse consequences from disclosing this information to others, thus heightening the level of ambivalence about further disclosure.

Concern about damaging one's interpersonal relationships is often a focus of discussion related to disclosure. Many worry that an early disclosure might drive a potential partner away before an opportunity for commitment to the relationship has had time to develop. On the other hand, delaying disclosure might be unfair to the other if in fact a commitment has already begun. Despite these misgivings, there is often a simultaneous sense of urgency to use whatever time is remaining in life to develop supportive and satisfying connections with others. Consequently, clients feel a heightened need to make the most of their time, leading them to re-examine their existing relationships and to consider withdrawing from those that do not seem fulfilling. For those already in a primary relationship, the antibody status and health of the partner can be an additional source of strain and potential isolation in the relationship.

Counseling Interventions

There is a role for both individual and group counseling in the care of people who are seropositive. Some clients use the knowledge of their antibody status as an impetus to seek in-depth kinds of counseling or psychotherapy.

Individual Counseling

For the client who has recently tested positive and who is experiencing a flurry of disturbing and disorganizing emotions, some form of crisis intervention is frequently indicated. This means providing support and validation for feelings, mobilizing resources for coping, providing educational information, and helping the client solve pressing situational demands.

The counselor can begin by normalizing the emotional "roller coaster" that is so commonly experienced. As many of these clients have had little if any opportunity to discuss their situation with anyone in depth, the experience of feeling heard, understood, and accepted by an empathic counselor who actively listens can be a significant starting point. Learning that many others have experienced similarly severe reactions to testing positive can also help reduce their sense of isolation.

The counselor should be sensitive to the possibility of suicidal ideation, though actual hospitalization of suicidal seropositive clients has been a rare occurrence in our experience. A useful initial response to such thinking is to normalize it by pointing out its commonness among seropositive individuals. When present, suicidal ideation should be monitored carefully and can be expected to subside as the client begins to adjust to the information and the sense of immediate crisis is alleviated.

Helping the client mobilize resources for coping can include identifying internal strengths and abilities as well as external supports, such as friends, family and social services in the community. Identifying effective coping strategies in past situations of high stress or crisis is also useful. Teaching coping strategies ranging from controlled breathing, visualization, or taking a walk in the park, to problem-solving approaches such as "taking things one step at a time," ensuring frequent rest periods or "mini vacations," and remembering other successes in coping with past adversity have all been used effectively.

Friends and family supports of the HIV-infected individual are often underutilized. This is sometimes due to the fear of a negative reaction or to the fear of overburdening them. The counselor can assist the client in realistically considering which friends or family members would be the most likely to respond in an accepting and supportive way. Referral to support services in the community, such as emotional support groups and AIDS informational centers, contributes further to the sense of having a range of resources from which to draw.

Finally, reminding clients who have recently tested seropositive that the emotional turmoil of the initial adjustment period is time limited can be extremely useful. It is critical that the counselor provide an opportunity for clients to recognize, express, and eventually accept the full range of feelings that are sparked by facing a life-threatening illness. When negative thinking predominates, however, and clients become trapped in a downward spiral of hopelessness, cognitive techniques can help to replace some of the dysfunctional thought patterns with more constructive ways of thinking. For example, the client who repeatedly thinks "I'm going to die, so I may as well give up," or "I am unacceptable now that I am seropositive," or "I'm failing if I don't keep a positive outlook *all* the time," can be helped to examine the dysfunctional nature of these thoughts and to recognize the potential for changing them. Efforts at altering dysfunctional thinking can contribute to a growing sense of being able to manage life's problems.

Role playing can provide a forum for the counselor to model effective communication and for clients to practice disclosing information about their antibody status in a supportive setting. Often the client's difficulty in disclosing antibody status to friends or family reflects problems with self-esteem associated with being seropositive. In such cases, it may be important to first address negative feelings before encouraging disclosure to others.

It is not uncommon for the counselor to encounter a client who is continuing to engage in potentially self-destructive behaviors such as drug or alcohol abuse, unsafe sexual activity, or poor daily health habits involving diet, sleep patterns, and so on. If these behaviors do not change during the course of counseling, firm but gentle confrontation of the behaviors is indicated. Sometimes providing information about the potential harm of such behaviors to an already vulnerable immune system can help motivate the client who is poorly informed. For others, being pushed to seriously examine such behaviors requires confronting the potential seriousness of the situation in a way which may have been avoided out of fear. Such fears need to be explored with careful timing and in an atmosphere of respect. In other cases, unhealthy patterns such as those involving diet, sleep, or substance use may reflect an underlying depression or crippling anxiety which inhibits the client from making important changes. In such instances, a referral to a psychiatrist for evaluation for medication should be made.

Throughout the work, it is important that the counselor convey a sense of hope and encouragement while at the same time allowing space for experiencing emotional pain and loss. The re-examination of basic values and priorities in life that many seropositive clients undergo can be framed by the counselor as an opportunity to enrich the quality of life. Giving examples of others in similar circumstances who have managed to survive and make progress over time can be inspiring. Supporting the client's right to engage in "healthy" denial—i.e., regularly taking breaks from dealing with emotionally painful realities—is also key. Finally, the value of using humor in a compassionate way cannot be overemphasized.

The crisis which most clients experience following an antibody-positive test result can be a source not only of emotional turmoil, but also of motivation for making significant positive changes. The confrontation with potential mortality brought on by the test result leads many individuals to a commitment to work through troubling personal issues which they previously lacked ability or motivation to address effectively. For such clients, a decision to enter longer-term psychotherapy may be an important step towards turning the crisis into a profoundly life-enhancing transition.

Group Counseling

Groups for seropositive individuals can be a tremendous help in reducing social isolation, bolstering coping resources and capacities, and providing support for making positive changes. The average client feels a sense of relief when hearing others describe similar experiences and emotional reactions to a seropositive test result. Many benefit from involvement in such a group concurrently with individual counseling, whereas others prefer only one or the other.

In some communities, there may be a variety of types of groups from which to choose, including short-term topic-focused groups, drop-in support groups, longer-term closed-membership support groups, and psychotherapy groups. Short-term topic-focused groups, often lasting six to ten weeks, tend to have the dual objective of offering interpersonal support as well as information relevant to coping with HIV and protecting oneself and others. Drop-in support groups generally offer the individual an opportunity for group support and educational information without having to make an ongoing commitment to attend. Such groups are particularly helpful to those with limited experience in therapeutic groups and who want to "test the water" before considering a longer-term support group. More traditional psychotherapy groups for individuals who are seropositive can offer an opportunity for greater depth of exploration of personal and interpersonal concerns than is possible in short-term groups. Choosing among these types of groups is usually handled best in a process which actively involves the client.

Countertransference Issues

A common feeling among counselors of seropositive clients is frustration over the tremendous ambiguity that must be faced in the work—ambiguity about HIV disease itself and about the appropriate therapeutic approaches to take. This ambiguity parallels that which the client is facing, and it can sometimes increase the empathy felt for the client. For the counselor who has particular difficulty accepting ambiguity, the risk of inhibiting the client's freedom to recognize and experience the uncertainty of the situation must be carefully watched. Often clients resist the painful awareness of this uncertainty by looking for clear-cut, instant answers. The counselor may, in turn, feel pulled to respond to this pressure by offering "quick fix" solutions.

Related to this is the pressure many counselors feel to become experts on HIV as a way to be better prepared to provide answers whenever the client expresses confusion. This can lead to spending considerable time and energy attempting to stay current about research and treatment issues. The overwhelming amount of information available places such a counselor at risk of becoming seriously overextended, and the counselor must be willing to accept his or her own limitations, including the limits of one's expertise. Often a critical element of being informed about HIV involves knowing which people or organizations to refer clients to for further information.

Counselors who are in so-called "high-risk groups" themselves face special countertransference issues. The gay counselor, for instance, is likely to have been directly affected in his personal life by the epidemic, thereby increasing the likelihood of a strong identification with the client's situation. This can both enhance and detract from the counseling relationship. It can serve to increase the capacity for empathy and the degree to which the counselor is perceived by the client as a potentially understanding helping figure. It can also lead to the counselor's becoming overinvested in the work, and eventually unable to continue the work because of emotional strain.

The antibody status of the counselor introduces another level of complexity. It is not uncommon for the seronegative counselor, whether gay or straight, to experience feelings of "survivor guilt." These feelings may be fueled by the client's anger and resentment at those who do not share the burden of being HIV infected. The antibody status of the counselor has implications in terms of perceived capacity for empathy and level of personal investment which are similar to those described above in the discussion about counselors' personal risk. An additional issue the counselor must consider is whether, and under which circumstances, to disclose his antibody status to clients who ask.

Finally, it is important that counselors be aware of the personal meanings attached to HIV as a result of their own past experiences, so as to decrease the likelihood of imposing these meanings on clients. For example, counselors who have friends recently deceased or ill with HIV disease may attribute more significance to a client's recent seropositive test result than the client is prepared to hear. It is also important that counselors carefully examine their own attitudes and assumptions regarding such issues as homosexuality, IV drug use, and death and dying, so as to minimize the chances of colluding unconsciously with any self-ridicule their clients may feel in terms of these issues.

Summary

Seropositive clients must cope with a range of painful emotions which typically accompany an antibody-positive test result, including fear, grief, anger, and sadness. They must also deal with decision making in a number of important areas of their lives in which there is a great deal of uncertainty. This includes uncertainty about medical prognosis, health care options, how best to spend one's time and plan for the future, and how to share the news of being seropositive with others. Furthermore, social ostracism and the strain often imposed by the antibody-positive test result on important interpersonal relationships may contribute to a plummeting self-esteem.

Counselors who choose to work with this client population face a demanding set of challenges. They must struggle with a high degree of ambiguity and with the difficulty of identifying clear guidelines for how to address the client's needs and how to measure progress. The counselor's own attitudes and anxieties about AIDS and HIV must also be channeled in a healthy direction. Ultimately the counselor, along with the client, has an opportunity to develop an enhanced sense of purpose and meaning within a situation of crisis proportions.

■

Editor's Notes

Page 18. Since this chapter was written, medical research has shown that early treatment with antiviral medications and drugs to prevent the development of HIV-related conditions is safe and effective (see Appendix A: "Natural History of HIV Disease," page 358). In the past, the lack of consensus about how to approach HIV infection placed additional burdens on patients, who were often left with the anxiety of not knowing whether their doctors' advice was the "best" way to approach treatment (see Baker et al below). Early treatment also means that people with HIV must accommodate a routine of taking prescribed medications, keeping doctors' appointments, and submitting to regular immune system monitoring, which may evoke emotional reactions in response to changes in measures of immune system health.

Updated References

Baker RA, Moulton JM, Tighe J: Early Care for HIV Disease (2nd ed.). San Francisco, CA: San Francisco AIDS Foundation, 1992

■

David Silven, PhD, is a clinical psychologist and Coordinator of the Prevention/Education Program of the UCSF AIDS Health Project in San Francisco. Thomas J. Caldarola, MA, MFCC, is a counselor for the AIDS Prevention Project and AIDS Family Project at Operation Concern and a member of the UCSF Prevention Team, UCSF AIDS Health Project in San Francisco.

■

Cross-Cultural Counseling:
The Extra Dimension

Bart K. Aoki, PhD

    To be effective counselors for persons with HIV disease, it is important to consider how cultural influences shape individuals' responses to illness and their health-seeking behaviors in general. With its emphasis on treating a tangible "disease," the Western medical model often overlooks "illness," or the individual's perception of what is wrong, in favor of sophisticated technical procedures and laboratory tests. This lack of attention to the individual's experience of the problem is particularly noticeable to the individual who is culturally different.

    AIDS, like other illnesses, presents cultural variables that affect all aspects of being ill. These include the labeling of symptoms, how or when pain or other symptoms are communicated and to whom, and the notion of what doctors and helpers are expected to do. In some cultures, the subjective experience of pain triggers help-seeking behaviors, while in others, help is sought only when symptoms intensify to the point of interfering with daily responsibilities. Moreover, while many of those affected by HIV disease may appear highly acculturated or westernized, otherwise submerged cultural reactions and needs can surface intensely when faced by this life-threatening illness. At the same time, a helper's assumptions based solely upon a person's surname or skin color can prove alienating to an individual who is the product of generations of American life. This chapter addresses these and other cultural influences on the individual's adaptation to a diagnosis of HIV disease. (See Editor's Notes, page 33.) A case example is presented to begin the discussion.

Gordon

Gordon is a 37-year-old gay Chinese American who is employed as a school teacher. He is the only son of parents who were born and raised in Hong Kong. His parents now live in San Francisco near his two older sisters, both of whom are married. Gordon has been homosexually active for several years and though his homosexuality is not known at school, his family is aware of his lifestyle. His family never discusses the fact that Gordon is gay, and Gordon has chosen not to discuss it with them. However, he has been ill for several months; recently his physician told him that he has AIDS. His family physician is also Chinese, and he relays this information to Gordon's parents without consulting Gordon. He refers Gordon to a psycho-therapist when Gordon expresses despair over his situation and thinks of killing himself.

When thinking of Gordon and the pressures upon him, cultural issues in understanding and helping him adjust to his diagnosis become paramount. Since he is both Asian and a gay man, Gordon has already had to struggle with the process of reconciling his sexuality with a culture which values the family as the most important social unit throughout life. In the context of his culture, he knows that his behavior reflects upon the entire family and that his primary obligation, especially as a son, is to perpetuate the family through his marriage and children. When Chinese parents produce a child who is homosexual, the implication is that they have failed in their role and that the son is rejecting both the importance of his family and his culture. In effect, especially if the child is the only son, his homosexuality is seen as the death of the family.

To cope with his conflicting personal priorities, Gordon has always observed his family obligations to the fullest, short of agreeing to marriage. At the same time he also exercised a great deal of personal freedom in his social and sexual life. The fact that he now has AIDS, however, has caused culturally specific, but previously dormant, issues to surface. While his parents and sisters continue to express worry and concern about his condition, including admonishing him to take care of his health, they also reacted initially with feelings of shame over the community's awareness of his illness and his related but undisclosed homosexuality.

While many Asian cultures carry the expectation that families will care for those who are seriously ill, HIV disease challenges some of these values. In certain Asian cultures the death of a child prior to the parents' is seen as the epitome of an affront to family obligations. In spiritual terms, it is the worst of omens. In addition to his own personal fears in facing a life-threatening illness, Gordon has had to confront what would be the ultimate failure: leaving this earth before his parents. Even more difficult for Gordon was his awareness of the practice adhered to by many traditional Chinese families that forbids parents from visiting an ailing child and from attending an offspring's funeral because of its tainted quality. Although Gordon's family had visited him in the hospital, his awareness of these practices led to acute fear of his being left alone in the end stages of his illness. Gordon wants and needs his family's support, yet he also understands their need to withdraw from him.

Other Views of Dependency

It is typical of Western cultures to place a high value on individual autonomy and independence and to equate these attributes with ideal maturity and health. Faced with an AIDS diagnosis, many are concerned with the potential for prolonged dependency upon others. This concern often triggers enormous discomfort, but it can also serve to spur efforts towards maintaining an independent and self-sufficient level of functioning.

In those who are culturally different, dependency often carries with it a different meaning. In some cultures lifelong mutual and family interdependence may be valued more highly than self-reliance and autonomy. For the Asian or Hispanic person with HIV disease, for example, a ready reliance upon health providers or specific family members to the exclusion of more independent activity could be consistent with cultural patterns and actually serve to enhance that individual's sense of well-being. Given past experiences with hostile and discriminatory institutions, many who belong to minority cultures may limit comfortable expressions of vulnerability and dependence to family and friends who have proven their trustworthiness over years of shared experience. Additionally, the absence of true peer support networks outside major urban settings for those who are both gay and culturally different may have forced lifelong patterns of highly selective dependence. This response adds another dimension to the AIDS patient's reactions to this illness by people with AIDS. Thus, the experience of dependence and expressions of dependency are often at opposing extremes in culturally different people with AIDS.

Questions of Control

Related to dependency is the issue of control, an issue that has clear cultural roots; it arises in various forms when an individual is faced with AIDS. HIV disease raises the fear that control over one's life and bodily functions may be lost eventually, and it naturally triggers often desperate efforts to maintain or regain a sense of control.

Western cultures value exercising control over external forces, including life's events and other people. Consistent with this is the high value placed upon self-assertion in American culture. Seen as highly positive is a community's organizing to influence the system in proactive ways and patients asserting their needs to health care workers to ensure timely and effective care. These are culturally supported attempts to gain control within an inherently out-of-control situation.

Other cultures, however, place primary value upon the exercise of control over the self as opposed to the imposition of control over others. Persons influenced by these values may prefer internal psychological coping mechanisms, particularly the control of thoughts and emotions and may actually view self-assertion as selfish or foolish. This culturally bound pattern has a host of implications for the PWA. For example, patients who prefer to maintain self-control in the face of highly emotional issues may, despite being frustrated or confused, be hesitant to assert themselves with providers. Others, having experienced years of powerlessness in an oppressive system, may prefer as protection to devote their psychological resources to self-control rather than risking exposure to further frustration. Thus what may appear to be an attitude of fatalism among those with AIDS who are culturally different can have multiple underpinnings related to culture as well as to minority group status.

Culturally Sensitive Interventions

As counselors become more aware of the cultural influences on the behavior of people with HIV disease, they will want to determine how to respond in an appropriate and useful way.

First, cultural knowledge of the client is crucial at the very beginning of the relationship to gain rapport and build trust with the person with AIDS. It is based upon a recognition and an affirmation of the cultural fabric of that person's life. In particular what needs to be understood is the specific culture's expectations of a credible helper. In Latin cultures, for example, personal informality combined with an explicitly demonstrated respect is critical to build initial trust. Black clients may be more comfortable in relation to someone of a different background when a level of respectful distance is maintained and combined with inherent acknowledgement of equality in the relationship. Asian Americans are often most comfortable when a respectful indirectness of communication is an inherent part of the relationship.

For persons with AIDS of certain cultures the credibility of the helper is facilitated by an overt expression of authority, while in others the authority and expertise is implicit and serves as a backdrop for familiar and personal interactions. This process also applies when discussing issues of sexuality and drug abuse with someone of a different culture. For certain individuals an authoritative approach that couches the issue within a technical or medical framework is most comfortable. On the other hand, when familiarity in the helping relationship is more the norm, then "talking dirty" and the use of slang terms for sex and drugs may enhance the counselor's credibility and ultimate impact on the patient. Thus the helper's expertise itself will be expressed differently in the process of establishing the credibility and rapport necessary for an ongoing relationship. In Gordon's case it was necessary for the therapist to display respect for his need to maintain control over his emotions by not prodding him to discuss directly issues that would overwhelm and embarrass him. At the same time the therapist needed to communicate an implicit understanding of the value of self-control, of the legitimacy of his family concerns above and beyond his friends, and of his discomfort and distrust of the counseling process.

Once the counseling relationship itself has begun to develop in a culturally consistent way, knowledge of the specific culture can be directly applied to learn more about the meaning and evolution of the person's current difficulty. The emotional struggles in confronting and dealing with any one of the myriad issues triggered by HIV infection develops within its cultural context. It is necessary to make sense of the pain or conflict and to be able to articulate it with the PWA in a way that is most tangible and useful. In defining the problem, the person with AIDS may focus on not being able to cope, on falling apart every day and feeling unable to be with friends or at work without emotionally breaking down. Another may feel depressed about having perceived a basic loss of respect within the community or having lost a warm sense of family as a result of a father's detachment when learning of the AIDS diagnosis. Some individuals experience most urgently a re-emergence of feelings of self-hatred triggered by an increased separation and alienation from society. For many patients anger will be directed at the caregiver due to immediate frustrations and to years of feeling oppressed for their cultural and sexual differences. In Gordon's case, he could not articulate the central issues at first. Because of this, the therapist had to understand that one of the more immediate concerns for him was to control some of his emotions so that he could think clearly and feel better about being with others, particularly his family. The broader concern that developed was Gordon's sense of having failed his family by his sexuality, his illness, and his impending death.

Helping the person with AIDS occurs within the context of a culturally meaningful understanding of the problem at hand. This includes helping the client to recognize dormant cultural strengths and to apply these to the current situation. Cultural strengths often available to the person with AIDS include promoting family relatedness and loyalty, and the re-establishing of a specific pattern of autonomy and self-sufficiency often lost in the midst of the multiple crises of AIDS. The helper's role is to appreciate and revive these strengths. Once this has occurred through the ongoing relationship, specific challenges to attempt new or modified strategies for living and coping are met with renewed motivation and hope for success. In relation to Gordon, the therapist was able to help him re-interpret his pain as being an indication of his importance in the family and to encourage him to remember and re-activate his old methods of belonging and contributing to the well-being of family members. For Gordon this also meant drawing up his will in a way that considered everyone and spending more time with his parents in their daily activities.

Summary

Working therapeutically with those who are HIV infected poses multiple challenges, especially cross-cultural ones, as the epidemic continues to spread. The preceding discussion has focused on some of the issues all counselors will need to understand and to apply to be most effective with people with AIDS.

First, they should understand that the experience of "illness" is influenced culturally. People of color carry varying levels of cultural influences depending upon their level of acculturation and life experiences in American society. They express and understand pain differently and may rely upon helpers in different ways depending upon some of these variables.

Second, it is important for caregivers to appreciate that cultural factors influence significantly two broad psychological issues inherent in reaction to a life-threatening illness: dependency and control. While self-reliance and assertiveness might be expected as a Western ideal, individuals of different cultures and those whose historical experience includes generations of discrimination and racism will feel and express dependency and control in widely varying ways.

Finally, with an acknowledgement and awareness of some of the cultural dynamics at play, the counselor can apply this understanding to facilitate the entire therapeutic process. Establishing rapport through the building of the helper's credibility in cultural terms, defining a mutual and culturally relevant understanding of the current issues, and ultimately facilitating change through enhancing rather than negating cultural strengths are specific phases of this helping process.

Given the highly emotional nature of the work with people with HIV disease, it is unavoidable at times that the counselor's own cultural biases will emerge and rigidify in reaction to the threat confronting the patient. This can make the work both highly challenging and rewarding as one's own cultural dynamics are illuminated through the process. The necessity of increased consultation and supervision will be felt more keenly with these clients. In certain situations it may be necessary to refer to a counselor who may be more prepared to respond to the individual's needs; recognizing the wisdom of such a move is an inherent part of the challenge of working with the HIV infected. More counselors will be able to meet these challenges with care and professionalism when they achieve a better understanding of the relevance of these specific cultural issues to the therapeutic process.

■

Further Readings

Jue S: Identifying and meeting the needs of minority clients with AIDS, in Responding to AIDS: Psychosocial Initiatives. Silver Spring, Maryland, National Association of Social Workers, Inc., 1987

Sue S, Zane N: The role of culture and cultural techniques in psychotherapy: a critique and reformulation. Am Psychologist 1987; 42:37-45

Weisz JR, Rothbaum FM, Blackburn TC: Standing out and standing in: the psychology of control in America and Japan. Am Psychologist 1984; 39:955-969

Editor's Notes

Page 26. Because of the rising prevalence of HIV infection among people of color (see "Ethnic Minorities, HIV Disease and the Growing Underclass," page 230), the issues raised by cross-cultural counseling become increasingly important. While relatively little has been written about this complex issue, the articles below from our monthly newsletter are among the best we've seen.

Updated References

Marin B: Hispanic culture: effects on prevention and care. FOCUS: A Guide to AIDS Research and Counseling 1991; 6(4):1-2

de la Vega E: Homosexuality and bisexualtiy among Latino men. FOCUS: A Guide to AIDS Research and Counseling. 1989; 4(7):3

McLaurin P, Juzang I: Reaching the hip-hop generation. FOCUS: A Guide to AIDS Research and Counseling. 1993; 8(3):1-4

■

Bart K. Aoki, PhD, is a clinical psychologist currently affiliated with the Asian American Recovery Services, Inc., and St. Mary's Hospital in San Francisco.

II
HIV Counseling: Tests and Treatments

■

T-Cell Tests and Other Laboratory Mysteries

John F. Krowka, PhD

Laboratory tests of blood samples are an essential part of the medical evaluations of HIV. The nature of these tests and their uses, however, are a great mystery to many people. Knowledge of immunological tests is useful for health care providers and patients to make informed decisions regarding the progression of HIV-related disease and the use of experimental drug treatments. As most HIV-infected individuals are expected to develop symptoms of HIV disease or AIDS in the natural course of HIV infection (1), many people are eager to "do something" to at least slow this destructive process. Thus, an understanding of laboratory test results can help HIV-infected people to confront realistically their prognosis and lead them to become active participants in monitoring the effects of various treatments or behavioral changes on their health.

This review describes laboratory tests used to determine the effects of HIV on the immune system and to detect the presence of virus in the blood. In particular, "helper T-cell" and "HIV p24 antigen" tests, commonly used as predictors of the progression of HIV disease, are discussed in detail. Because many HIV-infected individuals are currently taking the antiviral drug zidovudine, also known as azidothymidine (AZT or Retrovir), a brief description of the laboratory tests to detect common harmful side effects of zidovudine therapy is also presented.

Although laboratory tests are important, they are not a substitute for physical examinations and evaluations of a patient's medical history. Health care providers may find that discussions with patients about laboratory test results and symptoms of disease are useful for reassuring patients that they are receiving the best available strategies for the management of HIV infections.

Detection of HIV's Effects on the Immune System

Many abnormalities in the immune systems of HIV-infected individuals have been detected by laboratory analysis (1,4). A list of tests commonly used to detect these abnormalities is shown in Table 1. Although many types of abnormalities have been associated with progression from initial infection by HIV to AIDS, a reduction in the number of helper T-cells is the most frequently used prognostic indicator in individuals at risk for developing AIDS. The testing of helper T-cells at multiple time points is useful particularly in detecting trends and rates of immunological deterioration. However, helper T-cell tests are not a surrogate marker for HIV infection, and results of these tests should be evaluated with regard to the patient's HIV antibody status.

HIV Antibody Tests

HIV infection stimulates the immune system to produce antibodies that specifically bind to this virus in a lock-and-key fashion. The sensitive and specific tests to detect antibodies to HIV (5) are an essential first step in the medical evaluation of individuals who may be HIV infected. Some recently infected individuals may not yet produce any detectable antibodies to HIV (5,6). Therefore, two negative HIV antibody tests, at least six months apart without exposure to HIV in between, are usually adequate to show that an individual has not been infected by HIV. In some patients with advanced AIDS, antibodies to HIV may not be detectable. In situations where a negative HIV antibody test is questionable, the p24 antigen test or other methods to detect HIV may be warranted. Although decreasing levels of antibodies to some HIV proteins have been associated with disease progression (7), these tests are rarely used as prognostic indicators for individual patients.

Helper T-Cell Tests

All individuals who test positive for the presence of antibodies to HIV should have helper T-cell tests performed to evaluate the degree of damage done to their immune system by HIV. It is essential that health care providers understand these tests, especially since the tests are being used more frequently.

The immune system has evolved to eliminate microorganisms and cancer cells from the body. This defense system is composed

Table 1. *Laboratory Tests Commonly Used in the Evaluation of HIV-infected Patients*

Lab Test	Normal Range in HIV Antibody-Negative Adults	Units of Measure in Blood[a]	Values Indicating A Need for Medical Intervention
Total Lymphocytes	1,108 - 4,338	cells/mm^3	NE[d]
Total T-Cells	754 - 2,720	cells/mm^3	NE
Helper (CD4+) T-Cells	459 - 1,535	cells/mm^3	<200[e]
Suppressor & Cytotoxic (CD8+) T-Cells	229 - 990	cells/mm^3	NE
CD4+/CD8+ Ratio	1.1 - 2.8	—	NE
Beta$_2$ Microglobulin (β_2M)	<2,000	μg/ml	NE
Platelets	140,000 - 450,000	Platelets/mm^3	<20,000 - 50,000
HIV Antigen[b]	<33	U/ml	>33 andincreasing over time
White Blood Count	3,940 - 9,230	cells/mm^3	NE
Total Neutrophils	1,800 - 6,800	cells/mm^3	<500
Hemoglobin[c]	13.5 - 17.5	g/dl	< 8 - 10
Hematocrit[c]	41 - 53	%	<24 - 30
Creatine Phosphokinase (CPK)	32 - 267	U/L	>534

a. mm^3=cubic millimeter; μg/ml=micrograms/milliliter (ml); g/dl=grams/100 ml; U/ml=Units/ml; U/L=Units/Liter
b. Levels of HIV antigen <33 U/ml are considered to be negative.
c. Normal values for adult females may be slightly lower.
d. NE = Not established.
e. Individuals with less than 200 helper T-cells per mm^3 are at very high risk for developing AIDS and may be eligible to receive the anti-viral drug zidovudine. It is **not** known, however, if zidovudine is beneficial to asymptomatic or mildly symptomatic HIV-infected individuals.

of various types of white blood cells (WBC) that have distinct and coordinated functions. In each cubic millimeter (mm^3) of blood there are an average of 6100 WBC. About 38% of the WBC are called lymphocytes. The lymphocytes that mature in the thymus gland before being released into the blood are called T-lymphocytes or more simply, T-cells. The total numbers of WBC, lymphocytes, and T-cells are relatively normal in many HIV-infected individuals. Some patients with AIDS, however, may have low numbers of one or more of these cell types. Tests to determine the levels of these three cell types are generally not useful as indicators of HIV-related disease progression, but they are often performed to provide a more complete picture of the immune systems of HIV-infected individuals.

One type of T-cell, the helper T-cell (also called a CD4 or T4 cell), provides essential support for many of the other cell types in the immune system. Although helper T-cells usually do not eliminate directly foreign microorganisms and cancer cells from the body, without their assistance many of the other cell types of the immune system are unable to function effectively.

Helper T-cells are a major target for infection by HIV. Located on the outer surface of HIV is an "envelope" protein that physically complements the structure of the CD4 protein, found on the surface of helper T-cells and some other cell types. These two proteins fit together in a lock-and-key fashion, allowing HIV to select and infect these cells. After binding to the CD4 surface molecules, HIV enters these cells and can multiply. The newly produced HIV then enters other helper T-cells and progressively destroys them.

Helper T-cells constitute only about one-sixth of all WBC, but their destruction by HIV cripples the defense capabilities of the entire immune system. The CD4 protein is also found on the surface of another type of WBC, called a monocyte or macrophage. Infection of monocytes by HIV may also play an important role in the immunological impairment of HIV-infected individuals (2). Unlike helper T-cells, monocytes are not readily destroyed by HIV infection. As a result they may serve as a reservoir for the spread of the virus throughout the body.

Lab tests have been developed during the last decade to count helper T-cells in blood samples. In these tests, the red blood cells are removed and the remaining white blood cells are mixed with a fluorescent antibody that binds to the CD4 protein on helper T-cells and monocytes. Under ultraviolet light, these labelled cells glow brightly and can be counted using a microscope or by semi-automated methods. The larger labelled monocytes can be distinguished from helper T-cells by their size. Variations in the details of this procedure may cause differences in test results from different labs. It is, therefore, important to have helper T-cell tests performed in the same lab every six months, or more frequently if disease symptoms are progressing, to assure accurate monitoring.

Approximately 500 to 1500 helper T-cells per cubic millimeter (mm^3) of blood constitutes the range in people who have not been infected by HIV (Table 1). The immune system is dynamic, adapting the numbers of some cell types in its arsenal to meet the body's ever-changing defensive needs. As a result, the numbers of helper T-cells and other cell types may vary somewhat from day to day, even in HIV antibody-negative individuals.

Studies of gay men in San Francisco show that there are subnormal numbers of helper T-cells (less than $500/mm^3$) in many HIV-infected individuals (1,4). The numbers of helper T-cells in HIV-infected infants and hemophilia patients vary greatly, but they are also often below $500/mm^3$. In both gay men and hemophilia patients, the numbers of helper T-cells are associated with the duration of time since exposure to HIV (1,8). In San Francisco, HIV-infected gay men lost a median of 107 helper T-cells per mm^3 each year (1). Individual patients, however, may vary greatly from this rate of decline. The loss of helper T-cells may also be more rapid in the later stages of HIV infection. In general, most HIV-infected individuals suffer severe losses of their helper T-cells with the passage of time (1,2,3,4).

The decline in helper T-cells is associated often with HIV-related symptoms of disease in infected individuals. These symptoms include persistent fevers, fatigue, weight loss, oral lesions, diarrhea, neurologic manifestations and other symptoms of ARC. These symptoms occur in HIV-infected individuals with 400 or more helper T-cells/mm^3 but are more frequently observed in persons with lower numbers of helper T-cells. Many studies indicate that HIV-infected people with less than 400 helper T-cells per mm^3 are very likely to develop AIDS (1,3,4,8). Studies in San

Francisco showed that the three-year actuarial progression rate to AIDS was 87% in HIV-infected gay males with less than 200 helper cells per mm^3. It was 47% in those individuals with 200 to 400 helpers/mm^3 and 16% in HIV-infected gay men who had more than 400 helpers/mm^3. Higher helper T-cell counts are also associated with longer survival times in patients already diagnosed with AIDS.

The association of low numbers of helper T-cells and the appearance of HIV-related disease symptoms is not absolute. Some asymptomatic HIV-infected individuals have less than 200 helpers/mm^3. In these cases, helper T-cells are useful to detect individuals at very high risk of developing AIDS who would not be identified by their medical history or physical examinations. In rare cases, some persons with AIDS may have more than 500 helpers/mm^3. Thus, a relatively high helper T-cell count in an HIV-infected individual does not guarantee the absence of physical symptoms of HIV-related disease. The progressive decline of helper T-cell numbers in many HIV-infected individuals cannot be charted along a straight line. Many "peaks and valleys" are seen in helper T-cell counts during the years after HIV infection. However, as time progresses, the peaks become fewer and the helper T-cell counts tend to remain low and continue to decline.

Given the grim prognosis of the natural course of HIV infection, many individuals are seeking treatments to intervene in this process. The antiviral drug zidovudine is now available by prescription at the discretion of the patient's physician. It is generally recommended for patients diagnosed with AIDS and HIV-infected individuals with less than 200 helper T-cells/mm^3. Its use in asymptomatic or mildly symptomatic HIV-infected individuals with helper T-cell counts above 200/mm^3 is controversial. Although zidovudine has proven to be useful in some patients with AIDS or symptomatic HIV infection (9,10), it is not known if this drug, or any other, can slow down the progression to AIDS in HIV-infected asymptomatic individuals. Studies are currently in progress to address this issue. Individuals with helper T-cell counts between 200 and 400 cells/mm^3 may benefit from the additional information provided by the p24 HIV antigen test or the beta$_2$ microglobulin test as discussed later in this review.

Helper T-cell tests may be useful as an indicator of immunological improvements in HIV-infected individuals, including those who are receiving zidovudine or other therapies. In some individuals who are taking zidovudine, slight or variable improvements in the numbers of helper cells may make it difficult to evaluate the possible benefits from this drug on an individual patient basis. If helper T-cell levels continue to decline in the presence of increasing symptoms of HIV infection or side effects of drug therapies, modifications of these therapeutic procedures may be indicated. Although helper T-cell levels may continue to decline in patients taking zidovudine, it is impossible to know if this decrease would be more rapid without this drug. Therefore, a decreasing CD4 level is not generally a sufficient reason for stopping zidovudine therapy in individual patients.

Other Tests to Measure the Effects of HIV

Cytotoxic (killer) and suppressor T-cells are two types of T-lymphocytes that characteristically have the CD8 protein but not the CD4 protein on their surface. Cytotoxic T-cells are important in killing virus-infected cells and cancer cells. Suppressor T-cells are important regulators of other cells of the immune system; they attempt to prevent the generation of immune responses that might harm healthy cells. Using methods similar to those described above for helper T-cells, elevated levels ($>1000/mm^3$) of CD8 cells (mainly killer T-cells) are detected frequently in HIV-infected individuals (1,2,3,4,8). These elevated levels of CD8 cells are associated with increased risk of developing AIDS in HIV-infected individuals (1,3). However, elevated levels of CD8 cells are also seen in HIV antibody-negative individuals who have been infected recently with other viruses such as influenza or cytomegalovirus (CMV) (2). Thus, elevated levels of CD8 cells are not associated uniquely with HIV infections and are not used generally as indicators of HIV-related disease progression.

The ratio of CD4 and CD8 cells (Table 1) is characteristically, but not uniquely, subnormal in HIV-infected individuals. Therefore, this ratio is also not useful as a prognostic indicator. Increases in the levels of CD8 cells, however, may indicate an adaptive response of an immune system attempting to control viral infections. In AIDS these adaptive responses are ineffective, and the levels of CD8 cells may fall to normal or subnormal levels (Table 1).

A relatively small protein called beta$_2$microglobulin (β_2M) is a normal component of cells and is present in the serum of healthy HIV antibody-negative individuals at concentrations below 2000 micrograms per milliliter (μg/ml) (1,11). Elevated levels of β_2M (more than 3000 μg/ml) are observed in HIV-infected individuals and are strongly associated with progression to AIDS in this group (1). Thus, β_2M tests may be useful indicators of immunological deterioration in HIV-infected individuals. Elevated levels of β_2M also occur in HIV antibody-negative individuals with some types of cancer, autoimmune diseases, and in acute infections by CMV or other viruses (1,11).

Platelets are fragments of cells called megakaryocytes that play an important role in blood clotting. In healthy HIV antibody-negative adults, there are between 140,000 and 450,000 platelets in each mm^3 of blood (Table 1). In some HIV-infected individuals, the concentration of platelets may become dangerously low (less than 20,000-50,000/mm^3). These individuals with very low platelet counts are susceptible to bleeding disorders, and therapy with zidovudine or other drugs may be necessary.

Functional abnormalities have been detected in helper T-cells, CD8 cells, and monocytes of infected individuals (2). Defects in both helper and cytotoxic functions have been reported. These tests are useful in basic research studies to elucidate the mechanisms by which HIV destroys the immune system. They are not, however, generally used to detect HIV-related disease progression in individual patients.

Detection of HIV

In addition to the previously described tests to detect HIV's effects on the immune system, other tests have been developed to detect directly this virus or its components in blood, other body fluids or tissues. These tests may be useful to detect HIV-infected individuals with questionable HIV antibody test results or in basic research.

HIV p24 Antigen Tests

The p24 antigen test has been developed to detect a specific protein subunit of HIV. Physicians currently use it in the evaluation of HIV-infected patients (12,13). The molecular weight of this HIV protein is approximately 24,000 times the weight of a hydrogen atom (24 kilodaltons) and accordingly is called p24. "Antigen" denotes its ability to be recognized as foreign by the immune system. The p24 antigen is also called a "core" protein because it is located in the interior of HIV, surrounding the genetic information contained in ribonucleic acid (RNA). The test to detect the p24 antigen is a modification of the ELISA used to detect antibodies to HIV. This p24 test is called a "sandwich" ELISA or "antigen capture" assay because the p24 of HIV is trapped between two antibody molecules.

The p24 antigen test does not directly measure infectious HIV, but it is a relatively good index of the HIV burden being carried by infected individuals. This sensitive test can detect as little as 30 to 50 picograms (trillionths of a gram) of p24 antigen in a milliliter of serum. Values in this test that are less than 33 Units/ml indicate that HIV p24 is not detectable (Table 1).

Within weeks after HIV infection, p24 antigen is often detected in blood (13). After acute HIV infection, p24 may remain detectable in blood for months (12,13). The persistence or reappearance of the p24 antigen is associated with clinical, immunological, and neurological deterioration (1,12,13). HIV-infected individuals who have detectable p24 antigen in serum are at a higher risk for developing AIDS than those who do not. HIV-infected asymptomatic individuals with normal numbers of helper T-cells often do not have detectable p24 antigen in their serum (14). Therefore, the p24 antigen test is frequently not useful in this group. More than one-third of the patients already diagnosed with AIDS or those who are symptomatic may also have undetectable levels of HIV antigen in their serum (15). This finding indicates that a "negative" p24 antigen test result is not a guarantee of good health.

Individuals with physical symptoms of HIV-related disease or helper T-cell counts less than $400/mm^3$ may benefit from the additional information provided by the p24 antigen and $ß_2M$ tests. Elevated or increasing levels of p24 antigen in conjunction with other laboratory or clinical evidence of an advancing HIV infection may indicate a need for the initiation or modification of therapy. The p24 antigen test may also be useful for infants or accidentally exposed health care workers in whom HIV infection is suspected.

Other Tests to Detect HIV

Laboratory tests to detect HIV by the presence of its characteristic "reverse transcriptase" (RT) protein were important in identifying the role of this virus in AIDS. Using sensitive culture techniques, HIV can be detected in the blood of more than 80% of healthy HIV-infected individuals by the RT test (16). The labor-intensive and expensive RT test to detect HIV in blood or cultures of body fluids is currently important in basic research studies, but it is used rarely in the medical evaluation of HIV-infected individuals. In infants born to HIV-infected mothers and after accidental exposure of health care workers, RT tests and the culture of blood cells may be used to determine infection.

Other tests have been developed to detect the genetic information of HIV contained in its nucleic acid (5,17). A powerful new assay, called the polymerase chain reaction (PCR) test, is able to detect very small amounts of HIV's nucleic acid by an amplification technique (17). Additional research is needed to standardize the PCR test and to reduce the incidence of "false positive" results. The PCR test may be useful in basic research and in screening HIV-infected donors at blood banks, but it is used rarely to evaluate HIV-infected patients. In cases where the results of HIV antibody or p24 antigen tests are inconclusive, the PCR test may provide useful additional information.

Detection of Common Side Effects of AZT

The toxic effects of zidovudine on the production of red blood cells can result in the development of anemia in some HIV-infected individuals (9,10). Laboratory tests to determine the concentration of hemoglobin, a protein in red blood cells that transports oxygen to the tissues, are regularly performed on blood samples from patients taking zidovudine to detect anemia. In adult males the normal range of hemoglobin concentration in blood is between 13.5 and 17.5 grams in each deciliter (100 milliliters) of blood (Table 1). The normal range in adult females is slightly lower.

The hematocrit test is also used to detect anemia. Blood is composed of red blood cells, WBC, platelets and plasma. The hematocrit test measures the percentage of blood volume occupied by the red cells. The normal range for the hematocrit test is between 41% and 53% (Table 1). In patients taking zidovudine, hemoglobin levels below 8 to 10 grams per deciliter or hematocrit levels below 24% to 30% indicate a need for a dose reduction or discontinuance of zidovudine therapy. Blood transfusions may also be administered as therapy for anemia.

Another side effect of zidovudine seen in some HIV-infected individuals is neutropenia (9,10), a reduction in the production of a type of WBC called neutrophils. The normal range of neutrophils is between 1800 and 6800 cells/mm^3. When neutrophil levels fall below 500/mm^3, dose reduction or discontinuance of zidovudine is recommended. Additional precautions to prevent infections in patients with neutropenia may also be warranted. Neutropenia or anemia may also occur in AIDS patients who are not taking zidovudine. In general, these tests to detect neutropenia and anemia are necessary to compare the harmful side effects of zidovudine to its benefits.

Some HIV-infected patients may develop muscle pain or weakness as a side effect of long-term zidovudine therapy. Laboratory tests to determine the levels of an enzyme called creatine phosphokinase (CPK) are performed commonly on blood samples from patients experiencing these symptoms. The range of CPK concentrations in the sera of healthy HIV antibody-negative individuals is between 32 and 267 units/liter. If the CPK concentration is greater than 534 u/l, discontinuance of zidovudine therapy may be recommended.

Conclusion

Laboratory analysis can provide useful information regarding the progression of HIV infection and the benefits or harmful side effects of experimental drugs. All individuals who have a positive HIV antibody test should also have their helper T-cells counted to evaluate the approximate degree of damage done to their immune system by HIV. Some HIV-infected individuals may also benefit from p24 antigen or ß$_2$M tests. Patients taking zidovudine need to have hemoglobin and hematocrit tests as well as neutrophil counts performed in order to detect anemia, neutropenia or other side effects of this drug. All of these tests are most useful when evaluated by a knowledgeable physician in the context of other symptoms of HIV infection.

Some HIV-infected individuals with relatively normal laboratory values and without physical symptoms of HIV-related disease may wish to wait until more is known about experimental therapies before beginning treatment. Other individuals with documented decreasing helper T-cell counts and increasing levels of HIV p24 antigen or β_2M may wish to begin treatment. Counseling is advisable for HIV-infected individuals to understand the results of these tests and to use them to their advantage in monitoring disease progression.

■

References

1. Moss AR, Bacchetti P, Osmond D, et al: Seropositivity for HIV and the development of AIDS or AIDS related condition: three year follow up of the San Francisco General Hospital cohort. Br Med J 1988; 296:745-750

2. Krowka JF, Moody DJ, Stites DP: Immunological effects of HIV infection, in AIDS: Pathogenesis and Treatment. Edited by Levy JA. New York, Marcel Dekker, 1988; 257-303

3. Polk BF, Fox R, Brookmeyer R, et al: Predictors of the acquired immunodeficiency syndrome developing in a cohort of seropositive homosexual men. N Eng J Med 1988; 316:61-66

4. Lang W, Anderson RE, Perkins H, et al: Clinical, immunologic, and serologic findings in men at risk for acquired immunodeficiency syndrome. JAMA 1987; 257:326-330

5. Jackson JB, Balfour HH: Practical diagnostic testing for human immunodeficiency virus. Clin Micro Rev 1988; 1:124-138

6. Ranki A, Krohn M, Allain JP, et al: Long latency precedes overt seroconversion in sexually transmitted human-immunodeficiency-virus infection. Lancet 1987; ii:589-593

7. McDougal JS, Kennedy MS, Nicholson JK, et al: Antibody response to human immunodeficiency virus in homosexual men. J Clin Invest 1987; 80:316-324

8. Ragni MV, Winkelstein A, Kingsley L, et al: 1986 update of seroprevalence, seroconversion, AIDS incidence, and immunologic correlates of HIV infection in patients with hemophilia A and B. Blood 1987; 70:786-790

9. Creagh-Kirk T, Doi P, Andrews E et al: Survival experience among patients with AIDS receiving zidovudine. JAMA 1988; 260:3009-3015

10. Dournon E, Rozenbaum W, Michon C, et al: Effects of zidovudine in 365 consecutive patients with AIDS or AIDS-related complex. Lancet 1988; ii:1297-1302

11. Burkes RL, Sherrod AE, Stewart ML, et al: Serum beta-2-microglobulin levels in homosexual men with AIDS and with persistent, generalized lymphadenopathy. Cancer 1986; 57:2190-2192

12. Goudsmit J, Paul DA, Lange JM, et al: Expression of human immunodeficiency virus antigen (HIV-Ag) in serum and cerebrospinal fluid during acute and chronic infection. Lancet 1986; i:177-181

13. Allain JP, Laurian Y, Paul DA, et al: Long-term evaluation of HIV antigen and antibodies to p24 and gp41 in patients with hemophilia. N Engl J Med 1987; 317:1114-1121

14. Krowka JF, Stites DP, Moss AR, et al: Interrelations of lymphocyte subset values, human immunodeficiency virus antibodies and HIV antigen levels of homosexual males in San Francisco. Diagnostic and Clin Immunol 1988; 5:381-387

15. Krowka JF, Stites D, Mills J, et al: Effects of interleukin 2 and large envelope glycoprotein (gp120) of human immunodeficiency virus (HIV) on lymphocyte proliferative responses to cytomegalovirus. Clin Exp Immunol 1988; 72:179-185

16. Ulrich PP, Busch MP, El-Beik T, et al: Assessment of human immunodeficiency virus expression in cocultures of peripheral blood mononuclear cells from healthy seropositive subjects. J Med Virol 1988; 25:1-10

17. Kwok S, Mack DH, Mullis KB, et al: Identification of human immunodeficiency virus sequences by using in vitro enzymatic amplification and oligomer cleavage detection. J Virol 1987; 61:1690-1694

■

John F. Krowka, PhD, is a Research Immunologist at SyStemix in Palo Alto, California.

The Decision to Test: A Personal Choice

Robert Marks and Peter B. Goldblum, PhD, MPH

The debate surrounding HIV antibody testing continues to surprise many health practitioners who are trained to use every means available, even imperfect ones, to diagnose and treat illness. But as with so many facets of the AIDS epidemic, antibody testing raises new issues and draws attention to old questions of quality and value of life. At the same time, the debate challenges the assumption that complete knowledge about one's health is an appropriate goal no matter what the cost, and brings into sharp focus the politics of health care.

Beyond the public policy debate, which has occupied the attention of politicians, doctors, and AIDS activists, is the personal decision individuals must make about taking the test. In this context, the debate becomes distant, and its issues become identified as the range of factors a person may consider in the process of reaching this decision. Chief among these factors are those related to medical treatment and legal protection.

On one hand is the societal notion that all disease be treated aggressively and that medical practice requires physicians to know as much as they can about their patients' health in order to facilitate treatment. On the other hand is the concern that since HIV infection and the people it most commonly affects are objects of stigma, antibody test results may identify them and expose them to discrimination. While each of these beliefs is compelling, the decision is actually far more complex and encompasses psychological, behavioral and financial components, in addition to legal and medical ones.

As researchers develop new tests to detect HIV infection and as medical professionals bolster arguments that early detection may lead to more effective treatment, community-based AIDS organizations have shifted from their previously neutral stances and have begun to urge those at risk to take the test. Nonetheless, individuals may still be overwhelmed by the factors that influence the testing decision. This chapter will define the range of issues that may emerge as factors in an individual's decision making, and will suggest approaches for shepherding clients through this process.

This chapter does not deal with issues of test accuracy. Although researchers are confident that a positive antibody test result accurately detects HIV infection, recent studies have shown that a negative result does not necessarily mean that a person is uninfected. These studies have shown that, in rare cases, antibodies to HIV may not form for up to 42 months after infection (1,2) and that people who test positive for HIV antibody may revert to seronegativity over 2.5 years (3). (See Editor's Notes, page 58.)

Experts emphasize that most people will develop antibodies within six months of infection, or at least within one year, and will remain seropositive. Still, a few who test negative may, in fact, be infected, and it is unclear how many people fall into this category. This information raises a number of questions regarding behavior that need to be explored as a component of post-test counseling.

Legal Issues

The most commonly endorsed protections against HIV-related discrimination are the use of anonymous testing and the passage of laws to prohibit discrimination in employment, housing, insurance coverage and medical care against people who are HIV infected or even suspected of being infected. Some suggest that people avoid testing altogether unless their results are anonymous or until such antidiscrimination protections have been adopted.

But even these measures have shortcomings. In order for test results to be useful in facilitating treatment, individuals must be prepared to sacrifice anonymity and disclose this information to their doctors, and potentially to permit their doctors to disclose this information to other medical personnel. Individuals grappling with the testing decision must evaluate the cost to themselves of this disclosure, and weigh this cost against the potential benefits of treatment.

There are positive legal ramifications of HIV antibody testing. Knowledge of HIV antibody status may influence an individual's choices about travel, employment, and medical and life insurance coverage. For instance, when considering a change in employment or insurance coverage, one might hesitate to make this change if HIV antibody positive. Employers, insurance companies, the military and the government may be able to force a person to be tested and may use test results in discriminatory ways. It may be in one's best interest to seek anonymous or even confidential testing, before being forced to test, in an attempt to maintain control over this information.

Medical Treatment Issues

Individuals must consider the life-threatening impact of HIV infection and the potential access to treatment that antibody testing offers. During the past few years, there have been advances in the development and use of new treatments, ranging from FDA-approved drugs such as AZT, aerosolized pentamidine and gancyclovir, to experimental drugs that may be effective in fighting HIV directly, enhancing immunity, and treating opportunistic conditions. Confirmation of HIV infection may lead to the initiation of these interventions at an early stage in the infection, even before the occurrence of symptoms.

Many physicians believe that early intervention may be crucial to successful long-term treatment of HIV infection. For instance, there are good data showing that among people with AIDS, early treatment with AZT leads to longer survival. There is also clear evidence that among HIV-infected patients with falling T-cell counts, the use of aerosolized pentamidine prophylaxis leads to a decreased incidence of *Pneumocystis carinii* pneumonia.

The greatest inducement to test originates from the inspiration of these proven benefits and the potential benefits of promising treatments, combined with what amounts to an instinctive reaction among those infected to do what is best for their bodies. In addition, the latest theories about treatment suggest that the negative side effects of any particular drug may be alleviated by using several drugs in concert (4, 5).

For those who are concerned about the drawbacks of antibody testing, but who are committed to pursuing treatment, other screening methods—using markers such as T-cells, p24 antigen and beta$_2$ microglobulin—may be preferable. These markers, when surveyed over time, are correlated more closely than HIV antibody with the development of symptoms and are therefore more helpful in making treatment decisions. Most physicians, however, will suggest that an antibody test precede these other tests.

Although the medical evidence provides hope that HIV may soon become the "chronic manageable condition" that the most optimistic commentators have predicted, the data are not conclusive. For example, there is no firm evidence that AZT is effective in asymptomatic people with HIV infection. Also, AZT-resistant strains of HIV have been isolated in patients who have undergone long-term treatment with the drug, and some researchers are concerned that drug resistance may be a problem with many HIV-inhibiting treatments. Finally, roughly 20 to 25 percent of people with HIV infection cannot tolerate the toxic effects of AZT. Individuals may consider such potential treatment issues when facing the decision of whether or not to test. (See Editor's Notes, page 58.)

Economic Issues

While advances in early treatment offer good reasons to be tested, the expense of most of these treatments may become an obstacle to many HIV-infected people, particularly people of color, women, and people who have lost their jobs and medical insurance. Comprehensive and continuing quality health care is crucial to the success of treatment and this, too, is expensive.

For people who cannot afford AIDS treatments, or even routine health care, the exhortation to be tested may be meaningless at best, and unethical at worst. People in this group should ask, how can I pursue early treatment and receive quality health care with limited resources? If the options for treatment are minimal and the decision to test is based primarily on the availability of treatment, a person may want to reconsider the decision to test.

In addition, individuals who decide to test may want to consider delaying testing until they are employed, and have secured health insurance and housing. The psychological and legal ramifications of a positive test result may be easier to manage if a person has a stable source of income and health insurance.

Behavioral Issues

HIV antibody test results will have a behavioral and psychological effect on people who test. In terms of behavior, individuals should ask themselves, how does a test result, either positive or negative, affect my health care habits, life-style choices, and sexual behaviors?

A positive test result may encourage individuals to make changes in their lives—in terms of diet, exercise, drug and alcohol use, and level of stress—that may enhance their immunity and diminish the effects of HIV infection. For example, seropositive people may be more motivated to cease drug, alcohol or cigarette use, to improve their eating habits to ensure their diets include all necessary nutrients, and to exercise to improve bodily functioning, maintain mobility, bolster mood and reduce stress. A positive result may induce individuals to seek the advice of physicians about medical conditions they have ignored in the past, but which may need particular attention because of the effects of HIV infection.

Testing also provides crucial behavioral information for those who must make informed decisions about having children. Test results also are important for those women with a history of risk who must make decisions about breast-feeding and infant inoculation.

Finally, several studies have shown that a positive test result may motivate individuals who continue to engage in high-risk behaviors to practice safer sex and cease needle sharing during intravenous drug use. Other studies, however, have shown that knowledge of antibody status does not affect the rate of reported high-risk sexual activity (6). Furthermore, knowledge of negative test results may offer individuals a false sense of security and be perceived as permission to engage in unsafe behaviors.

Psychological Issues

Ultimately, psychological issues have the greatest effect on a person's decision to test, and some say that these should be the most important factors. In the early days of testing, before there was clarity about either transmission or treatment of HIV, the decision to test was made largely on the basis of whether it "felt" better to know or not to know. While issues of treatment, discrimination, money and behavior mitigate and inform any feelings people may have about whether or not they want to know their serostatus, feelings are still central to the decision. A person's ability to live with his feelings and reactions after making a decision must be central in discussing the debate.

For many, the most compelling reason to be tested is simply to know because, for them, not knowing may be psychologically detrimental. For others, even those who would and could afford to take advantage of early treatment, the most compelling reason to avoid testing is to avoid the knowledge of infection and the devastating psychological effect it may have on them.

Both situations may bring on a series of negative psychological reactions: nightmares, sleep disturbance, depression, suicidal behavior, anger, self-imposed withdrawal and social ostracism, relationship problems, and a preoccupation with unrelated or minor bodily symptoms. For many people, the process of deciding to test or not to test may be an exploration of how much they need to know the results and how they will react to a positive test result. At the same time, some may decide that knowledge, even of infection, will reduce anxiety of uncertainty and, in the case of a positive test result, may offer people a sense of control over their destinies.

There can also be negative psychological effects for those whose tests are negative. These negative effects may be similar to the effects of surviving holocausts, wars and natural disasters. Some who are seronegative, particularly members of communities embroiled in fighting the epidemic, may feel guilt and isolation from the community. For many, there may be psychological safety in the uncertainty of knowledge of serostatus.

Finally, it is important for people who test to have support during the time they struggle with the decision to test and following testing and the receipt of results. For some individuals, the decision to test or not to test may jeopardize this support. If rejected for their decisions, where do these people turn at a time when they may need this support most, at a time when they may be most vulnerable to depression, guilt and suicidal feelings? Should a person who anticipates losing this support not be tested?

In the end, those who are choosing psychological health over potential physical health must confront these questions and contradictions. The resolution is not a blanket statement to that person,

"You should be tested, therefore be tested," but instead, "What do you need to think about and resolve in order that testing, and possibly treatment, become viable options?"

The Counseling Process

For some, it may be difficult to untangle the range of thoughts and feelings related to the testing decision. Counseling may help individuals approach this process coherently and with confidence. The primary role of the counselor is to help define the complex areas of concern to clients. In preparation for providing counseling, mental health professionals must first become familiar with the testing options, what the tests measure, their levels of accuracy, the potential benefits and risks of knowing one is infected, and the cross-cultural and regional variations that affect factors related to testing. It is important for counselors to maintain current information about these testing issues.

As with any counseling issue, it is crucial for counselors to limit their input regarding their own beliefs about whether to test, in order to allow clients to come to their own decisions. While misinformation about the tests must be corrected, clients' choices must be interpreted in terms of their values and problem-solving styles.

The testing decision should be seen as an integral part of an overall medical and health promotion plan, and should be accompanied by information about community resources for those who test positive. Counselors should help clients develop a healthy skepticism of the rhetoric that surrounds the testing debate and assist them in identifying the biases that most educators, counselors, physicians and AIDS activists bring to a discussion of an individual's decision to test.

The first step in helping someone decide whether to be tested is to determine that person's level of risk for HIV infection. This can be accomplished by evaluating, for the past 15 years, that individual's history of unprotected sexual activity, IV drug use, and blood transfusion or use of blood products. Next, the counselor should assess the individual's knowledge of HIV and its transmission and, if necessary, should offer basic AIDS education prior to a discussion of testing. Finally, the counselor should discuss testing and how it fits into an overall strategy for AIDS prevention and HIV infection management.

If a decision to test is made, counselors should help their clients prepare for emotional reactions to both positive and negative results, for disclosing the results and for using the results to motivate healthy behavior. Counselors should be prepared to encourage those clients who choose not to test to re-evaluate their decision periodically as social, medical, economic and psychological criteria change.

Benefit-Risk Analysis

Clinicians should take responsibility for providing a structure for facilitating the decision-making process. One process that has been used successfully is based on a "Benefit-Risk" analysis. The client lists the potential benefits and risks of being tested. Each benefit is scrutinized to determine whether it can be accomplished using a method other than antibody testing that does not have a concomitant risk. For example, if an individual wants to be tested to lower the risk of contracting HIV through sexual contact, an understanding that following safer sex guidelines is recommended for those who test negative as well as for those who test positive may obviate the person's need to take the test.

If a greater overall benefit has been established to proceed with the test, a careful review of risks must be undertaken. In some cases perceived risks are in fact groundless, such as the fear that someone could obtain a person's name from an anonymous test site. Other risks can be reduced somewhat by careful planning. For example, an individual's concern about how his or her partner will handle test results may be resolved through discussions with the partner prior to testing.

After a careful examination of the benefits and risks, the final choice—an educated decision—is the client's alone to make. If a client chooses to take the test, the counselor and client should explore the client's feelings and thoughts in preparation for receiving test results. For example, clients can be encouraged to imagine their reactions to being given a positive result. Despite planning and discussion in the practice sessions, however, unexpected reactions may occur. Therefore, a plan for additional emotional support during the time prior to getting test results should be discussed. In addition, clients would benefit from counseling sessions scheduled shortly after receiving the test results so that they have a chance to fully discuss their reactions. Such follow-up counseling may help clients incorporate test results into a plan of action.

Conclusion

Individuals considering HIV antibody testing must be encouraged to make informed choices about testing and to explore all of the factors involved; they should be prompted to question the assertions of both those who advocate and those who discourage testing. Ultimately, both advocates and opponents must accept that the decision to test is an individual one, a personal choice.

Individuals faced with the decision, and counselors and educators charged with facilitating the decision process, should view the test as one of several approaches to cope with the epidemic, rather than a goal in and of itself. This process must go beyond the testing debate and even AIDS itself, to help clients see testing in the context of broader issues such as their beliefs about medicine, death, quality of life, religion and spirituality, and politics. Counselors must acknowledge the incredible challenge HIV infection poses, recognize the variety of ways people will choose to meet this challenge, and encourage clients to deal with this challenge in the way that is most beneficial given the individual's psychological state, spiritual beliefs, medical condition, financial outlook, and social support.

All of us must be prepared to accept an individual's choice to avoid treatment as a spiritual choice, not of death versus life, but of one way of living versus another. The choice to live without the effects of potentially toxic treatments and a strict regimen of drug intake, doctor's appointments and tests, is a legitimate one even if it means an individual may be choosing to die an earlier death. At the same time, the choice to use unproven and potentially toxic treatments must be recognized as a reflection of a fundamental will to live.

Testing is a means to an end, and people who face the decision to test should be clear what ends they are seeking. Counselors can facilitate this process by defining testing as one of many tools that may help clients make life decisions in the face of the epidemic.

■

References

1. Loche M, Mach B: Identification of HIV-infected seronegative individuals by a direct diagnostic test based on hybridization to amplified viral DNA. Lancet 1988; ii: 418-421
2. Imagawa DT, Lee MH, Wolinsky SM, et al: Human immunodeficiency virus type 1 infection in homosexual men who remain seronegative for prolonged periods. N Eng J Med 1989; 320(22):1458-1462
3. Farzadegan H, Polis MA, Wolinsky SM, et al: Loss of human immunodeficiency virus type 1 (HIV-1) antibodies with evidence of viral infection in asymptomatic homosexual men. Ann Intern Med 1988; 108:785-790
4. Broder S: Anti-retroviral therapy: past, present and future. Plenary speech at the V International AIDS Conference, Montreal, June 1989
5. Merigan TC, Skowron G, Bozzette SA, et al: Circulating p24 antigen levels and responses to dideoxycytidine in human immunodeficiency virus (HIV) infections: phase I and phase II study. Ann Intern Med 1989; 110:189-194
6. Ostrow DG, Joseph J, Kessler R. et al: Disclosure of HIV antibody status: behavioral and mental health correlates. AIDS Education and Prevention 1989; 1(1):1-11

Editor's Notes

Page 50. In 1991, David Imagawa—whose study found the 42-month lag in antibody development—stated that in attempting to replicate his study he was unable to isolate HIV from any but one of his original subjects (see Imagawa et al below). Standard HIV antibody tests continue to reliably detect HIV infection six months after exposure.

Page 52. The practice of using more than one antiviral drug at the same time, as well as using them in sequence, is becoming the standard of care. (See Appendix A: "Natural History of HIV Disease," page 358.)

Updated References

Imagawa DT, Detels R: HIV-1 in seronegative homosexual men. N Engl J Med 1991; 325:1250-1

■

Robert Marks is the Editor of the UCSF AIDS Health Project publication Focus: A Guide to AIDS Research and Counseling. *Peter B. Goldblum, PhD, MPH,* is former Deputy Director of the AIDS Health Project, on the faculty member of the Pacific Graduate School of Psychology, and co-author of Strategies for Survival: A Gay Men's Health Manual for the Age of AIDS.

■

Experimental Treatments and Counseling Issues

William J. Woods, PhD

Almost from the very beginning of the AIDS epidemic, hopes and expectations have been placed on promising treatments. Though the media continually reminds us that AIDS has "no known cure" and is "100 percent fatal," those closer to the epidemic realize that the true picture is not quite so simple.

With increasing knowledge about the disease, its cause, and its many manifestations, patients and their health care providers now face increasingly complicated medical options and decisions related to HIV infection. For many, these expanded treatment options result in more conflict and confusion than comfort.

Conflicts and Confusion

Previously only people diagnosed with AIDS struggled with the decision to take drugs; now people at all points along the spectrum of HIV infection face this dilemma. At least four recent developments pressure seropositive individuals to consider treatments: 1) several studies indicating that over time, most seropositive people will develop symptoms; 2) recommendations by treatment information groups, AIDS organizations, and several physicians for testing and early treatment intervention; and indirectly, 3) efforts to lobby the government and pharmaceutical companies for treatment research, and 4) the large number of treatments both studied and supplied for HIV or its related opportunistic infections. With the passage of time, this pressure increases as evidence supports earlier intervention and the efficacy of some treatments.

Despite these developments, there is no consensus on major issues related to experimental treatment. Discussion of these issues is influenced by segments of at-risk populations as well as the established medical and political forces responsible for the testing and marketing of treatments. Without consensus on treatment approaches and timing, individuals infected with HIV often feel that time is running out while they struggle with a decision. Often the individual is left wondering which treatment to use given certain known side effects, or which drug is more important to take given that some cannot be taken together. They must also ask, "Who do I believe," and "Who do I trust?" The different messages from community groups, AIDS educators, physicians, and friends often vary widely; individuals are left to sort out not only what treatments to take, but what information to trust.

Treatment Classifications

There are several treatment alternatives which an individual infected with HIV may consider. These include antivirals, immune stimulants, and prophylactic treatments for specific opportunistic infections. Antivirals are expected to improve the medical condition of the individual by fighting HIV at some stage of its reproduction. By this interference, the antiviral slows the progress of the infection.

Immune stimulants rebuild what the virus has destroyed, since HIV causes destruction of immune cells. Though many immune stimulants are currently under investigation, there is controversy about their use. For instance, some physicians theorize that immune stimulants may provide fuel for the virus by stimulating the cellular machinery that facilitates viral replication. There is also debate about the quality of the new cells produced in terms of their ability to fight the virus. General consensus among health care providers and treatment advocates suggests that antivirals should be used before starting any of the immune stimulants.

There are many therapies which show promise for preventing the onset of certain opportunistic infections, specifically, aerosolized pentamidine for *Pneumocystis carinii* pneumonia and clofazimine for *mycobacterium avium-intracellulare*. These drugs can usually be prescribed by a physician outside a clinical trial.

Many people infected with HIV, hoping to increase fighting power of a given treatment, take more than one drug at a time; but these combinations may be antagonistic. For example, ribavirin should not be taken with AZT because it has been shown (in vitro) to interfere with AZT's activity in fighting the virus. This is also a problem when one must decide which drug is more important to take. For example, DHPG (for CMV retinitis) cannot be taken with AZT, and thus many face the choice of continuing on AZT and going blind or saving their vision and risking a more rapid destruction of their immune system.

Treatment Options

There are five viable treatment options for people infected with HIV: 1) obtain prescriptions from private physicians for treatments already approved for use with either HIV-associated or other illnesses, 2) enter a clinical drug trial, 3) join a "buyers' club" or "guerrilla clinic" (organized individuals who provide as yet unproven treatments and information), 4) import treatments not yet approved in their own country, or 5) "wait and see." Many of these options are unavailable to most people with HIV in developing countries.

Most physicians are comfortable with either prescribing a drug approved by the Food and Drug Administration (FDA) or entering a patient in a clinical trial, since they consider these options responsible and reasonable. Nevertheless, people entering clinical trials need to be aware that they may get, unknowingly, a placebo or another drug of unproven efficacy. For example, many asymptomatic men with low T-cell counts began taking AZT under a physician's care. Others have been referred to clinical trials across the country for the same treatment, but with the benefits and risks of being in a clinical trial.

The widespread use of experimental drugs outside of clinical trials creates concern that the validity of trials has been compromised. Often, if participants determine that they are on the placebo or the unproven, experimental treatment, they decide to use other treatments as well or instead, without informing the researchers. Individuals considering participation in a clinical trial should understand fully the elements of the study and commit themselves to observing the restrictions of the trial. An example of this case has been seen in the AZT trials. Some patients pooled their drugs in an effort to increase the odds that each would get some AZT. The unfortunate consequence is that nobody wins; AZT may or may not have been useful, and the study which might have answered the question has been weakened. The lack of national health care in the U.S. has been implicated in this dilemma, since it is usually those without resources who feel the most need to enroll in research to obtain treatment and medical care.

Using experimental treatments outside of supervised clinical trials is less comfortable for many people. Much of the media coverage of these alternative treatments implies that they are underground, illegal or black market. While there may be some cases in which people are engaging in illegal activity, the vast majority of those acquiring, importing and using these treatments are doing so legally. To continue to treat such use as legally questionable is misleading and unfair since it further burdens the individual's already difficult medical situation. For patients, the clear advantage to obtaining experimental treatments outside of supervised clinical trials is knowing they are getting the specific substance under investigation rather than a placebo. Also, many people cannot or do not meet the demand of the clinical trial, but they believe a drug might make a real difference; for them using treatments outside a clinical trial is the only viable option.

Finally, many individuals consider all the options and choose to "wait and see." This option will some day become untenable and ill-advised. An interim period during which some advocate strongly against this choice has already begun. Still others will argue for it. However, there are many possible reasons for this decision, even if only for a short time: getting lost in the thicket of decision making, procrastinating, using denial as a primary coping skill, or deciding that the potential risk of taking a particular treatment is greater than the potential benefit. At this point all treatments are experimental. Even the highly toxic AZT, though approved by the FDA, remains experimental, since little is known about its long-term use or its usefulness for people who are infected but asymptomatic. Since AZT is highly toxic, even someone who is eligible to receive it may choose against it. Though it is just a matter of time before some treatment is shown to be better than none, individuals still choose to wait for evidence that a particular treatment does in fact make a difference and is safe to use. As more treatments become available, it is more typical that those choosing to "wait and see" are those with few financial resources; they just cannot afford the other options. Furthermore, people with HIV in developing countries generally do not have any access whatsoever to these options.

Counselors can help ensure that clients make informed choices that fit their understanding of the disease and their view of how to be responsible for their health. These clients need support and encouragement to take as much time as they need to make the decision and to do so without undue influence from others.

Risks and Benefits

Counselors can help clients to assess the benefits and risks of using experimental treatments.

Benefits to taking experimental treatments include:

1. the possibility that one is, in fact, slowing the disease progression;

2. a sense of doing something, of taking responsibility, to slow the progress of HIV;

3. lessening isolation by feeling a part of a "social movement," and not being "left behind"; and

4. the positive psychological effect of observing possible improvements.

Risks to taking experimental treatments include:

1. wasting time, energy and money on useless treatments;

2. losing hope if a treatment used proves to be ineffective;

3. creating tensions between the patient and physician in treatment decisions;

4. toxic drugs may do more harm to the individual than to HIV; and

5. drug combinations may do nothing or, instead, worsen the condition.

Structure of the Decision-Making Process

The first stage of decision making is to acquire information. Clients should consider seriously the following important questions as suggested by Delaney et al regarding any treatment information: 1) What evidence is there that the product works? 2) What is known about its side effects? 3) What is being done to get the product licensed for use? 4) What are the motives and background of the suppliers? 5) What does the official medical establishment think of the solution being offered? 6) Who can I talk to who has used the product, and how long have they used it? Also, most people will want to consider how much time and money will be needed to use a treatment. Stretching limited resources for unproven treatments may be detrimental to the overall quality of life—at least as important as quantity of life to some.

After learning about various alternative treatments, individuals might need assistance with several areas: 1) determining what other information is needed before a decision can be made, 2) guidance in decision making, 3) establishing a follow-up review date to consider whether circumstances have changed, and 4) discussing under what circumstances treatments would be pursued (for example, increased anxiety or appearance of new symptoms).

For those who decide to pursue treatment options, the process depends on the person's medical status. If infected, they should establish the medical facts as soon as possible: What do antibody, antigen and T-cell count test results suggest about their medical status? Those who choose to wait until after a diagnosis of AIDS or of symptomatic HIV disease should continue to learn about treatment alternatives as well as the signs and symptoms of the various opportunistic infections. The decision-making process is dynamic due to the changing nature of the information base. The individual should work with a physician who is willing to assist with this process and to monitor the use of all treatments used.

Action Plan

Because working closely with a physician is imperative for anyone using treatments, clinicians will need to assist in identifying available and knowledgeable physicians for their clients. Most physicians are willing to work with their patients to try to understand the very complicated situation of HIV infection and treatment. Mental health professionals may be useful resources in teaching patients and physicians to negotiate these new, more active and responsible roles.

Depending on the treatment regimen chosen, the task of acquiring the treatment can range from very simple to very difficult. AZT is now a prescription drug, as are many of the other available experimental treatments. However, practitioners may find that clients must deal with the stress of challenging insurance companies' denial of coverage for these treatments. Clinical trial partici-pation can also provide easy access to the treatment, depending on the site of the trial. However, many of the available experimental treatments are more difficult to acquire. Some require contacting special groups organized to make the product available, while others require relatively frequent travel to foreign countries. Finally, the cost of treatment itself or of obtaining it may be prohibitive.

Support from other people who are seropositive, or who have AIDS or symptomatic HIV disease, can be an important part of both the decision making and action plan. Most large cities have organizations and support groups where people with similar health status can meet and share information and experiences. These meetings can help to reduce the sense of isolation and fear.

Conclusions

Decisions about medical interventions for HIV require knowl-edge of one's own medical status, information on available treat-ment options, and awareness of the mechanisms for appropriate use and monitoring of treatments. Until definitive medical answers for treatment are found, the individuals faced with these decisions will look to professionals for assistance in this important decision-making process.

Some of the militancy that many gay men express about the AIDS treatment issue is due to their perception, and emerging scientific opinion, that without an effective treatment a whole generation of gay men will likely die of AIDS. There is a sense that the whole community, an extended family, will be lost. Many minority communities express similar sentiments. Thus, health care providers and their clients continue to place their hopes and expectations on promising treatments. Clinicians, then, should see their role not only as one of providing information and struc-ture for the decision-making process, but also as one of promoting and maintaining hope.

■

Suggested Readings

Delaney M, Goldblum P, Brewer J: Strategies for Survival: A Gay Men's Health Manual for the Age of AIDS. New York, St. Martin's Press, 1987

Helquist M: The Helquist report: experimental treatments. *The Advocate*, Dec. 8, 1987

Information and Resources

AmFAR Directory of Experimental Treatments for AIDS and ARC - 40 W. 57th St., Suite 406, New York, NY 10019; 212-333-3118

Project Inform's Hotline - 347 Dolores Street, San Francisco, CA 94110; US: 800-822-7422; CA: 800-334-7422

AIDS Treatment News - P.O. Box 411256, San Francisco, CA 94141; 415-282-0110

Gay Men's Health Crisis - 132 W. 24th St., New York, NY 10011; 212-807-6664

New York PWA Coalition - Box 234 70-A Greenwich Ave., New York, NY 10011; 212-995-5846

■

William J. Woods, PhD, is a research fellow with the UCSF Center for AIDS Prevention Studies. He is also the former Project Manager of Project Inform, a national information clearinghouse for experimental treatments for people concerned about AIDS.

■

How to Evaluate Experimental Treatments

John S. James

Editors' Introduction

Most health care providers will encounter sooner or later a client or patient concerned about AIDS. Certainly any health care professional who works with people who are seropositive or who have HIV disease will find that clients struggle with questions about what they can do to stop the disease. With so few effective and approved treatments available—and with those beyond the resources of many individuals—clients will seek other remedies. They will ask for help from physicians, nurses, clinic staff, and counselors: What can I do? Should I take this treatment I heard about? How can I decide what drugs are safe to take?

Mental health practitioners should recognize that these clients will be exposed to, if not inundated with, opinions and articles about HIV treatments. There exists an extensive information-sharing network including treatment newsletters, hotlines, magazine columns, and anecdotal reports to advise an individual seeking treatments. Practitioners do not need to be aware of each new treatment development or theory, but they can be important resources for their clients if they understand the issues well enough to help clients in their decision making.

The following article focuses on unapproved treatments for HIV infection and AIDS. It poses questions for clients to consider with their health care providers before starting any new treatment regimen. The author, John S. James, is the Editor and Publisher of the San Francisco newsletter AIDS Treatment News.

Note on terminology: In the following discussion, non-approved treatments are divided into "experimental" and "complementary." Experimental treatments are those obtained through sanctioned clinical trials. "Complementary" means those treatments which have come into use through non-official channels. Essentially the only official channel is pharmaceutical companies obtaining FDA approval and then promoting their product with FDA-sanctioned claims.

At first glance it may seem impossible for a lay person to evaluate intelligently unapproved treatments. The established procedure for proving a new drug safe and effective takes about eight years for human testing alone (AZT, approved much faster, was a unique exception), and the process usually costs $80 million or more. When experts disagree, and major institutions spend years and millions of dollars to evaluate a drug, how can an untrained individual make a rational personal decision?

Practical considerations make the situation different from what it seems. Persons with serious illness will in fact make treatment decisions. Some patients choose to leave everything to their physicians; others want to inform themselves and work with their physicians in making decisions. Many of these patients also want to consider participating in clinical trials of experimental treatments or using complementary treatments which they obtain on their own. Hopefully, patients who choose the latter option will do so with the knowledge and ongoing monitoring of their physicians. Those individuals who cannot tolerate AZT may see non-approved treatments as their only hope.

Experimental Treatments

Experimental treatments offer several advantages: medical and scientific supervision in sanctioned trials, review procedures and informed consent intended to protect human subjects, and enough scientific rationale to justify expenses to its sponsor. But clinical trials also have drawbacks for volunteer subjects. For example, the therapies being tested are often inherently more dangerous than the untested complementary therapies adopted by adherents. Subjects may receive a placebo in a clinical trial and receive no direct benefit when they need it. Almost always subjects are required to forego other treatments to avoid "contaminating" the data. The other possible treatments may be medically indicated otherwise. Finally, most people cannot participate in trials due to geography, numerous medical exclusion criteria, difficulty in finding out about the trials, physicians' reluctance to refer patients to a medical center for study if they will lose those patients from their private practices, and, ultimately, the limited number of open slots in the trials.

Potential volunteers should note the differences between "phase I," "phase II," and "phase III" trials. Phase I (dosage and toxicity studies) are the first human trials once laboratory and animal tests have been completed. Placebos are not used in this phase; but doses may be much smaller, or considerably larger, than believed optimal. Volunteers may face the added risk of being among the first to use a substance.

Phase II trials (efficacy testing) commonly use a double-blind design, meaning that neither subjects nor doctors conducting the study know whether the medication being given to a particular patient is the drug being tested, or a "control" which is often a placebo. Fortunately, new study designs often avoid a placebo and use a known drug, such as AZT, as the control.

A placebo may be acceptable if the study design prevents harm to subjects receiving it. For example, if the study's "endpoints" include worsening values on blood or immunological tests, subjects can be removed from the study before serious illness develops—whether they were taking the placebo or the experimental drug if it did not work for them. Many studies, however, have used only serious illness or death as endpoints, meaning that the researchers try to keep subjects on the placebo or drug regimen until damage develops, despite worsening values on blood work.

Phase III trials (large-scale efficacy studies) can involve hundreds or even thousands of subjects at different medical centers. Generally, placebos or other controls are used. These trials can continue for several years.

Phase IV trials (post-marketing surveillance), a newer concept not yet applied to most drugs, involves careful monitoring after a drug has been approved for marketing to look for rare side effects. This phase matters less to subjects, since individuals do not volunteer for phase IV; they obtain the drugs by prescription and purchase them like any others. Federal health officials are considering proposals to speed access to drugs for serious or life-threatening conditions by eliminating phase III and replacing it with phase IV and an expanded phase II. Phase III testing usually delays drugs for several years, yet it rejects few of the drugs which have passed phase II.

Volunteers in clinical trials should also ask whether they are guaranteed continuing access to the drug, if it works for them, after the trial is over. It may take years following the study before the drug is approved for marketing. During this time the volunteers could probably not obtain it, unless the manufacturer promises to supply it. Many studies adopt an "open label" status after each volunteer finishes, meaning that subjects can receive the drug if they want it, without the risk of getting a placebo, whether they received the drug or the placebo in the trial itself. Open label status benefits the volunteers, and it also benefits the trial sponsors by letting them collect data on longer-term administration.

Complementary Treatments

Complementary treatments, which have attracted a substantial grassroots following, are usually fairly safe. The community of people interested in HIV treatments shares information extensively, and acceptance of a treatment does not occur without substantial prior experience with human use. This informed community never tries a new chemical not taken by humans before, and members almost never use prescription drugs without a physician's supervision. Unless this community accepts a treatment, patients are unlikely to hear of it—except through commercial promotion.

Complementary treatments usually have NOT been rejected by the mainstream of medical opinion. Instead, they have simply been ignored. Usually there is more scientific evidence for these treatments than against them.

Since the officially sanctioned medical and pharmaceutical system of drug testing often does not pursue low-cost, safe, and available therapies, these have become starting points for grassroots treatment movements as well as for promotions by the health food industry. Often there is no reason to think that some of these treatments do not work; in fact, some admittedly sketchy evidence suggests that they might be effective against HIV infection.

Judging Complementary Treatments

Individuals usually become aware of complementary treatments through word-of-mouth. Interested individuals can learn to ask—and be encouraged to ask by their counselors—certain questions and to apply criteria to help weigh the credibility of the statements they hear about treatments. Even when answers cannot be found, the questioning and investigation can lead to valuable information and better judgment about a proposed therapy.

Some Questions to Ask

Is someone trying to sell you something? Rejecting all treatments for which the answer is "yes" would leave few options remaining. But potential users of a treatment should consider the motives of those who are providing it.

The danger of commercial promotion is that it can encourage drugs that may not be safe or effective. To prevent this abuse, officially approved treatments have passed extensive tests to justify the uses for which they are indicated and promoted. Treatments not approved for any medical use lack this critical protection.

Potential users should realize that the books and magazines sold in health food stores promote specific products. Some of the information may be legitimate and valuable, but none of it should be taken at face value without further research. Since most people will not do their own research in the scientific literature, or by sending products to testing laboratories for analysis, self-help groups like HIV-positive "buyers' clubs" can be valuable resources.

Does a product contain secret ingredients? Secrecy allows promoters to overstate and oversell without independent analysis and evaluation. Valuable treatment approaches are more likely to result from open, public discussion than from somebody's secret concoction.

Do promoters use pseudoscience to help sell the product? Pseudoscience uses technical words in ways unconnected with any recognized discipline. The issue here is not fairness toward new ideas but honesty in argument. Users may reasonably choose to accept unorthodox ideas over conventional ones, but they should not be deceived about the difference. They can seek help from friends, AIDS self-help organizations, or physicians if they do not have the background to evaluate the terminology themselves.

In all cases, individuals should ask for evidence to support claims about treatments. They should ask whether there is any evidence or independent analysis in support of the treatment. Is there any independent case for the treatment? Written evidence is most important. Do any articles published in mainstream medical journals support the case that the treatment might be helpful?

Are the journals "refereed"? The leading journals, such as *The Journal of the American Medical Association* and *The New England Journal of Medicine*, submit articles to several specialists for pre-publication review. These referees can suggest changes, or they can reject the article entirely. This peer review system takes time, but it helps avoid mistakes and usually blocks faulty research from publication. Only articles are reviewed this way; letters to refereed journals are not, and they carry less weight.

Articles in popular health books and magazines can vary greatly in quality. Readers can check whether the articles include references to medical or scientific articles so that independent researchers can confirm claims. Sometimes individuals will see unpublished drafts or manuscripts circulated by treatment promoters. These have less credibility than published articles.

In addition to written evidence, individuals should inquire whether the person promoting a treatment can support claims of effectiveness in other ways. For example, have they used the treatment themselves, finding that it worked for them? Do they personally know people who used the treatment successfully? How many? Under what conditions did they use the treatment? What other treatments were they using at the time? Interested parties should also determine whether the promoter has any commercial interest in the treatment.

Treatment Strategy Questions

Individuals should develop a treatment strategy to help them determine the potential costs and benefits of a treatment.

What is lost if the treatment fails? If a treatment is safe and ineffective and does not cause the individual to forego other treatments such as AZT, there is little harm in trying it.

How long will it take to determine if the treatment is working or not? A therapy treatment to give tangible results within weeks can be dropped if it doesn't. These have a major advantage over those treatments which require use for months or years. Blood tests, or other medical tests such as a skin immune assay, should be monitored as indicators of effectiveness.

The strategy that seems to work best for many individuals is to try different treatments, giving each one at least a few weeks to work, and keeping those which appear to help them. They should keep detailed written records of what they do and what changes in symptoms or medical tests they observe. Response to treatments is highly individual for HIV and AIDS; at this time there is no way to predict who will find success with which treatments.

Fortunately, there are many relatively harmless complementary options from which to choose; if one does not work, others can be tried. Individuals who want to explore complementary therapies can pose questions like those suggested above to improve their decision making about these. These questions can help them consider relevant factors which might otherwise be overlooked.

■

John S. James is the Editor and Publisher of the San Francisco newsletter AIDS Treatment News.

III
Counseling for
AIDS Prevention

AIDS Prevention Counseling in Clinical Practice

Michael Shernoff, MSW, ACSW

The majority of mental health professionals have received relatively little or no training in human sexuality or sexuality counseling. Therefore it is not surprising that as a group, psychotherapists are often uncomfortable discussing sexual matters with clients. The HIV health crisis brings this issue sharply into focus and challenges all clinicians to learn how to discuss sexual behavior in a candid and accurate manner. Most importantly, therapists must learn how to counsel clients on specific ways to prevent the transmission of the virus that causes HIV disease.

This new responsibility has implications for mental health professionals. First, they must learn exactly how HIV is transmitted and about safer sexual practices (see Addendum). Second, clinicians need to examine their own biases regarding sexuality and sexual orientation (i.e., homosexual, bisexual and heterosexual); and third, clinicians need to consider the impact of these issues on the therapeutic alliance. This chapter will focus on a discussion of the impact of HIV prevention counseling on the process of psychotherapy and will give suggestions for helping clients who are having difficulty adopting safer sex practices.

To assess whether clients are at risk for HIV disease, practitioners need to ascertain their current and past sexual practices. Simply asking "Are you gay?" is not sufficient. Many men who have sex with men do not label themselves as homosexual and certainly do not identify as part of the gay community. Therefore, questions regarding sexual practices need to be asked in accepting, nonjudgmental and gentle ways that do not use labels. For instance, one way to inquire about this area is: "As an adult, have you ever had any sexual contact with another man?" If the answer is "yes," then asking "When was the last time?" can provide useful and pertinent data about the individual's risk for being exposed to HIV.

Counseling Issues

Discussing sexual issues can be uncomfortable for the clinician. The urgent need to ensure that people eliminate high-risk sexual behaviors, however, requires that all mental health professionals begin to introduce an aspect of sex education into clinical practice.

The issue of sexual practices in relation to HIV prevention needs to be raised with every individual. It may be best to introduce this issue in one of the early sessions as part of the initial psychosocial evaluation, taking cues from the client about how quickly to focus on these issues. Introducing the topic can be achieved by asking questions such as: "How do you feel about the fact that HIV is sexually transmitted?" "How did you feel when you first heard that you might have to change your sexual patterns in order not to contract HIV?" "When you think about 'safer sex,' what thoughts and feelings do you have?" Therapists need to ask clients, "What are you doing to protect yourself and your sexual partners from becoming infected with the virus that causes AIDS?"

There are understandable concerns about introducing this topic into treatment. Questions of whether the interview content becomes overstimulating or "inappropriately eroticized" have to be judged on a case-by-case basis. In addition to the therapist's discomfort with the area of sexuality, many clients are also not comfortable with issues of sexuality and may feel intruded upon or angered by this discussion.

Questions of this kind often provoke profound feelings on the part of the client; these may include intense anger and sometimes relief. Anger may arise because any discussion of the subject of AIDS may challenge the client's denial and demonstrate that the therapist believes it is a relevant issue. Anger can also derive from transferential issues if the client perceives the questions as negative parental injunctions. An exploration of these negative transferential feelings can provide a fertile ground for discussions of sex and sexuality in general, taking care of oneself, self-image and the consequences of impulsive behavior. When relief is expressed, it is most often due to the feeling that this highly charged issue can be discussed openly at last.

Once the subject of sex is successfully introduced and agreed upon as an issue for discussion, the next step is to elicit feelings about changes in sexual behavior the client will likely need to make. Asking which specific behaviors will be missed and exploring feelings about this situation has proven very useful in furthering the discussion. Therapists should encourage clients to be behaviorally specific about sex in this discussion. It is also helpful for the therapist to validate feelings of sadness, anger and mourning that can accompany an exploration of this issue.

Many important issues are raised as a result of these discussions: feelings about past sexual experiences or styles, thoughts about the various roles sex may have played in the individual's life, including the possible use of sex as a defense against feelings of anxiety, depression or intimacy, and memories of past sexual partners.

These discussions can help individuals make the transition to a state in which adherence to safer sex practices becomes easier. One method of helping clients accomplish this is to elicit feelings that reflect which aspects of safer sex they actually enjoy.

An additional tool that has proven especially helpful in therapeutic settings is a chart that illustrates the spectrum of sexual practices grouped from low to high risk (see Addendum). This can be a particularly useful technique for the clinician who is not comfortable asking clients directly about specific sexual practices.

Eroticizing Safer Sex

Many professionals who discuss high-risk behaviors have counseled clients to reduce their number of sex partners. In and of itself, this is not particularly helpful nor accurate advice. An individual can be the receptive partner in anal or vaginal intercourse with an exclusive person who is HIV positive and as a result be at higher risk for becoming infected than if he or she has engaged in mutual masturbation with several different partners. For example, a study of female sexual partners of HIV-infected individuals reports that these women became infected after repeated exposure to one man (1). Thus, they may have falsely assumed they were not at risk for becoming infected because they had only one sexual partner.

In the age of AIDS, it is clear that safer sex practices need to be considered seriously by all sexually active people, regardless of age or antibody status. If two people follow the guidelines for low-risk sex, there is no reason why they cannot enjoy a creative, healthy sex life, whatever their antibody or current health status. However, clients often are unsure about the specifics of safer sex and may believe that low-risk sex is dull or boring. To integrate safer sexual practices into their lives, clients have to believe that low-risk sex can be sexually satisfying. Therapists can have their clients practice a number of helpful exercises to achieve this aim.

One simple method is to ask clients to reflect upon the very specific erotic ways they like to touch or be touched—ways that will not put the client or a partner at risk for transmitting HIV. If verbally reporting this information to the therapist produces too much anxiety or discomfort, the client should be given the option of simply writing down a list and keeping the contents private. However, the feelings that arise from doing the exercise should be discussed.

Clients invariably report that this exercise prompts thoughts of various approaches to foreplay they have always enjoyed. Additionally, they frequently develop some innovations as well. If an individual has a sexual partner, the suggestion can be made that they set aside time to practice erotic ways of touching or being touched that are not high risk for transmitting HIV. Traditional sex therapy techniques of focusing on sexual exercises that stop short of actual penetration are useful for helping clients gain confidence in this area and for learning how to degenitalize sexual activity.

The next step is to ask the client to imagine, discuss or write down a list of erotic but low-risk ways of performing specific sexual acts such as mutual masturbation, oral sex, intercourse, or eroticizing condom use. This allows the client to discover a variety of satisfying, fun and low-risk ways to remain sexually active that are still available to them.

Helping people learn to verbalize where they want to be touched, how they like to be touched, what they would like to do with their partner and what they do not wish to do can be important steps towards sexual assertiveness training and enhanced sexual enjoyment. These skills become essential in the face of an epidemic that is sexually transmitted.

Condoms

Since research has demonstrated that the **correct use** of condoms can reduce the risk of transmitting HIV during intercourse (2,3,4,5,6), clinicians need to elicit feelings about condoms and their use from clients.

It is true that some sensitivity is lost when using a condom. This needs to be acknowledged by the therapist, and any feelings that arise need to be discussed. It is important that therapists ask clients to consider how they can incorporate erotic use of condoms into foreplay.

At the same time, it is critical to remind clients that using condoms cannot guarantee absolute safety and protection. Therefore a variety of options needs to be explored. For example, sometimes clients need permission from the therapist to say "no." They need to learn they can refrain from engaging in anal or vaginal intercourse completely if that makes them feel safer. They also need to know that some people use two condoms at the same time and that other people practice withdrawal even while wearing a condom.

Mental health professionals should become familiar with the steps for correctly using a condom in order to help clients with any questions they may have.

If it appears inappropriate to discuss the specifics of condom use with the client directly, then literature should be provided which gives complete instructions (7,8,9,10). It might also be added that for many men an unexpected benefit in using a condom is that intercourse is prolonged, since the loss of sensitivity from the condom causes a delay in reaching orgasm.

Some clients will also need help feeling comfortable in talking to prospective partners about safer sex. Providing individuals with the opportunity to role play situations in which the client initiates a conversation with a prospective sexual partner about safer sex is a useful way to help the client gain confidence in integrating these skills. People need to be reminded that they do not need to apologize about introducing the topic of safer sex.

Conclusion

All people, but especially health care professionals, need to be concerned about stopping the spread of AIDS. The mental health professional has a special opportunity to correct misinformation, encourage adherence to safer sex practices, and help clients work through the feelings that occur by having to make changes in sexual behavior due to the AIDS epidemic. With accurate information, mental health professionals are in a unique position to help clients make intelligent choices about how to be sexually active and sexually responsible while remaining sexually satisfied.

■

Addendum

No-Risk Sexual Activities involve no exchange of blood, semen, vaginal secretions, urine or feces and pose no risk of transmitting HIV. These include:

- flirting
- fantasy
- solo masturbation
- hugging, body rubbing
- dry kissing
- massage
- showering together
- mutual masturbation with external orgasms
- light S/M without bleeding or bruising
- phone sex
- talking "dirty"
- watching another person
- being watched

Probably Safe Sexual Activities are safe as long as the barrier used remains intact; there may be danger of transmitting HIV if the barrier slips or breaks. Using barriers correctly increases the safety. These include:

- **Anal or Vaginal Intercourse with a Condom: using a water-based lubricant** is even safer if a spermicide is also used. Withdrawal before ejaculation increases safety.
- **Fellatio with No Exchange of Semen:** a condom can be used and/or ejaculation can take place outside the mouth.
- **Cunnilingus or Analingus (Rimming) through a Barrier:** a latex sheet (dental dam) or light plastic wrap over the vulva or anus.

- **Sharing Sterile Sex Toys:** cover the toy with an unused condom or latex barrier and put a new one on before sharing it with someone else.
- **Brachioproctic/Brachiovaginal sex (fisting) with a Latex Glove:** will protect the hand of the inserter, but this practice can still cause damage to internal tissues.

Possibly Risky Sexual Activities are those during which exchange of body fluids might create some danger of transmitting HIV, but from which no known cases of transmission have occurred to date. These include:

- **Deep Kissing,** particularly if there are cuts or sores where blood might be present in the mouth.
- **Oral, Anal or Vaginal Intercourse Without a Condom and Withdrawing Prior to Ejaculation.**
- **Cunnilingus** may be most risky when the woman is menstruating.
- **Sharing Sex Toys or Enema Equipment** which have come in contact with vaginal secretions, semen or blood.
- **Fisting** if the hand has cuts or sores on it. The risk is increased if internal tears are produced and there is subsequent intercourse.
- **Mucous Membrane or Broken Skin Contact with Urine or Feces.**
- **Rimming** can spread bacteria, viruses and parasites that are harmful to one's health.

Risky Sexual Activities are clearly linked to HIV transmission in **some** cases.

- **Fellatio** with ejaculation in the mouth can be dangerous for the receptive partner.

Definitely High-Risk Sexual Activities are known to provide a major route of transmitting HIV. These include:

- **Anal and Vaginal Intercourse Without a Condom and Internal Ejaculation** is most risky for the receptive partner, but is dangerous for both partners.

References

1. Padian N: Male to female transmission of HIV. J Am Med Assoc 1987; 258(6):788-790
2. Conant M, Haddy D, Levy JA, et al: Condoms prevent transmission of AIDS associated retrovirus. J Am Med Assoc 1986; 255(13):1706
3. Goldsmith MF: Sex in the age of AIDS calls for common sense and condom sense. J Am Med Assoc 1987; 257(17):2261-2264
4. Rinzler CA: The return of the condom. American Health 1987; New York Times, March 16, 1987, Section A, p. 17

5. Hicks DR, Martin LS, Getchell JP, et al: Inactivation of HTLV-III/LAV: infected cultures of normal human lymphocytes by nonoxynol-9 in vitro. Letter, Lancet, Dec. 21-28, 1985, 2:1422
6. Bruce V: Nonoxynol-9 and HTLV-III. Lancet, May 17, 1986; 1:1153
7. Palacios-Jimenez L, Shernoff M: Facilitators Guide to Eroticizing Safer Sex: A Psychoeducational Workshop Approach to Safer Sex Education. New York, Gay Men's Health Crisis (GMHC), 1986
8. Breitman P, Knutson K, Reed P: How To Persuade Your Lover to Use A Condom...And Why You Should (Complete Information and Advice About Condoms). San Francisco, New York Publishing, 1987
9. Gay Men's Health Crises (GMHC): The Safer Sex Condom Guide For Men and Women. New York, GMHC, 1987
10. Douglas PH, Pinsky L: The Essential AIDS Fact Book: What You Need to Know to Protect Yourself, Your Family, and All Your Loved Ones Including Clear and Direct Talk About Safe Sex. New York, Pocket Books, 1987

Further Reading

Hunt M: Sexual Behavior in the 1970s. Chicago, Playboy Press, 1974
Hyde JS: Understanding Human Sexuality. New York, McGraw-Hill, 1982
Kinsey AC, Pomeroy WB, Martin CE: Sexual Behavior in the Human Male. Philadelphia, W.B. Saunders Co., 1948
Palacios-Jimenez L, Shernoff M: AIDS: Prevention is the only vaccine available, an AIDS prevention education model. Journal of Social Work and Human Sexuality 1988; 6(2):135-150

■

Michael Shernoff, MSW, ACSW, is Co-Director of Chelsea Psycho-therapy Associates in New York City.

A Group Model for AIDS Prevention and Support

John R. Acevedo, MSW

The primary purposes of AIDS risk-reduction groups are to provide accurate information about AIDS risk reduction, inform group members about strategies for coping more effectively with the changes brought on by the AIDS epidemic, and promote individual social support.

This chapter will describe a group model for AIDS prevention and risk reduction. This particular model combines a cognitive-behavioral educational approach with a brief therapy, problem-solving orientation. The model was developed by the AIDS Health Project over the past four years' experience with gay and bisexual men at risk for contracting HIV. The model has been adapted to address the needs of other populations: those aware of their antibody status, people with symptomatic HIV disease, women at risk, and couples. Following a general discussion of the background and development of this approach, a description of the mechanics of organizing and facilitating a group will be presented.

Background and Development of the Group Model

A short-term group approach for AIDS prevention was selected, given the success of short-term cancer-related group work, experience of the medical self-help movement, and cognitive-behavioral psychology. This approach offers time for group bonding while prohibiting the development of dependence on the facilitator or other group members. In addition, there is adequate time for the presentation and practice of new skills. The short-term approach is also cost-effective in reaching a larger number of individuals.

Group members are encouraged to develop a wholistic view of health which involves defining a healthy state as more than simply the absence of disease. Rather, a healthy state is one which involves adopting positive health habits as well as considering a wide range of issues such as social support, personal values and attitudes, and spirituality. In addition, participants are taught risk reduction strategies and ways to improve their overall health. Considerable emphasis is placed on reducing stress, depression, isolation, and the use of drugs and alcohol, while encouraging proper nutrition, relaxation, social support, and a sense of having some control over one's life.

Both closed and open group formats can be helpful. The major advantage of the closed group model is the continuity of structure and group participants. This facilitates the building of trust in group members and provides a counterpoint to the chaos of medical, physiological, and emotional uncertainty so often present in the lives of those affected by HIV. Group members come to expect the same people being present each week, allowing everyone to get to know each other better.

Open, drop-in groups offer an immediate service to those who may be waiting to enter a closed group. They may provide adjunctive services to individuals requiring more than once-a-week intervention, and may give "as needed" support for people unable or uninterested in committing to a closed group. No intake or screening is required to enter a drop-in group. The open group format provides clients an opportunity to try a group experience without making any greater commitment than showing up at the appropriate time. Finally, open groups usually also allow participants to determine their own topic for discussion.

Groups can be designed for participants dealing with a range of concerns, though in our experience, some issues have surfaced repeatedly. These include stress reduction and management, how to eroticize and maintain safer sex practices, how to understand changing medical conditions, and how to talk to others about these issues. Other groups address the specific needs of individuals who share some common characteristic—for example, those with more severe symptoms of HIV infection or those who are HIV positive. The decision to separate groups by medical status was based on conflict between clients in early groups. One ill client in a group of men who were relatively healthy stated, "This is hard. You're talking about safer sex techniques, and I'm wondering if I'll ever have sex again."

Groups were also separated by gender in an effort to meet the needs of a growing population of women at risk. Women frequently are more isolated than gay men because fewer of their peers are affected by the AIDS epidemic. Consequently, women often have greater concerns about confidentiality, reproductive health, and limited sources of community and family support.

Format and Member Selection Criteria

The most common format for a psychoeducational AIDS risk reduction group used by the AIDS Health Project is a closed eight-week group focusing on one or more of the issues above. (See the Addendum at the end of the chapter for a list of sample group materials and outline.) Members for the groups are obtained through a network of referral agencies, professional therapists and physicians in the community. Once referred, each prospective group member is interviewed by a staff clinician, and a psychosocial assessment is made. Information about substance use, sexual behavior, and psychosocial functioning is obtained. Clients are informed about the various groups available, and a mutual decision is made about joining the group that best meets the clients' needs. Clients with major psychiatric disorders or substance addictions are referred to other community resources.

The following psychological criteria are used as general guidelines for appropriate referrals to groups: non-psychotic, non-suicidal, non-acting out, not currently abusing substances, and motivated to participate in the group. The intake clinician recommends that people with symptomatic HIV infection be under the care of a physician. Frequently, those with severe symptoms are also encouraged to be in individual therapy.

If individuals and their partners are both interested in participating in a group, they are advised that couples should not attend the same group unless it is specifically a group for couples. Couples tend to withhold information in the group to protect themselves. In addition, a couple may shift the group focus from the individual group members to problem solving for the couple. Couples who insist on being together often have other issues.

While most individuals will self-select into the appropriate group, some will need guidance. Occasionally, a second session is needed to explore the individual's decision or to obtain more information.

Goals and Objectives

Specific goals of an AIDS risk reduction group include 1) to provide education regarding the multidimensional aspects of health and HIV infection; 2) to improve stress management, coping, and communication skills; and 3) to expand the individual's social support and use of community resources.

Groups should provide a safe place for the exploration of thoughts and feelings. Members are given a list of ground rules and guidelines designed to establish that safety. For example, all members must agree at the first session to protect confidentiality and not to tolerate physical violence. (See Addendum for a list of standard ground rules and guidelines.)

Group Structure and Role of the Facilitator

Each session of any given group has a specific structure. Most sessions include welcome and announcements, a brief stress management and centering exercise, and a structured opportunity for members to say how they are doing. This is followed by educational material on the particular topic for the week, guided exercises, discussion, and group processing. Sessions end with a relaxation exercise, guided imagery, or visualization.

Consistency in the group structure provides stability as a counterpoint to AIDS-related confusion and uncertainty. However, some members can be expected to resist this group structure and challenge the facilitator.

The facilitator is responsible for maintaining the structure and schedule of the group, as well as for promoting adherence to ground rules and guidelines. The role of the facilitator is similar to that of a classroom teacher, guiding the group through different tasks as the group progresses. The facilitator opens and closes the session, presents educational material, coordinates discussion, and makes appropriate interventions, while actively participating *with* the group. The ability to shift from educator to clinician requires practice.

Facilitators need to feel comfortable with a greater degree of disclosure than in a traditional therapy group. Clinicians may want to speak to some of the issues raised in the group, commenting on how the issue was resolved or dealt with in their lives. This is most often productive when the facilitator uses examples from the material presented and illustrates the usefulness of a particular technique in dealing with a specific issue. The facilitator who remains totally neutral or undisclosing may sometimes inhibit group process.

Gay facilitators of gay groups can serve as role models for change when they share some of their own experiences and feelings in the group. However, it may be best for the facilitators to remain more distant from the material being presented and discussed. For example, it is inappropriate for facilitators to participate in partner safe-sex negotiation exercises with clients. Participating in this kind of exercise is a setup for problematic sexual transference.

Facilitators need to confront members who expect facilitators to "fix" a problem or concern. Group leaders must often acknowledge a client's feelings of powerlessness while encouraging members to try out new solutions to their problems. Reflecting the issue back to the group may promote problem solving and may illustrate the support available in the group.

It is also recommended that groups have two facilitators. In this way, responsibilities can be shared, and one facilitator is always free to observe group process. If groups are to be co-facilitated, leaders need to clearly discuss and agree upon who will be responsible for which aspects of group structure and process.

Managing Problematic Clients

Individual sessions are routinely offered to clients felt to have continued difficulty in the group. Clients are told that experiences in the group may stir strong feelings and reactions, and that the leaders are available for individual consultation if needed. This message acknowledges the complex issues that may arise in the group and reinforces the idea that support for potentially overwhelming feelings will be provided. At times, group members may require special attention and pose potential problems. Strategies for dealing with these situations are suggested below.

1. **The suicidal client:** Differentiate between suicidal thoughts and suicidal plans. Normalize the feelings. Suicidal thoughts are normal for individuals facing life-threatening illnesses; what to do with these thoughts can be a problem solving task for the group. Limit setting is mandatory, and establishing a

no-suicide contract with individuals may be necessary. For those with persistent suicidal ideation, a referral for individual psychotherapy should be made. After obtaining consent, the leader should discuss the client's continuing in the group with the individual and the therapist.

2. **The angry client:** Angry feelings need to be acknowledged and accepted. While anger is a natural and common reaction to situations like AIDS that make us feel powerless, it is not acceptable to threaten individuals or the group, and strong limit setting may be necessary. Refer to the ground rules. Use the group's structure as an anchor and return to the focus on the session's topic.

3. **The substance-abusing/using client:** Refer to group ground rules. If clients attend the session drunk, high on drugs, or with alcohol on their breath, take them aside and ask them to leave, reminding them of their agreement not to use substances before attending the group. Invite them to return the following week. Follow-up consults are advised. The client may be reacting to group material or issues raised during the group process. Facing HIV issues is frightening for many clients, and substance use is a common coping strategy. Make referrals for substance abuse treatment, and educate clients about the impact of substances on the immune system. Examine with both the individual and the group how getting high can inhibit judgment and facilitate denial.

4. **The sexually inappropriate client:** Set limits of acceptable behavior and remind the group that one ground rule was not to become sexually involved with others in the group. Acknowledge that being attracted is a normal human reaction. Ask the group to explore how sexual relations among group members would affect the ability of the group to function. Facilitate discussion of "why people have sex" to examine underlying issues.

Other important strategies that the group facilitator may find helpful in promoting group interaction are listed below.

1. **Acknowledge the demand.** Clients who are intrusive or dominate the session may be asking permission to talk about a difficult subject without knowing how to broach the topic.

Acknowledging the demand can take the emotion out of the request and promote group trust. However, limits must be respected, and after some discussion the facilitator should put some closure to the issue and return to the material being discussed.

2. **Reflect the question back to the group.** The client may be speaking for the group, and the issue can be diffused by asking the other group members to respond to the question. This technique can serve to clarify whether the issue is an individual or a group concern.

3. **Identify underlying themes.** For example, if suicide is raised as an issue and the group seems uncomfortable discussing it, the facilitator should look for underlying themes. Feelings of powerlessness, sadness, and loss of control are group concerns. The facilitator may or may not choose to comment on these underlying themes.

Summary

This model for AIDS prevention and risk reduction combines a cognitive/behavioral educational approach with a brief, problem-solving orientation. It is important to appreciate that different people will respond differently to the challenges of AIDS risk reduction and that a variety of approaches may be needed. The strength of the psychoeducational group model lies in its adaptability to these differing needs. The model also helps group members learn specific skills and techniques to manage stress, depression, anger, and the uncertainty of the illness, while strengthening social support systems and knowledge of community resources.

■

Addendum

Sample group materials have been included to illustrate the educational group format used by the AIDS Health Project. The materials are those used in a group for gay men with symptomatic HIV infection. This group was selected as an example because it demonstrates common themes seen in groups coping with various stages of HIV disease: definition of illness, care for self, emotional stress, disclosure, sex and relationships, impact on meaning and purpose of life, and planning for the future.

Included are group goals, ground rules, and a sample outline of issues to be covered.

Goals of the Symptomatic HIV Group

1. To assist individuals coping with initial and ongoing reactions to a diagnosis of symptomatic HIV disease;

2. To enhance coping and communication skills and to help clients make decisions about disclosing their diagnosis;

3. To provide a supportive environment for the exploration of thoughts, feelings, and information;

4. To explore new ways of improving quality of life, leisure time, and creativity;

5. To help clients gain an understanding of the personal meaning of having symptomatic HIV disease.

Group Ground Rules and Guidelines

1. Confidentiality. To develop trust and openness, we need to respect what people say about their personal lives. Personal information stays in the room. It is all right to share educational information and your own reactions with others.

2. No alcohol or drugs during the day of the group meeting. We want you to be able to hear what is presented; alcohol and drugs distort perceptions. Physician-prescribed medications are allowed. However, individuals are encouraged to report to the group leader changes in medications which could affect behavior in the group.

3. No physical violence or sexual behavior between group members.

4. No verbal abuse. People may disagree or get angry; that is understandable. It is not all right to be verbally abusive, and the leader(s) will help group members be constructive with their anger or disagreements.

5. Group members will agree to attend all eight sessions.

6. If an absence is unavoidable, contact the group leader. Please try to give 24 hours' notice if possible.

7. The group will start and end on time.

8. The structure of the group will be maintained.

9. This is not a therapy group, but a place to learn new information and develop new skills. This group is not intended to tell you what you "should" do. Also, this is not a group to find a lover, boyfriend, or sex partner.

10. Participate and disclose at your own rate. If anyone has difficulties with a specific exercise, talk to the group facilitator.

11. One person should talk at a time.

12. Emergencies: crisis sessions are available. An AIDS diagnosis during a group does not disqualify an individual from continuing. The member can remain in the group for all eight weeks, at which time appropriate referrals can be made.

Symptomatic HIV Group Outline

Week #1 **Ground Rules and Guidelines**

Introduction and expectations: What do you want from this group?

What is symptomatic HIV disease? How has symptomatic HIV disease affected your life?

Week #2 **Treatment Regimens**

How are group members taking care of themselves?

Daily Life Regimen/Health Resources: Choose one and talk about its impact.

Week #3 **Feelings and States of Mind: Stress and Depression**

Define stress and depression; connect with loss.

Examine and discuss prevention versus reduction.

Examine and discuss cognitive approaches to depression prevention such as: time out, thought stopping, humor, affirmations, and limit setting.

Introduce stress management techniques: breathing, meditation, etc.

Week #4 **Whom do you tell? Whom have you told?**

Share with the group the best disclosure experience.

Whom have you avoided telling and why?

Examine correlation of disclosure with homophobia.

Stress management techniques.

Week #5 **Sex and Relationships**

Why do people have sex? Examine reasons and discuss how other needs can be met without sex.

Who's having sex? Discuss.

What is safer sex?

Optional: Role playing negotiating safer sex.

Partner exercise with condoms.

Week #6	**Feelings and States of Mind: Anger**
	Examine messages one receives about anger.
	Identify people, places, and events that make one angry; validate the right to be angry.
	Identify healthy ways to express anger.
	Anger visualization: discharging anger.
Week #7	**Meaning and Purpose: Creativity and Spontaneity**
	Discussions:
	How do you spend your time?
	What is the purpose of life?
	What are the most important values to you?
Week #8	**Where do we go from here?**

Suggested Readings

Stress Management: Group Leaders Guide. Compiled by Marcia Quackenbush. San Francisco, UCSF AIDS Health Project, 1987. (Available from the AIDS Health Project, Box 0884, San Francisco, CA 94143-0884.)

Stall RD, Coates TJ, Hoff C: Behavioral risk reduction for HIV infection among gay and bisexual men. Am Psychologist 1988; 43:878-885.

Joseph J, Montgomery C, Kirscht J et al: Perceived risk of AIDS: assessing the behavioral and psychological consequences in a cohort of gay men. J Appl Psych 1987; 17:231-51.

Vitiello WR: Group work with people with ARC: a conceptual framework. FOCUS: A Guide to AIDS Research and Counseling 1987; 2:1-2, UCSF AIDS Health Project.

■

John R. Acevedo, MSW, the former Coordinator of the AIDS Prevention Program, UCSF AIDS Health Project, is an independent consultant with a private practice in San Francisco, California.

Do Groups Work?
Evaluation of a Group Model

Jeffrey Moulton, PhD, David Sweet, MA,
Gamze Gurbuz, BA, and James W. Dilley, MD

The urgency of the HIV disease epidemic precluded early systematic evaluations of programs that serve the needs of people with HIV infection and those fearful about contracting AIDS, the "worried well." The basic evaluation issues for these AIDS education and prevention programs are whether the interventions help to ameliorate distress, increase knowledge of HIV prevention, and assist individuals to change high-risk sexual behaviors.

The UCSF AIDS Health Project has developed an eight-week group education model based on a cognitive-behavioral approach to HIV prevention and risk reduction. This chapter reports the evaluation results of this group model based on data collected from 1986 to 1987.

These evaluation results should be understood in the context of the psychosocial sequelae associated with the continuum of HIV infection. This chapter addresses the issues most relevant to seronegative gay men and those along the continuum of HIV infection, from the asymptomatic seropositive to the symptomatic individual, since the educational support group focussed on the needs of these men.

Individual Psychosocial Consequences of HIV

Knowledge of seronegative antibody status results in significant reductions in the distress seen among the worried well (1). However, persons notified of their seronegative status often continue to see themselves at risk for HIV infection despite this news (2). Seronegative individuals have the essential task of protecting their status by maintaining safeguards to prevent future exposure (3,4). Experiencing "survivor guilt" in the midst of continuing loss of peers usually leads to distress.

Seropositives who are asymptomatic or have early manifestations of HIV infection are growing in number, with estimates of more than one million in the U.S. alone. Among asymptomatic individuals, knowledge of a seropositive status may result in increased levels of stress and depression (5,6). However, those who have early symptoms of HIV infection may conclude that they are HIV infected prior to actual notification of an antibody test result (1). For these individuals, distress is more likely related to symptomatology and the expected and perceived outcome of the disease rather than notification of the result itself. Reports of projected disease outcome for seropositives reveal a bleak picture (7). It appears that most seropositive individuals will develop clinical manifestations of HIV infection over the course of their lives in the absence of prophylactic treatments. Resulting psychological distress and increased use of mental health and primary care services should be expected.

Longitudinal psychosocial studies of persons with AIDS and symptomatic HIV infection (8,9) have found psychological distress greatest among symptomatic individuals when compared to the seropositive without symptoms or to people with AIDS. Persons with HIV-related symptoms may suffer from cognitive impairment (10) and physical incapacitation which may be as debilitating as that seen among persons diagnosed with AIDS. A lesser degree of empathy, as well as the fewer clinical and social services available for symptomatic individuals, often leads to alienation among those without a formal diagnosis of AIDS.

Methods

One hundred sixty gay and bisexual male clients participated in the evaluation. Each attended one of three groups: a support group for symptomatic people, an educational group on "hot and healthy sex," or a stress management group. These eight-week groups were led by a mental health clinician and consisted of 10 to 12 individuals. Group members completed pre- and post-intervention questionnaires which surveyed the following variables: psychological distress, knowledge of HIV risk activities, social support, coping skills, current mental health needs, alcohol and drug use, and sexual practices.

Results

The respondents represented a group of predominantly white (87%), gay men in their mid-thirties who were knowledgeable about their antibody status or the current state of their health. More than 25% of the respondents were seropositive; another 25% had been diagnosed with symptomatic HIV infection. More than 33% did not know their antibody status, and the remaining 11% reported a seronegative status.

Prior to the intervention, respondents were asked about the extent to which they engaged in high- and low-risk sexual practices in the past year. Approximately 60% reported "almost always" or "always" engaging in safer sex activities. Slightly more than 30% said they practice safer sex "seldom" or "half the time." Nine percent reported abstaining from sex altogether.

When asked what factors had influenced a compromise in safer sex standards in the previous twelve months, respondents selected the following reasons:

a) I lack self-control (40%);

b) I was more aroused than usual (37%);

c) My partner was more of a "turn-on" than usual (32%); and

d) I was lonely (32%).

Substance use was another reason given for a compromise in safer sex standards, although it was reported to be a less frequent factor. Drug and alcohol problems, however, were major issues for this group of clients. More than 50% reported current or past substance use problems as measured by the Michigan Alcohol Screening Test.

Respondents rated their perceived degree of risk of HIV infection on a scale of one to ten, where one was "no risk," five was a "50/50 chance," and ten was "certain to develop AIDS or ARC" (the term used at the time for symptomatic HIV infection). Excluding symptomatic clients or those with AIDS, nearly half rated their chances of developing symptoms as five or greater. When excluding persons with AIDS only, two-thirds rated the likelihood of their developing AIDS as greater than five.

Many clients had developed methods for coping with distress before they entered the educational support groups. Active behavioral and cognitive methods were significantly correlated with reductions in hopelessness over the course of the group intervention. Behavioral coping strategies included improving diets, forming a personal plan of action about AIDS, being involved in political activities, and learning more about HIV antibody testing and possible treatments for HIV infection. Cognitive strategies included thinking about AIDS concerns on a one-day-at-a-time basis, thinking more about the meaning of life, and considering how others in similar situations might respond. Taking responsibility for maintaining and perhaps improving one's health status was another important and significant factor which correlated with reductions in distress.

To assess changes over the life of the group in terms of psychological distress, knowledge about AIDS, and risk behavior, pre- and post-intervention scores were compared. Across all measures of psychological distress, statistically significant reductions occurred at the post-intervention assessment, even for those individuals who had already developed their own coping strategies. For example, we found reductions in hopelessness as measured by the Beck Hopelessness Scale, as well as reductions in all subscales of the Profile of Mood States measuring depression/dejection, fatigue/inertia, tension/anxiety, anger/hostility and confusion. No significant increases in the already high level of knowledge about HIV transmission were noted after the intervention. However, statistically significant increases in the frequency of safer sex practices and reductions in unsafe sex practices were reported at the post-group assessment.

Discussion

The psychological and social impact of the AIDS epidemic on those who have been the most affected has been enormous, and is summarized briefly below. Individuals in our evaluation sample are men along the continuum from those concerned about becoming infected, to those who are infected but are asymptomatic, to those with symptoms of HIV disease. The psychosocial concerns of these different groups accelerate with time.

Summary of Study

Certain methodological issues must be considered when reviewing this type of evaluation research data. For example, the absence of a control group limits our ability to determine with certainty that changes in distress and behavior are due to the group intervention and not some other influence. In addition, the data reflect self-reported changes by the participants. Therefore, it was not possible to determine more objectively whether the group intervention resulted in reductions of risk behavior and HIV transmission.

These results indicate that this group intervention model is effective in ameliorating psychological distress, assisting in behavior change, and encouraging health promotion practices. These data and the clinical experience of the group facilitators suggest that clients need supportive interventions to assist them in maintaining commitments to HIV risk reductions. The data also suggest the need for mental health interventions directed at the emotional distress clients are likely to experience as a result of an ever worsening manifestation of the HIV epidemic. Finally, attention to the effect of substance use and abuse is critical in the group model.

The Future

While there has been an unprecedented change in behavior among most individuals at risk of HIV disease in San Francisco (11) and other cities, there is a continued need for community structures which support that change. The task of prevention education may be as great as any faced to date. It is important to note that despite the very real changes in behavior that have occurred, continued high-risk sex is reported among some groups (12) and a steady number of individuals continue to seroconvert each year (13). Some groups have been particularly hard to reach with prevention messages, including youth and those in ethnic minority communities. Prevention education programs must continue to be modified and refined to meet the changing mental health and prevention needs of all people at risk (14).

In the future, programs must also conform more closely to the recommendations of the National Academy of Science report which suggests that measures to help in the planning and provision of psychosocial care for persons affected by AIDS infection (15) must be evaluated properly. Among the measures recommended were 1) to assess the efficacy of psychosocial interventions for those seronegative and seropositive individuals with "psychopathological" reactions to having AIDS or symptomatic HIV; 2) to develop and test educational materials for use with those stressed by HIV-related disorders; and, 3) to assess the impact of psychosocial interventions on high-risk individuals in efforts to limit the spread of HIV.

Furthermore, the experience of the AIDS Health Project indicates that ongoing monitoring of psychosocial programs for persons affected by HIV is essential, due to the constant need to refine programs so they remain relevant and effective in a rapidly changing environment. Specifically, there are unique aspects of the HIV epidemic that place special demands on services delivered by psychosocial programs. First, the changing demographic nature of groups affected by the epidemic requires psychosocial services specifically relevant to each population. Second, the changing clinical picture of HIV disease reveals the increasingly grim prognosis for the natural course of HIV infection. Individuals who take tests to determine the health of their immune system are more able to monitor the course of their infection. Services to seropositive individuals must attend to these increased levels of anxiety and fear associated with the knowledge of their antibody and immune function status. Finally, the changing nature of the social context of the epidemic takes a heavy toll on the mental health of many individuals. The prolonged and unremitting exposure to death and dying within communities hard hit by the epidemic has led to special problems associated with grief and bereavement (16). Additionally, the vicissitudes of public opinion and legislative action may also affect psychological outcome.

HIV prevention programs must address the large-scale social and psychological ramifications of continuous loss. For those infected with HIV, expanded mental health care and substance abuse programs are a necessity, and evaluation of such programs plays a critical role in the future development of increasingly sophisticated prevention interventions in HIV disease.

Given the usefulness of the psychosocial interventions employed by the AIDS Health Project and the expected continued need for such services, there is strong support for the increased use of this model in providing services for all groups at risk for HIV infection.

■

References

1. Moulton JM, Stempel R, Bacchetti P, et al: Psychological consequences of HIV antibody test notification. Poster presentation, Fourth International Conference on AIDS, Stockholm, Sweden, June 12-16, 1988

2. Stempel R, Moulton JM, Kelly T, et al: Patterns of distress following antibody test notification. Poster presentation, Third International Conference on AIDS, Washington, D.C., June 1-5, 1987

3. Holland J, Tross S: The psychosocial and neuropsychiatric sequelae of the acquired immunodeficiency syndrome. Ann Intern Med 1985; 103:760-764

4. Morin SF, Charles KA, Malyon AK: Psychological impact of AIDS on gay men. Am Psychologist 1984; 39:1288-1293

5. Coates TJ, Morin SF, McKusick L: Consequences of AIDS antibody testing among gay men: the AIDS Behavioral Research Project. Poster presentation, Third International Conference on AIDS, Washington, DC, June 1-5, 1987

6. Pindyck J, Avorn P, Cleary P, et al: Notification of Anti-HTLV-III/LAV Positive Blood Donors: Psychosocial, Counseling and Care Issues. World Health Organization report on AIDS. Geneva, World Health Organization, 1986

7. Moss AR, Bacchetti P, Osmond D, et al: Seropositivity for HIV and the development of AIDS or AIDS related condition: three year follow up of the San Francisco General Hospital cohort. Br Med J 1988; 296:745-750

8. Tross S: Psychological and neuropsychological functions in AIDS patients. Poster presentation, International Conference on AIDS, Atlanta, GA., April 14-17, 1985

9. Temoshok L, Sweet D, Moulton JM, et al: A longitudinal study of distress and coping in men with AIDS and AIDS-related complex. Poster presentation, Third International Conference on AIDS, Washington, D.C., June 1-5, 1987

10. Temoshok L, Canick J, Moulton, et al: Distress, coping and neuropsychological status in men with ARC: longitudinal studies. Poster presentation, Fourth International Conference on AIDS. Stockholm, Sweden, June 12-16, 1988

11. McKusick L, Coates T, Stall R, et al: Psychological and behavioral predictors of AIDS risk reduction. Poster presentation, Fourth International Conference on AIDS, Stockholm, Sweden, June 12-16, 1988

12. Bye L: The Third Probability Study of an Urban Male Community: Designing an Effective AIDS Prevention Campaign Strategy for San Francisco. San Francisco, Communication Technologies, 1987

13. San Francisco Department of Public Health: AIDS in San Francisco: Status Report for Fiscal Year 1987-1988, and Projections of Service Needs and Costs for 1988-1993. A report prepared by the San Francisco Department of Public Health for the San Francisco Health Commission, March 15, 1988

14. Baker R, Moulton JM, Gorman M: Epidemic of Loss: AIDS in San Francisco's Gay Male Community, 1988-1993. San Francisco AIDS Foundation, San Francisco, 1988

15. National Academy of Sciences: Confronting AIDS: Directions for Public Health, Health Care, and Research. Washington, DC, Institute of Medicine, National Academy of Sciences, 1986

16. Martin JL, Dean L: The secondary epidemic of AIDS-related bereavement. Poster presentation, Fourth International Conference on AIDS, Stockholm, Sweden, June 12-16, 1988

■

*Jeffrey Moulton, PhD, is Program Evaluator, UCSF AIDS Health Project, and Director of Psychological Services, HIV Evaluation and Treatment Unit, Letterman Army Medical Center in San Francisco. **David Sweet, MA,** is an Assistant Research Psychologist at the University of California San Francisco. **Gamze Gurbuz, BA,** is a graduate student at the California School of Professional Psychology in Berkeley and Research Assistant, UCSF AIDS Health Project. **James W. Dilley, MD,** is an Assistant Clinical Professor of Psychiatry, UCSF School of Medicine, and Director of the UCSF AIDS Health Project.*

Being Seronegative in a Seropositive World: A Personal Perspective

Ronald D. Moskowitz

As more people decide to take the HIV antibody test, a population of gay men who know they are seronegative, but don't quite know how to live with that fact, increases daily. Surrounded by lovers, friends, and colleagues who are ill or dying, many seronegative men stifle disclosure of their test result and struggle with getting on with their lives.

One might imagine that these lucky men would be cheered and gratified by the good news—and most of them are, at least initially. But instead of remaining joyful, many are surprised to find that they, as well as their friends and loved ones, have major problems in coping with their new status. A great many accept the news with disbelief; others react with various forms of anxiety, fear and guilt. Still others, remembering their sexual activity of the past or the recent illness or death of a sexual partner, reject the news as "a mistake" and accept it only when retesting one or more times confirms the initial results.

Although reports indicate that gay men in San Francisco, for example, are divided equally between those who are seropositive and seronegative, many who in this city test negative feel isolated from the majority of the gay community. These men find talking about being negative to other gay men difficult, since the latter may be positive and may consider remarks as "bragging" or elitist. Yet many gay men hope to find a partner who is also negative, though they feel inadequate about broaching the subject of anti-body status. A new etiquette is being developed as seronegative gay men cautiously find ways to locate others of similar status without offending friends and acquaintances who are untested or who have tested positive.

Some seronegatives search the bars or other pickup spots, believing they can have sex with anyone as long as they practice safer sex. Yet these men freely concede that they would prefer not to fall in love with someone who is positive. When it comes to a lover, they would prefer someone who has also tested negative.

Still others have decided to give up their sexual activity and have become celibate or even chaste. Some say they are following this route as a temporary measure until they meet the man of their dreams. Others have simply abandoned hope of both sex and love until some vaccination or cure for AIDS is found.

There are still others who worry so much about staying sero-negative that their fears and anxieties have led them to be sexually dysfunctional.

A serious problem facing these men is "survivor guilt," which causes extreme depression for those who have lost one or more partners and large numbers of close friends.

Understandably, the resources of the community are focused on those most directly affected by the epidemic. Seronegative men frequently feel their problems are minuscule compared to those of the infected, and they are reluctant to come forward and seek help from mental health professionals already inundated with sero-positive and diagnosed people.

To assist in drawing them out, a "personals" advertisement was placed by this writer in a San Francisco gay newspaper. A box number was given, and those replying were asked to send their name, address and telephone number. The ad read:

HIV NEGATIVE GROUPS

Testing negative is great but can present problems of its own. Some have become so fearful, they have all but given up sex with others. Many, watching their friends and loved ones die, are burdened with what psychologists call "survivor guilt." Support groups to deal with these problems and others are forming.

Within a few weeks there were several dozen replies. Here are some excerpts:

"I was considering an ad like the one you placed but I didn't know if there was really anyone out there who felt the way I do or take it quite as earnest. Seems like being negative is becoming more of a minority issue every day, especially in my neighborhood (the Castro, a pre-dominantly gay neighborhood). I have yet to meet another negative."

"I have dealt with the passing of more than sixty friends and three relationships. Guess I've passed the point of watching everyone fade away. I'd really welcome meeting some new friends with at least their health status in common."

"I am HIV negative and would like to meet other men who are going through 'withdrawal.' My sex life has just been (to) jack off for several years and I feel (it is) very difficult to meet men and try to make relationships."

Letters were sent to those who replied, along with a questionnaire asking about meeting times and places, and types and lengths of meetings preferred. The replies indicated that most preferred to meet weekly for two to three hours somewhere in San Francisco, and most preferred a health professional as group leader if the cost did not exceed $5 or $10 per person per session. Some said they would not be interested in the meeting if any fee were charged.

The San Francisco AIDS Foundation supplied a meeting room, the AIDS Health Project furnished one of its volunteer licensed psychologists to act as group leader, and ten men appeared for the first meeting. They agreed to meet each Wednesday for eight weeks and then decide whether to continue.

One thing became evident the first night: all the men discussed their seronegative status openly and comfortably—many for the first time since they received their results. The homogeneity of the group gave its members license to talk about a vital part of themselves that they had buried deep inside, almost as though it were something to be hidden in shame. The men expressed this feeling during the meetings that followed as well.

As the meetings continued from week to week, people who were quiet at first began to open up and talk about their individual problems. The psychologist who was our group leader would employ, from time to time, structured activities to help deepen our discussions.

It soon became evident that because they were seronegative, few of the members were having much sex and that even fewer were enjoying what little they did have. Surprisingly, the men disagreed about what constituted "safe sex," even though every member of the group said he had read literature or had been counseled on the subject. Some members said they were afraid of sexual contact with anyone who was not seronegative. Even those who didn't share that view conceded they would prefer to fall in love with a seronegative person rather than a seropositive one. The group agreed to invite the San Francisco AIDS Foundation to send a speaker to a future meeting to enlighten them and standardize their information about "safe sex."

Two weeks later two experts from the AIDS Foundation joined the group, and the entire two-hour meeting was focused on safe sex, including a condom demonstration and questions and answers. Although one physician member of the group questioned the necessity of the session, virtually all the others applauded it. The group learned that it is possible to have enjoyable and safe sex without knowing the antibody status of your partner if safe sex guidelines are followed.

Besides giving its members a comfortable forum and some of its members "authorization" to have sex again, the group was helpful in other ways.

Since most meetings were held at members' homes and refreshments were served afterwards, a camaraderie developed among the members, some of whom often telephoned each other and met during the week to discuss problems and common interests. One member, who had a kidney stone attack during a meeting, was escorted to a nearby hospital emergency room by three concerned group members.

The gathering also provided a ready-made pool of prospective seronegative sexual partners. In fact, some group members did socialize together, others dated, and there were a few sexual liaisons—though none was officially reported during group meetings.

At the eighth session of the group, the members decided not to continue meeting on an official basis. During the eight-week meeting period, however, many more responses to the advertisement came in, along with applications from other seronegatives who had heard about the support group from its members. These new men were referred to the AIDS Health Project, which acknowledged the demand for seronegative groups and recognized the success of the initial group. Additional groups for these seronegatives were formed and continue to meet on a regular basis.

■

Ronald D. Moskowitz is a Sausalito writer and educational consultant. He has been Education Secretary to Governor Edmund G. Brown, Education Editor of the San Francisco Examiner and the San Francisco Chronicle, and Associate Director of the Education Commission of the States.

IV
Substance Abuse and AIDS

■ **The Epidemiology of HIV Among Intravenous Drug Users**
John A. Newmeyer, PhD

■ **Mental Health Complications of Substance Abuse**
Glen Fischer, Sally Jo Jones, and Jack B. Stein, MSW

■ **Strategies for Working with Substance-Abusing Clients**
Barbara G. Faltz, RN, MS

■

The Epidemiology of HIV Among Intravenous Drug Users

John A. Newmeyer, PhD

Substance use increases an individual's vulnerability to HIV in three major ways. First, a person who shares hypodermic equipment with someone infected with HIV is at risk. Secondly, someone who becomes intoxicated may lose inhibitions against risky practices—for example, neglecting the use of a condom during a drunken sexual encounter. Thirdly, a number of substances, such as alcohol and cannabis, may have direct immunosuppressive properties. If one is already HIV infected, heavy use of an immunosuppressive substance might accelerate the collapse of helper T-cell activity. Further research is needed in all these areas. The primary purpose of this chapter is to focus on the "direct contagion" aspect of substance abuse and AIDS.

The risk behavior involves the sharing of contaminated injection equipment, the syringe and the needle, the "cooker" (the container in which the drug is dissolved in water), and the "cotton" (the material used to strain the drug solution as it is drawn up into the syringe). Even the rinse water employed by the user can be a source of infection. A distinction should be made between the act of intravenous drug use and the population of "intravenous drug users." There are about 1.2 million Americans who used drugs intravenously more than ten times during 1987 (1). These persons, who will henceforth be termed "IVDUs," were at great risk for HIV transmission because of their potentially high incidence of unsafe practices. People who rarely inject are at some risk, but their risk for HIV infection will not be addressed in this chapter. (See Editor's Notes, page 117.)

AIDS and IVDUs in U.S. Cities

More than 22,000 heterosexual IVDUs had been diagnosed with AIDS in the United States by October 1989. This group represented a steady 17% of the nation's AIDS caseload for the five-year period 1982-1987. Among new cases reported in 1989, however, that proportion rose to 23%. By contrast, the proportion of the caseload consisting of gay males dropped from the usual 72-73% to below 64% during 1989. This may reflect an earlier adoption of risk reduction among gay men than among IVDUs.

An extraordinary aspect of the HIV epidemic among IVDUs is its very uneven geographical distribution. As of October 1989, New York City alone had reported some 35% of all American cases of AIDS among heterosexual IVDUs. Studies of IVDU populations in various cities completed in late 1987 and early 1988 documented a pattern of HIV antibody seropositivity heavily biased toward the Northeast (see Table 1).

For 14 of these 16 cities, survey data from gay male samples were also available. All but one of these showed seroprevalence proportions in the range from 23% to 52%. The pattern of HIV infection for gay men, at least in these cities, appears to be more widespread and homogeneous than that for IVDUs. An obvious explanation is as follows: many gay men travel frequently, and they were likely to have visited such "HIV epicenters" as San Francisco and New York during the early 1980s. This factor allowed HIV to get a strong early start in almost all gay male communities. IVDUs, by contrast, tend not to travel nor to interact very much with gay men, thus delaying the start of HIV spread in most IVDU communities, especially those that were distant from the New York epicenter.

Table 1. HIV Seroprevalence Among Heterosexual IVDUs in the U.S. (1987-1988).

City	Seropositive	City	Seropositive
New York City	50%	Los Angeles	4%
Boston	28%	Milwaukee	2%
Baltimore	25%	Albuquerque	1%
Chicago	25%	Minneapolis	1%
Philadelphia	19%	Seattle	1%
San Francisco	16%	Kansas City	0%
Atlanta	10%	Louisville	0%
Denver	5%	St. Louis	0%

AIDS and IVDUs in Europe

The distribution of AIDS among IVDUs in Europe shows even more striking temporal and geographical disparities. In 1984, barely 1% of the European AIDS caseload consisted of IVDUs. Beginning in that year, however, IVDU numbers increased much more rapidly than those of the other major populations at risk; for example, there was a 222% increase in their caseload between 1986 and 1987. By the first quarter of 1989, IVDUs represented fully 34% of the new AIDS cases being reported. The overall total of IVDU AIDS cases was approaching 6,000 by April of 1989.

Italy and Spain have been especially hard hit, with 66% and 61% of their AIDS caseloads, respectively, ascribed to intravenous users. The proportion is 25-30% for Austria and Switzerland, approximately 16% for France, perhaps 11% for West Germany, and under 10% for all other countries. Italy, Spain, and France have among them fully 85% of all AIDS/IVDU cases in Europe. The Far East also has a significant problem among IVDUs. In Thailand, where the purity and availability of heroin is legendary, HIV seropositivity increased from 14% to 43% in a single year among IV drug users attending methadone clinics in Bangkok. Similar steep rises have also been recorded in Hong Kong and Singapore. A few samplings of IVDUs for antibodies to HIV also suggest strong geographical differences, as seen in Table 2.

Table 2. HIV Seroprevalence in European IVDUs

		Seropositive
Countries:	Italy	37%
	Switzerland	27%
	Greece	<5%
Cities:	Milan, Italy	80%
	Edinburgh, Scotland	50-60%
	Amsterdam, Netherlands	29%
	Dublin, Ireland	16%
	Naples, Italy	12%
	London, England	5-10%
	Hamburg, W. Germany	7%
	Stockholm, Sweden	7%*

* (heroin users 45%, speed users 5%, mixed users 13%)

These findings demolish the hopeful theory that "HIV won't spread among IVDUs who have access to legal injection equipment." That theory had been credible in the 1983-1985 period, when New York (with its stringent laws against possession of paraphernalia and its many "shooting galleries") seemed to be the only area of the world with a large AIDS problem among its IVDUs. But it is now obvious that HIV had spread quite widely in cities such as Milan and Amsterdam, where over-the-counter needle availability existed. "Needle exchange programs" may have some effect on the rate of increase of IVDU cases, but there is little expectation that this strategy will stop the practice of sharing equipment or stop the rise of HIV infection. It is likely that most IVDUs in most parts of the Western world share contaminated injection equipment often enough to assure rapid spread of HIV, as well as other diseases such as hepatitis. Regions without much HIV disease among IVDUs probably have been spared solely because the virus has only recently been introduced into the area.

The New York Experience

New York City is the best place to observe the full extent of the AIDS epidemic among IVDUs. It is no longer the only metropolis where the prevalence of HIV has reached the 50% range, but the city was evidently the first to have done so. Retrospective testing of IVDU blood samples shows that HIV may have infected half of New York's IVDUs by as early as 1982. Follow-up studies of HIV-infected persons demonstrate that progression to full-blown AIDS actually accelerates in the sixth through tenth years after infection (2). Thus, it is not surprising to find that New York City has already (November 1989) reported more than 8,100 AIDS cases among heterosexual IVDUs (3).

The New York experience permits the following observations:

1. An IVDU diagnosed with AIDS has a short life expectancy because diagnosis usually occurs rather late in the course of HIV infection and because *Pneumocystis carinii* pneumonia is the first manifestation far more frequently than Kaposi's sarcoma which, although lethal, has a slower course of disease progression.

2. In stark contrast to the gay male community, the IVDU population has not been able to muster self-help programs for its

stricken community. Nearly the entire burden of their care has fallen upon public agencies.

3. Public agencies are overwhelmed with a tidal wave of sick and dying IVDUs. Facilities and personnel are strained to the limit and, perhaps more significantly, they have been slow to adapt to the demands of coping with "misbehaving dope fiends" instead of the middle-class gay men with AIDS.

4. The morbidity and mortality of IVDUs is probably much worse than the AIDS caseload figures indicate. Medical examiner data of the New York City Department of Health indicate that huge numbers of New York IVDUs are dying of diseases which are linked to HIV infection without ever having been diagnosed with AIDS. Dr. Rand Stoneburner estimates that the true number of IVDU cases in New York is 100% to 150% higher than the officially reported numbers.

5. Widespread HIV infection of heterosexual IVDUs has resulted in similarly widespread infection of their sexual partners and their babies. Through 1987, about six times as much infection of this sort was ascribed to IVDUs as to gay or bisexual men, even though the latter group was four times as numerous in the AIDS caseload (4). It thus appears that the average IVDU is at least twenty times as likely as the average gay man to spread the virus in this "secondary" fashion—even though one-quarter to one-half of "gay" men are also heterosexually active. Hence, San Francisco, where fewer than 2% of the AIDS caseload consists of heterosexual IVDUs, has had almost no cases of AIDS among heterosexual partners or infants.

Dire Forecasts

What does the future hold for the world's intravenous drug users? One thing is clear: even if by some miracle no more become infected, there are likely to be tens of thousands more who will develop AIDS in the next few years. The table of HIV infection rates in IVDUs suggests that most American cases in 1988-1994 will be concentrated in the cities along the northeast corridor, plus Chicago and perhaps Detroit. A crude epidemiological method (which nonetheless seems to be the best one available to date) can be used to gauge the magnitude of the problem at hand:

1. The Drug Abuse Warning Network (DAWN) collects statistics on reported emergency room incidents and overdose deaths involving intravenous drugs. These data allow us to estimate the relative number of IVDUs in various metropolitan areas using the assumption that each 1,000 IVDUs will generate overdose problems at the same rate in every city.

2. New York is used as an "anchor" for prevalence estimates. The number of IVDUs in New York has been measured fairly precisely at about 200,000. It is assumed that a metropolis that has had one-tenth as many overdoses as New York has about .1 x 200,000, or 20,000 IVDUs.

3. Estimates of the seroprevalence of HIV exist for IVDU populations of most major American cities. These can be multiplied by the IVDU prevalence estimates to arrive at an estimate of the number of seropositive IVDUs. Most cities can be pretty well discounted, in that their seropositive rates are so small.

4. This method yields an estimate that in early 1988 there were about 190,000 HIV-infected IVDUs in the U.S. Nearly half of these were in New York City.

5. The number of new AIDS cases that will be generated by this infected population depends on the "age" of that infection. For example, various cohort study data indicate that about 2% will progress to AIDS in the third year following infection, and about 7% in the seventh year. Making certain assumptions about the distribution of infection of the 190,000 seropositive IVDUs allows us to predict that this population will generate some 12,000 to 14,000 new cases of AIDS each year between 1989 and 1994. IVDUs infected after early 1988 will only begin to add significantly to this caseload in 1993 or 1994. Of course, if effective measures for immune system modulation become widely available to seropositive IVDUs in the near future, the number of new cases could be considerably less than the above prediction.

The same predictive model could be applied to Europe. That continent, with about twice the population of the U.S., seems to have somewhat fewer active IVDUs. The data on IVDU prevalence and IVDU seropositive rates is less comprehensive than that for the U.S., but it is likely that the continent will be generating at least 5,000 new IVDU cases per year throughout the early 1990s—or about four times the case rate which prevailed in 1987.

AIDS Prevention and Care of IVDUs with AIDS

Clearly, the situation among IVDUs demands prompt and forceful action. There are two urgent needs: first, to prevent further HIV infection among IVDUs; and second, to enable already infected IVDUs to sustain their immune system health as long as possible and to avoid infecting their sexual partners and babies.

Fortunately, the prevention message for IVDUs is simple and consists of three exhortations: 1) "Stop shooting drugs." 2) "If you must shoot drugs, get your own works and don't share them." 3) "If you must share works, disinfect them with bleach between users." (Of course, IVDUs must also be encouraged to use condoms when engaging in sex.)

The first exhortation should be emphasized most. It is desirable that as many people as possible stop injecting drugs. However, IV drug use is generally an addictive behavior, sometimes strongly reinforced by peer-group or other pressures, and most areas lack the drug abuse treatment capacity to assist even half the IVDUs who might want treatment. Hence, it is important to recognize that a large number of IVDUs will continue their practices and not seek treatment.

There is a problem with the second exhortation: syringes and needles are not available over the counter in some states, and unauthorized possession can be grounds for arrest. "Works" are often scarce, and to obtain sterile equipment and not share it with other IVDUs requires the money and know-how to purchase them, either legally or illegally. Many IVDUs do not have this wherewithal; to counsel them with advice such as "get your own works and don't share them" is often akin to "let them eat cake" advice. Furthermore, even if works are abundant, there remain social and psychological reasons for sharing—for instance, as an expression of interpersonal trust or bonding.

Consequently, for a substantial number of IVDUs it is vital to use the third, last-ditch exhortation: disinfect between users. Bleach has been widely accepted as an ideal disinfectant because it meets the five key criteria of quickness, cheapness, convenience, effectiveness, and safety. The basic method of disinfection calls for two complete flushings of needle and syringe (and the "cooker" as well, if appropriate) with full-strength bleach, followed by two rinsings with water. This methodology is simple enough to teach with brochures, comic strips, billboards, or 30-second broadcast commercials.

An especially impressive model for education of IVDUs is provided by the Community Health Outreach Workers (CHOWs), a model used successfully in a number of cities. The CHOWs, who are hired for their ability to handle themselves "on the street," receive intensive training and work in one neighborhood of IVDUs. A CHOW takes care to become well known and trusted in the user community, then engages in one-to-one contacts with IVDUs to educate them about the nature of AIDS and the means to reduce risk. Providing ample supplies of one-ounce bleach bottles and condoms, plus repeated contacts with the same individuals, helps maximize behavior change toward safer practices.

When the three prevention exhortations are pursued vigorously (this may require considerable coordination and mutual respect between law enforcement agencies, drug treatment programs, and prevention outreach groups), real progress against the spread of HIV starts to occur within a fairly short time. Several surveys in San Francisco indicate that bleach disinfection was being practiced in the great majority of IVDU-sharing situations during 1987 and 1988, and the seropositive rate among IVDUs has not changed significantly (from around 15%) between late 1986 and early 1989.

The second task—to keep seropositive IVDUs healthy and prevent them from infecting their sex partners and babies—may be tougher than the task of preventing further needle contagion. It looks as if it will be much more difficult to imbue the condom-using habit among heterosexual, low-socioeconomic-status IVDUs than it was among gay men. It is also a tough job to convince drug users that taking the HIV antibody test is a wise diagnostic step and that, if they test positive, there are ways to maintain their health. The principal challenges are 1) to maintain conditions whereby antibody testing can be free, anonymous, and supported by sound pre- and post-test counseling; 2) to translate the message of HIV treatment information programs into a form that IVDUs can comprehend and respond to; 3) to advocate means of paying for the costly immunomodulator and antiviral therapies that seropositive IVDUs might choose; and 4) to help IVDUs and their sexual partners employ safer sex practices in situations which carry a significant risk of HIV transmission.

Summary

The HIV epidemic among the world's intravenous drug users is in a critical phase. It is clear that explosive contagion has occurred in several major IVDU locales, such as New York City, New Jersey, Italy, and Spain. An uneven pattern of HIV infection characterizes the remaining centers of IVDU activity. Ample evidence indicates that IVDUs in those centers are continuing the practice of sharing equipment, which may result in a duplication of the sad experience of New York City. However, the vigorous prevention work that has been pursued in San Francisco during the period from 1986-1988 suggests that needle-borne contagion can be slowed significantly.

The message about "safer needle practices" is a simple and straightforward one; the trick is to deliver that message to the at-risk population in a way that will lead to enduring behavior change. Repeated one-to-one encounters between outreach workers and IVDUs seem to be a key element of a successful strategy. Preventing heterosexual and parent-to-child transmission beyond the infected IVDU population appears to be much more difficult than preventing parenteral transmission among these same IVDUs. This is an area that will require ongoing intervention by the AIDS prevention team. Success is possible but requires the continued availability of resources.

■

References

1. Centers for Disease Control: HIV infection in the United States: a review of current knowledge. Mortality and Morbidity Weekly Report 1987 (Supplement 6); 36:1-48

2. Bacchetti P, Moss AR: Incubation period of AIDS in San Francisco. Nature 1989; 338:251-253

3. AIDS Surveillance Update, New York City Dept. of Health, November 1989

4. Newmeyer J: The intravenous drug user and secondary spread of AIDS. Journal of Psychoactive Drugs 1988; 20:169-172

Editor's Notes

Page 108. While the statistics in this chapter are dated, the basic prevention approaches discussed remain current. Note also that in some areas such as San Francisco, where prevention efforts were mounted early and have been consistently applied, the seroprevalence of HIV among injection drug users has remained fairly stable at 15% to 20%. In other areas, particularly other parts of the world such as in the far East, the seroprevalence among drug users has exploded.

Updated References.

Selwyn PA, Alcabes P, Hartel D, et al: Clinical manifestations and predictors of disease progression in drug users with human immunodeficiency virus infection. N Engl J Med 1992; 327:1697-1703

Chiasson MA, Stoneburner RL, Hildebrandt DS et al: Heterosexual transmission of HIV-1 associated with the use of smokable freebase cocaine (crack). AIDS 1991; 5:1121-6

Friedman S: Organizing drug users. FOCUS: A Guide to AIDS Research and Counseling 1991; 6(11):1-4

Hagen H: Studies support needle exchange. FOCUS: A Guide to AIDS Research and Counseling 1991; 6(11):5-6

Kaslow RA, Blackwelder WC, Ostrow DG, et al: No evidence for a role of alcohol or other pscyhoactive drugs in accelerating immunodeficiency in HIV-1 positive individuals: a report from the Multicenter AIDS Cohort Study. JAMA 1989; 261:3424-9

■

John A. Newmeyer, PhD, is an epidemiologist at the Haight Ashbury Free Clinics in San Francisco.

Mental Health Complications of Substance Abuse

Glen Fischer, Sally Jo Jones, and Jack B. Stein, MSW

The challenges brought to mental health professionals by HIV disease are enormous, and these continue to expand as the epidemic takes heavier tolls on additional populations. The thorniest parts of these challenges revolve around issues recognized as the nexus of the AIDS epidemic: sexually transmitted diseases and substance abuse.

HIV disease and substance abuse are linked in at least four inescapable, but not widely acknowledged ways:

- direct HIV transmission via sharing of intravenous (IV) drug works;
- sexual transmission of HIV from infected IV drug-using individuals to their partners and perinatal transmission resulting from high-risk behaviors of one or both parents;
- immune compromise from substance abuse as a co-factor in increasing the susceptibility to infection and in hastening the progression of HIV disease; and
- impairment of judgment that promotes continued or resumed high-risk behavior.

These associations have such an accelerating effect on the spread of HIV that all health care providers, including mental health professionals, must become engaged in the struggle to provide adequate and effective education and services to substance-using populations.

Substance Abuse: An Overview

Some mental health professionals are hesitant about working with substance abusers. People who are part of the drug "subculture" often manifest behaviors deviant to established social norms. As a result, they reinforce commonly held biases about them as a group. Furthermore, since substance abuse is a condition that is still not fully understood and because it is often associated with illegal and socially unacceptable behaviors, stigmatizing labels are often applied to those involved. For many, this response represents an attempt to gain a sense of control over a frightening presence in their midst.

There is a good deal of disagreement among those working in the field of substance abuse treatment about the ways in which substance abuse is defined and conceptualized. To assure clarity in this discussion and to ensure an understanding of these terms, we offer the following definitions:

■ **substance**: any chemical, whether licit or illicit; organic, distilled, or pharmaceutical, that affects an individual in such a way as to bring about physiological, emotional, and behavioral change;

■ **substance abuse**: the use of any substance in a manner that results in the individual's continuing or recurrent physical, mental, emotional, or social impairment.

Four conceptual models currently influence thinking about the phenomenon of substance abuse in the United States. Each of these varies in its etiological assumptions and implications for intervention.

■ **The Moral-Legal Model** — Drugs are either legal or illegal, socially acceptable or unacceptable. Those involved with illegal or socially unacceptable drugs are morally weak and/or criminal.

■ **The Psychosocial Model** — Drug use is a behavior that serves some function for the individual — for example, to alleviate an emotional problem or to maintain balance in a dysfunctional family.

■ **The Sociocultural Model** — Social pressure and repression— for example, poverty, poor housing, urbanization, and discrimination, forces drug use behavior.

■ **The Disease Model** — Drugs, including alcohol, are dependence-producing, and the individual user has a chronic and progressive disease.

If we move beyond causality and focus on intervention, it becomes apparent that the most useful understanding of substance abuse must be comprehensive and multifaceted, incorporating the most relevant aspects from each of these models. This approach conforms to the current professional view that every health condition is at once a physical, psychological, social, economic, and political phenomenon.

From this multidimensional perspective it is clear that the substance abuser's health can be significantly compromised:

- one's **physical condition** is habitually debilitated by poor nutrition, use of immune-suppressing drugs, bouts of infection and illness (especially sexually transmitted diseases), high stress, and physical addiction that takes precedence over all other life spheres;

- one's **psychological functioning** is dedicated to defending against intolerable feelings, largely rooted in maladaptive denial, fatalism, escapism, lack of self-esteem and feelings of personal power;

- one's **socioeconomic situation**, often involving criminal activities, precludes entitlement to social services and leads to chronic unemployment and poverty, with poor access to health services;

- **socioculturally,** one is alienated from community and family (itself often dysfunctional) and rejects all forms of authority and supports interpersonal relations that are limited in their ability to provide support; and

- **politically,** one has no power base from which to demand health rights.

Risk Reduction Counseling with Substance Abusers

Appreciating these dynamics is critical to working effectively with substance abusers on HIV-related issues. As a first step, service providers must examine and clarify their attitudes and values toward substance abuse as well as personal feelings about substance abusers.

In addition to these extremely difficult dynamics has been added HIV disease, yet another epidemic that is socially stigmatized, only partially understood, painful and deadly. The tools and strategies that exist in this area of human services are based on the experience of health behavior change in such areas as family planning and cardiovascular disease prevention. Additional insight comes from substance abuse treatment approaches that have evolved during the last 15 years and from innovative AIDS prevention work begun in the gay community.

Substance abuse is epidemic in the United States; eight out of every ten abusers are not in treatment for their chemical dependency. A majority of these express no desire to seek treatment. However, they do express a desire to avoid AIDS.

An effective strategy is needed for translating that desire into appropriate behavior change. Experience with behavior change, disease prevention, and health promotion indicates knowledge and education are essential for these processes to occur, but they are not sufficient in themselves. While new information about AIDS and HIV infection may be absorbed in an individual at risk, old values, judgments, feelings, and continued high-risk activities far outweigh attempts at substantial behavior change.

For example, among IV drug users, learning to clean "works" via bleaching is now well documented in several U.S. cities as the risk reduction behavior most amenable to change. The intervention is fairly straightforward. It is simple, inexpensive, fast, legal, and requires little unusual effort, since many users already flush their works with water to prevent clogging (2). Use of bleach, therefore, represents a first-line risk reduction practice. The nature of this practice poses few cognitive, attitudinal, or behavioral obstacles to change. The major barrier to wide-scale "needle hygiene" practices appears to be law enforcement and some substance abuse treatment professionals who view this type of intervention as adding to a criminal problem and do not promote or encourage its use.

Much more difficult to modify has been the sexual practices of drug abusers. Substance abuse treatment programs with gay men in San Francisco and New York City have provided leadership on this issue. These programs suggest that intensive psychosocial interventions are critical, especially those that target individual attitudes, interrelated behavioral patterns, and environmental influences. As noted in the foregoing section, these elements are likely to pose substantial impediments to health behavior change among substance abusers.

Service providers can initiate such interventions by actively engaging clients (in a process that helps them) to personalize their risks of HIV infection and transmission to others, to identify and rehearse practices that will reduce those risks, and to receive reinforcing feedback and continuing direction on the healthy changes initiated. Specifically, risk reduction counseling includes (3):

1. assisting the client to acknowledge the personal risks of HIV infection. This can be best accomplished by a complete assessment of:

   ■ drug use history and current substance use (4),

   ■ sexual practices,

   ■ nutrition, exercise, rest, and levels of stress.

2. explaining the range of changes that will reduce infection and transmission risks, addressing attitudinal and environmental obstacles (for example, feelings of having no control, resistance from partners) and rehearsing behaviors as needed; and

3. reinforcing changes in a way that helps the client to assume increasing control over health behaviors so that early accomplishments can be sustained and built upon.

In conducting risk reduction counseling, the mental health professional must constantly walk several tightropes. One such tightrope is drawn between providing straightforward information about the horror of HIV disease on the one hand, and attempting to instill deep-seated fear about the risks of substance abuse on the other. These types of fear tactics may be counterproductive for substance abusers, who, in the face of heightened anxiety, are likely to "shut down" and/or increase risk behavior.

Another such tightrope exists between conveying the urgency of adopting risk reduction behaviors as opposed to using coercive approaches that are likely to stimulate the substance abuser's resistance or undermine the personal sense of self-confidence needed to sustain behavior change. And of course, an overarching tightrope is to cast both substance abuse treatment and recovery and risk reduction as individually tailored processes and goals as opposed to all-or-nothing, overnight propositions that provide little hope of sustained behavior change.

A final note about risk reduction counseling with substance abusers relates to the promise of "peer educators." Given the success of this model in gay communities, and the drug abusers' antipathy for health "authorities," involving substance abusers in risk reduction support groups led by peers is gaining great currency in substance treatment. Identifying and referring clients to such groups may go a long way toward extending the effects of the mental health professional's interventions with substance abusers.

Providing Supportive Counseling to the Substance Abuser with HIV Disease

Individual psychosocial needs in HIV disease can be extreme, even when coping skills are highly developed and functional support systems are in place. Like any reaction to severe stress, adjustment to a diagnosis of HIV disease is governed by habitual coping mechanisms and psychosocial resources. In the case of active substance abusers, such mechanisms and resources are typically absent, severely strained, undeveloped, or maladaptive.

A useful model for understanding the process of adjusting to a diagnosis of HIV disease has been suggested by the "AIDS Situational Distress Model" developed by Dr. Stuart Nichols (5). This model describes four possible "stages" of adjustment to a diagnosis of HIV disease: crisis, transition, acceptance, and—for those in terminal AIDS—preparation for death. These four stages suggest supportive interventions appropriate to each stage.

The initial crisis of an HIV disease diagnosis is commonly met with denial as a defense against extreme anxiety. For substance users, since denial is already *the* psychological armor that allows continued use, many users remain in denial throughout the entire course of their HIV disease. Such denial often allows continued risk behavior, to self and to others, as well as thoughtless disclosure of HIV status to persons who have no "need to know." HIV infection may also force disclosure of previously disguised drug use to those needed for emotional support; the double stigma and ignorance about substance abuse and HIV disease may drive key people away. For the practitioner, maladaptive denial that leads to increased substance abuse should be challenged.

In the transitional stage, alternating waves of anxiety, anger, guilt, self-pity, and depression are typical. For the substance abuser, such feelings are historically mismanaged and intolerable. For those in recovery, this can be a thoroughly faith-shattering, regressive time. "Self-medication" with drinking and drugging and thoughts of suicide are common. To maintain control, the substance abuser may become particularly manipulative or may engage in more intense acting out. Helping professionals may become the brunt of all such adjustment reactions.

Gaining support from a family member or significant other of the substance abuser often requires task-oriented family therapy to address obstacles present from long-standing dysfunction. Enrolling a substance abuser in a buddy program or support group typically requires access to programs sensitive to the life-styles and special needs of substance abusers. For persons in recovery, Narcotics Anonymous and/or Alcoholics Anonymous chapters that have adapted their agendas to the issues of HIV-infected members are often the most promising options.

Achieving a level of acceptance of the new limitations and challenges that HIV disease brings and an ability to manage that state is a truly remarkable accomplishment for the substance abuser. Treatment strategies involve sustaining the client's accep-tance of his disease for as long as possible. Conflicts may arise around substance abuse and recovery goals, and these may need further examination and clarification.

Practitioners need to recognize that when the time for prepa-ration for death nears, substance abusers and their families are historically ill prepared to manage the feelings and tasks attendant to any loss, much less dying. The result can be an extremely taxing period for families and practitioners who must often be the pa-tients' advocates.

Conclusion

Mental health professionals will need to expand their role in providing supportive counseling and AIDS risk reduction coun-seling to substance abusers with HIV disease. These individuals and their families historically have been regarded as "tough clients" because of the nature of addiction and the multiple prob-lems addiction often brings to the individual. The emergence of HIV in this population only adds to these difficulties.

While these clients face multiple problems and can often be difficult to engage, many of the skills and techniques used daily by mental health professionals are useful in working with these "newer and tougher" clients. Finally, it should be remembered that in the treatment field, many caring and competent professionals are themselves recovering and sober, evidence that "tough clients" can become "tough professionals" who can do the "tough work" presented to them.

■

References

1. Bixler R, Palacios-Jimenez L, and Springer E: CARE—Comprehensive AIDS Risk-Reduction Effort: AIDS Prevention for Substance Abuse Treatment Programs. New York, Narcotic and Drug Research, Inc., 1987

2. Froner J: Street-based AIDS education, in Preventing AIDS in the IV Drug Using Community: An Orientation to Community Health Outreach. Falls Church, VA, The Center for AIDS and Substance Abuse Training, Fall 1988

3. Cook A, Fischer G, Jones S, et al: Preventing AIDS Among Substance Abusers: A Training for Substance Abuse Treatment Counselors. Falls Church, VA, The Center for AIDS and Substance Abuse Training, Fall 1988

4. Faltz B, Rinaldi J: AIDS and Substance Abuse: A Training Manual for Health Care Professionals. San Francisco, AIDS Health Project, University of California San Francisco, 1988

5. Nichols SE: Emotional aspects of AIDS—implications for care providers. J Substance Abuse Treatment 1987; 4:137-140

Further Reading

Selan B: HIVIES (HIV Information Exchange and Support): A Manual for Facilitators, Organizers, Group Leaders and Members. Chicago, Alcoholism and Drug Dependence Association, 1987

Shernoff M, Scott W: The Sourcebook on Lesbian/Gay Health Care, 2nd ed. Washington, D.C., National Lesbian/Gay Health Foundation, 1988

Siegel L (ed): AIDS and Substance Abuse. New York, Harrington Park Press, 1987

Audiovisual Resource

"Personal Perspectives on AIDS: Sibyl." Baltimore, HERO (Health Education Resource Organization), 1986. An 18-minute video exploring the psychosocial issues of an HIV-infected substance abuser.

■

Glen Fischer, formerly the Assistant Deputy Director of the New York State Division of Substance Abuse Services, is currently Director of the Center for AIDS and Substance Abuse Training located in Falls Church, Virginia. Sally Jo Jones coordinated the development of the National Institute on Drug Abuse's comprehensive AIDS and substance abuse curriculum from its inception in 1985, and is currently Director of the Center for AIDS and Substance Abuse Training. Jack B. Stein, MSW, formerly the Executive Director of HERO (Health Education Resource Organization) of Baltimore, Maryland, is now Deputy Director of the Center for AIDS and Substance Abuse Training.

Strategies for Working with Substance-Abusing Clients

Barbara G. Faltz, RN, MS

The combined issue of AIDS and substance abuse raises critical clinical, ethical, and personal issues for medical and mental health treatment providers. Because of the overwhelming nature of an HIV-related diagnosis, practitioners as well as their clients often feel a particular sense of hopelessness about the issues surrounding substance abuse. Difficulty in working with clients who abuse drugs or alcohol is compounded by the nature of the behavior which often accompanies such use: mistrust of health care and mental health agencies by clients, manipulation and a history of the provider's frustrating interactions with clients.

This chapter explores some common difficulties in providing counseling to substance abusers and offers approaches to them which are both effective and compassionate. It includes general guidelines for intervention. Attention is focused on assessment and referral of substance-abusing clients and on intervening with the clients who are in denial of their problem, manipulative or intimidating, noncompliant or who relapse into substance abuse.

Substance Abuse Assessment

A substance abuse assessment for persons with HIV concerns is an essential part of the initial psychosocial evaluation. It should include the amount, frequency and duration of use, and last use of all classifications of illicit drugs, mind-altering prescription medication, and alcohol. The following are common symptoms of a substance abuse problem to evaluate:

1. Emotional, social, relationship, employment, legal or other difficulties that can be linked to the use of alcohol or drugs;
2. Loss of control of frequency or amount of use;
3. Preoccupation with drug(s) or alcohol;

4. Self-medication for anxiety or sadness with drugs or alcohol;
5. Drinking or using drugs while alone;
6. Rapid initial intake of drugs or alcohol;
7. Protection of drug or alcohol supply—stocking up or hiding supply;
8. Tolerance to large quantities of alcohol or drugs;
9. Withdrawal symptoms; or
10. Blackouts (with alcohol abuse).

Considerations in Referring Clients for Treatment

When a client agrees to seek help for chemical dependency problems, several options are available. It is important to decide if the problem is primarily drug, alcohol, or polydrug abuse. Many programs are more appropriate for one or another problem. Another consideration is whether or not the person can stay clean or sober long enough to avail themselves of an outpatient clinic. Is their impulse control or social situation such that they need the safety of an acute inpatient facility, or are they ready for a longer term residential treatment program? At times clients may need detoxification before a rehabilitation program. For an opiate addict, the additional option of methadone maintenance treatment is available.

Another concern is the client's comfort with programs that are either gay identified, for women only, or identified with a particular religious or ethnic focus. This needs to be explored fully. The therapist's personal biases and desires for the client need to be shelved in order to ensure that the best program available is selected. For example, it is important not to insist that a gay or lesbian client "come out" in treatment or that he or she go to a gay-identified program if this is very anxiety producing. The first priority is the treatment of the chemical dependency.

Individual psychotherapy and couples counseling on a regular basis are usually not indicated in the early phases of treatment. The goal at this time is to treat the chemical dependency and not be sidetracked into other areas. After a usual period of at least three months of abstinence, other issues begin to be addressed. Chemically dependent clients who are also children or partners of alcoholics may need to be clean for a while before risking their recovery by uncovering and treating wounds from childhood.

The guidelines for referral discussed in this section are not meant to be rigid. Each client must be evaluated individually in order for the best treatment plan to be formulated.

Interventions to Avoid with Substance-Abusing Clients

Often an intervention with a substance-abusing client is ineffective because of a limited view of the nature of addiction. For example, if addiction is viewed solely as a moral issue, a practitioner may attempt to lecture on the evils of a particular drug or alcohol or to encourage the use of "will power" and cutting down on use. This, unfortunately, is not possible for one who no longer has the option of controlled use. Viewing addiction as a symptom of an underlying emotional disturbance can lead to trying to find the cause, hoping that the symptom will go away when insight emerges. Insight therapy often does not work while a person is still actively abusing drugs or alcohol. Insights which emerge during intoxication are usually forgotten or not acted upon. Likewise, viewing addiction solely as the result of environmental factors such as poor housing, political oppression, or poverty can lead to political activism, encouragement to change jobs, location or vocational rehabilitation. This approach again does not address the addictive pattern of substance abuse.

Additionally, health care and mental health practitioners may inadvertently assist the addiction process by minimizing or not talking about the abuse or its consequences. They may avoid confronting objectionable behavior. At times they can make excuses for the abuse, such as "if you had his/her partner, parents, children, you'd drink too." Often there is an attempt to save the client from feeling the results of his or her abuse and to "protect" the client from negative consequences of alcohol or drug use. When these sympathetic approaches do not work to curtail abuse, practitioners frequently become angry and frustrated with clients, often expressing blame or disappointment to the client or other colleagues that drug or alcohol use is continuing. There is a sense that one was victimized by the client's behavior— especially after exerting a special effort to be of help. Clarity, as to the nature of substance abuse, one's role in dealing with it, and checking one's countertransference issues can be helpful in avoiding many pitfalls in dealing with substance abusers.

Effective Interventions with Addictive Behaviors

It is possible to be both caring and effective in intervening with substance-abusing clients. The following are suggested guidelines for working successfully with this population:

1. Be willing to listen and encourage constructive expression of feelings.
2. Express caring and concern for the individual.
3. Hold the individual responsible for his or her actions.
4. Ensure consistent consequences for negative behaviors.
5. Talk to the individual about specific actions that are disruptive or disturbing.
6. Do not compromise your own values or expectations.
7. Communicate your plan of action to other staff members or professionals working with the client.
8. Monitor your own reactions to the client.

Using these guidelines can be helpful when approaching the client who denies a problem, the manipulative client, and the client who continues to abuse drugs or alcohol.

The Client Who Denies Substance Abuse

It is reasonable for a person to grieve about a diagnosis of a life-threatening illness such as AIDS. One may also deny that the threat is actually present. This usually continues until a person can begin to absorb the impact of the diagnosis. In the field of substance abuse treatment, "denial" is used as an umbrella term referring to a host of behaviors. Rationalizing use, minimizing harmful results, deflecting attention from one's own problem to society's or someone else's, and blaming childhood experiences are all common defenses against accepting the reality of a substance abuse problem. The client may also admit to a problem, claim that they can stop on their own, and thank you for pointing out the problem. Denial, although expressed in various ways, can be viewed as either the denial of the loss of control over use, the consequences of uncontrolled use, or both.

One doesn't have to give up fully this denial in order to believe that there may be a problem. Just the willingness to look at the situation may be what brings a person into treatment or to an Alcoholics or Narcotics Anonymous meeting. During a crisis in which a person seeks professional help, there is an opportunity to confront the denial that keeps the addiction going. Interventions that are caring, matter-of-fact, gently probing, and done with humor and directness are the most effective. Confrontation that is punitive or that attempts to elicit guilt feelings are most often destructive to the therapeutic relationship.

The immediate goal of an intervention is to link the current crisis or presenting problem to the continuing drug or alcohol use. This is the "missing link" in the mind of the client, who often wonders why multiple unfortunate circumstances happen to him or her as if by some Grand Scheme. "I always lose the one I love," or "Why do I always wind up with addicts?" and similar statements demonstrate the occurrence of drug and alcohol use, suggest a long-standing series of disappointments in life, and suggest a lack of insight.

Any presenting problem can be the event that brings a person into treatment and recovery. This is "hitting bottom," the time when it can no longer be denied that drinking or drug use is out of control. With early skillful intervention, this "bottom" can be "raised" so that a person need not wait until there are even more serious consequences of abuse before awareness of the problem emerges.

Manipulation Associated with Active Abuse

Dealing with active addiction is often frustrating. Manipulative behavior is part of this picture, and it usually has two aspects. The first is the manipulative behavior itself and the second is the request, either stated or implied, that the client is making. Flattery, intrusiveness, intimidation, inflammatory remarks, and bargaining are all common ways chemically dependent persons can alienate or attempt to manipulate therapists and health care workers.

One example of this behavior is the excuse that being gay, a member of a minority group, a person with HIV disease, or being in any other stigmatized group is a circumstance so unique that it cannot be addressed or understood adequately by the treatment provider. This gives the client the perfect "reason" to drink, to "not be understood" by staff, or to "be threatening" to staff. Being a "special case" can deflect from the main focus of the chemical dependency intervention.

Additionally, a client may appear overly helpless or compliant or, conversely, may repeatedly question your actions. Coupled with the denial of a substance abuse problem, there is often concurrent justification and rationalization of it and other actions. A client may state: "I'm so tense and worried that I need to drink," or "Everybody uses a little coke at parties." He or she may be evasive or avoid contact with the provider altogether.

The goal of these actions is the second aspect of manipulation—the request of the practitioner. Typical of the goals that a client hopes to achieve are acceptance of their drug or alcohol use, lack of confrontation, increasing the amount or strength of the medication prescribed, access to services or funds, or justification for continued use. Justification can come when the client "feels rejected" by a provider who may have been setting reasonable limits to manipulative behavior.

Practitioners dealing with the initial manipulative behavior need to ask themselves, "What does this person want?" This helps defuse the behavior. When it is established what the client hopes to accomplish, then it is up to the practitioner to decide what he or she wishes to do about the explicit or implicit request. The action taken by the provider should be based upon the merits of the request rather than on the initial manipulative behavior.

One particular problem area for staff members of an agency that can be generated by client behavior is "staff splitting" or attempting to turn one staff member against another. Comments such as "You know what he did to me?" or "You don't understand me, but she does," or "You are the only one who understands me," are examples of this maneuver. Frequent, regular staff case conferences and review of treatment plans are helpful in minimizing this behavior. Direct communication between staff members is essential to clarify the reality of the situation when there is an accusation by a client about another staff member or agency. This strategy can avoid needless distrust and negative feelings toward colleagues.

Noncompliance and the Use of Contracts

Use of contracts or agreements for complex problems such as pain management difficulties or noncompliance for substance abusers with HIV disease can be beneficial. When there is a dual diagnosis of AIDS and a substance abuse disorder, average effective doses of opiates or other psychoactive medication may be inadequate. If the prescription is appropriate, the client may be abusing it. A Medication Agreement entered into with the client focuses on an understanding between health care workers and the patient for the therapeutic use of medication (see Addendum). This agreement is meant as a guide to evaluating common behaviors that indicate medication abuse; agreements are made in a formal contract to address the problem.

Contracting in a similar fashion can be helpful in other therapeutic interventions with substance abusers. For example, drug treatment programs clearly state their expectations and regulations to clients in writing either as a contract or in a client handbook. Clients are asked to sign that they have read these so that there is no misunderstanding of policy. Contracting is also used for clients who relapse or who are noncompliant with substance abuse treatment policy. Improvement is expected within a stated time and expectations are clearly presented. Consequences for continued noncompliance are also clearly defined. Contracts can also be applied to situations in mental health and medical settings. For example, a medication agreement which can be useful with manipulative or drug-abusing patients is appended to this chapter.

The Client Who Continues to Abuse Drugs and Alcohol

The client who continues to drink or use drugs presents particularly difficult management problems. Whether he or she had been clean for some time and has relapsed or has continuously used, the psychosocial difficulties caused by the relapse are usually compounded. Practitioners facing continued abuse need to consider what actions are necessary in response to this behavior. Is the client jeopardizing therapy by appearing drunk or late to or belligerent in sessions? Can he or she avail themselves of housing, medical and social service interventions while under the influ-

ence? What, if any, effect does continued use have on the therapeutic relationship with an individual practitioner or agency?

Eventually, there are consequences of behavior that are unacceptable. Health care and mental health workers need to decide
what the limits for unacceptable behavior are and have policies for
themselves and their agencies in place. These need to be followed
fairly and consistently. Examples of limits include not allowing a
therapy session to continue if a person is intoxicated, not seeing a
client who is late, and discharging a client from a residential
housing program if he uses drugs on the premises. Every effort
should be made to confront the specific objectionable behavior,
relate it to continued substance abuse and, most importantly, offer
substance abuse treatment to the client. If this treatment is refused,
or the client is continuously noncompliant and still behaving in an
unacceptable manner, then he or she should experience the consequences of these actions.

Following through on an agency's stated policy or guidelines,
that are carried out evenhandedly, maintains the integrity of a program or agency. It gives clear messages to clients and a sense of
fairness. It also frees practitioners to be caring toward substance-
abusing clients because limits of what is allowable are clear. Going
beyond that point is "not in the job description."

The concept of "tough love" summarizes what setting limits
entails. The "love" comes from knowing that the client is not
responsible for a diagnosis of substance abuse, did not intention-
ally choose to become an addict, and is suffering from a chronic
progressive disease. It comes from knowing that there is hope for
treatment of a substance abuse disorder and that effective strategies are available in dealing with active use. The "tough" comes
from the knowledge that allowing unacceptable behavior to occur
sends the message that there are no consequences to such behavior. It comes from knowledge that people change by using
feedback from the environment and confrontation with reality. It
also comes from the feeling of self-respect providers have who
deal fairly and with integrity toward substance-abusing clients.

Summary

Some of the barriers and difficulties common to treatment of
substance abuse and HIV-related diagnoses have been detailed.

Practical strategies to improve the response of treatment providers in caring for this difficult population have been offered. While there are many problems associated with the dual diagnoses of substance abuse and HIV disease, practitioners can intervene effectively by first recognizing how their own values and anxieties impact upon substance abuse treatment approaches. Next, they can accept substance abuse as a problem that can be treated and that can be managed in a clinical setting by following guidelines that are appropriate and fair. Finally, they can evaluate the client's alcohol and drug abuse and plan for effective referral to appropriate community agencies treating substance abuse disorders.

■

Addendum

Medication Agreement

I, _____, REALIZE THE FOLLOWING PROBLEMS WITH MY CURRENT USE OF MEDICATION:

(Check if applicable)

1. Feeling tired or having a clouded mental state.
2. Feeling "hyperactive" or nervous.
3. Anticipating my next dose ahead of time.
4. Wishing for a higher dose or stronger medication.
5. Supplementing medication with alcohol or drugs.
6. Thinking of asking more than one doctor for medication.
7. Other _____

I AGREE THAT THESE PROBLEMS INTERFERE WITH MY TREATMENT, AND I COMMIT TO THE FOLLOWING AGREEMENTS:

1. Not to exceed the daily dose of medication prescribed.
2. To discuss any medication problems with my primary Health Care Worker.
3. Not to obtain medication from other sources.
4. Not to self-medicate with alcohol or drugs.
5. Other _____

Medication

Name	Dose	Frequency
_____	_____	_____
_____	_____	_____
_____	_____	_____

_____ _____ _____

Patient Signature   MD/Health Care Worker   Date

■

Barbara G. Faltz, RN, MS, is AIDS Services Coordinator at the Santa Clara County Bureau of Drug Abuse Services, San Jose, California.

V
HIV and the Psychiatric Patient

- **Neuropsychiatric Complications of HIV Infection**
  James W. Dilley, MD and Alicia Boccellari, PhD

- **HIV Disease and Suicide**
  Peter B. Goldblum, PhD, MPH and Jeffrey Moulton, PhD

- **AIDS Anxiety Syndromes**
  Charles R. Tartaglia, MD

- **Treatment of People with AIDS on an Inpatient Psychiatric Unit**
  Jay W. Baer, MD; Joanne M. Hall, RN, MA; Kris Holm, RN and Susan Lewitter Koehler, RN, MS

- **Caring for Patients with AIDS Dementia**
  Alicia Boccellari, PhD and James W. Dilley, MD

- **Educating Chronic Psychiatric Patients About AIDS**
  Amanda M. Houston-Hamilton, DMH; Noel A. Day and Paul Purnell

■

Neuropsychiatric Complications of HIV Infection

James W. Dilley, MD and Alicia Boccellari PhD

The psychiatric and neuropsychiatric complications of HIV infection are many and diverse, and it is the purpose of this chapter to discuss the most common among them. A brief review of the HIV-related mental health problems most commonly seen by health care professionals and recommendations about their care and treatment will be presented. In addition, a review of the effects of HIV infection on the brain will be offered, with an emphasis on the diagnosis and description of the AIDS Dementia Complex (ADC). (See Editor's Notes, page 151.)

Emotional Consequences of HIV Disease

The emergence of HIV disease as a fact of modern life has had an increasingly important influence on social and political discourse over the past eight years. Increasingly, the spectre of HIV has come to dominate the medical and public health arenas, both in the United States and around the world. This increasing political importance reflects the significant emotional and behavioral impact the presence of the disease has had on the individual.

Not everyone has been personally affected. For many, the consequences of HIV and the epidemic of loss left in its wake have gone largely unnoticed. These individuals have been spared largely because of circumstance: their lives have been untouched because of some confluence of factors having to do with their age, their family constellation, their geographic location, or even the status of their health. This ever smaller number has been only dimly aware of the AIDS epidemic. Life for them has been largely business as usual.

For many others, the fact of HIV has been unmistakable and devastating. It has meant having to face the deaths of many important others; it has meant watching these loved ones weaken and physically deteriorate; it has required major lifestyle changes, and coping with the loss associated with them; and it has caused serious re-examination of lifelong goals, a keen sense of mortality, and the need to live for today. Most of these individuals have been able to face these challenges and find in them a stimulus for change and personal growth. Others have become overwhelmed temporarily by the enormity of the losses or have lacked the personal skills to adapt to the required changes. These individuals deserve appropriate and sensitive professional help, and it is for them that this chapter is written.

Effect of HIV on Those Most Affected

Gay and Bisexual Men

The AIDS epidemic has had a profound behavioral and psychological effect on gay and bisexual men. Dramatic changes in sexual behavior among gay and bisexual men have been documented in New York, San Francisco, and Chicago. These studies, though differing in detail, generally utilized a longitudinal design that assessed changes in frequency of sexual activity, number of partners, and frequency of specific sexual practices known to be particularly high risk for HIV transmission. Data were collected through both subject self-report and face-to-face interviews. The results of these studies on some 1,898 men have been strikingly consistent: all report significant (50-80%) reductions in the numbers of sexual partners; significantly reduced frequency (60-80%) of the highest risk practices (anal intercourse receptive, oral-anal contact, and ingesting semen, either orally or anally); and increased condom use and adoption of safer sexual practices (1-3). However, a considerable proportion of subjects, perhaps as many as one in three, continues to engage in some high-risk practices.

Factors identified as important in successfully adopting safer practices were knowledge of AIDS risk practices and availability of social support (Chicago), ability to recall the image of deterioration of a person with AIDS, younger age, being in a primary gay relationship, and being newer to the gay lifestyle (San Francisco). In New York, men who identified themselves as being close to someone with AIDS reported a twofold greater reduction in the numbers of sexual partners than subjects who did not.

These major life changes and the threat of AIDS in the everyday lives of sexually active gay and bisexual men have not been without psychological consequences. In New York, asymptomatic at-risk gay men were followed as controls in a study on the psychological impact of AIDS and ARC on a total of 236 patients. These 139 men were "healthy" but clearly demonstrated above normal levels of distress. They were characterized as living in a "state of tempered vigil" about their health. Common coping strategies employed by these men included the use of risk reduction measures and frequently seeking medical attention. Fully 39 percent of this group qualified for an Axis I diagnosis of Adjustment Disorder with Depressed or Anxious Features on a structured DSM-III interview. Similarly, chronic stress effects were found in a sample of more than 5,000 asymptomatic, at-risk men in four cities (Baltimore, Chicago, Los Angeles, Pittsburgh). Compared to men at low risk, the sample showed significantly decreased levels of concentration, energy, and restful sleep. Furthermore, a recent increase in the numbers of gay men who report being angry at, or fearful of, society's responses to the AIDS epidemic has been reported. These men note fears of physical violence directed at them as well as the threat of such negative societal actions as being quarantined.

Intravenous Drug Users

Little has been written to date on the psychosocial impact of AIDS on the other groups hardest hit by the AIDS epidemic. Existing work with IV drug users has been primarily epidemiological and educational in nature, highlighting the need for greater awareness about AIDS risk reduction in the substance abuse treatment community. As the seroprevalence in this group continues to climb, one of the most commonly articulated messages is the various ways in which intravenous drug users serve as a conduit for further expansion of HIV infection in the community at large. The spreading of the virus through sexual contact, from mothers to newborns and through the sharing of needles, are all considerable public health hazards. The role of the mental health professional involved in drug abuse treatment will increasingly involve helping patients to understand these issues and to make appropriate behavioral changes. The need to make these changes will undeniably cause additional stress and anxiety among this population.

Hemophilics

The psychological impact of AIDS in this group of "high-risk" patients has been relatively unstudied. One 1987 study reported on the degree of AIDS anxiety in pediatric hemophilia patients (ages 7-19) compared with that found in non-hemophilic children drawn from private schools. The relationship of AIDS anxiety to AIDS information and psychosocial functioning was assessed by measures of self-esteem, trait anxiety, family environment and level of behavioral problems in the child. AIDS anxiety was not found to be greater among the hemophilia group, especially when they received AIDS education. However, self-esteem was found to be an important variable: low self-esteem was the most significant predictor of AIDS anxiety while high self-esteem correlated negatively. The authors concluded that their findings supported the need for greater AIDS education in this population.

Professionals working with the adult hemophilia community report high levels of stress and anxiety in their patients and their families. Among the most common concerns is the added threat that AIDS poses for the hemophilia patient dependent on blood products. As one man stated, "It is difficult to accept that the concentrate upon which our lives depend may very well be the greatest threat to our survival."

Neuropsychiatric Disorders in HIV Disease

The term "neuropsychiatric disorders" is used here to refer both to those problems of mood regulation which are primarily psychiatric—that is, not caused by any known underlying medical condition and assumed to be in response to psychosocial stressors; and those problems of thinking that are assumed to be a direct consequence of HIV infection of the brain. Drawing this distinction may be problematic because the two areas may overlap: a person who has developed significant cognitive impairment, or problems in thinking, can also be depressed; similarly, a person who is acutely and painfully anxious may not always think clearly. However, for ease of presentation, these problems will be discussed individually and treated as separate entities. The reader should bear in mind, however, that the distinction is drawn here more sharply than may always be warranted clinically.

Psychiatric Disorders in HIV Disease

Anxiety disorders are probably the most frequent psychiatric complications of HIV disease in both those who are uninfected but at high risk as well as those who have symptomatic HIV disease. Supportive individual and group psychotherapy are important interventions for these patients, and helping them establish greater social support is very often sufficient to improve these symptoms.

Some patients develop chronic anxiety states in which almost continuous conscious worry dominates their thinking, either about the development of future symptoms, or chronic preoccupation with existing illness. These patients can be very difficult to treat, and some relief is frequently gained only through the use of medication. Teaching active coping skills, such as relaxation training, hypnosis, and visualization are also sometimes helpful in giving the patient a greater sense of control and in reducing painful anxiety.

Depression in people with AIDS and those with symptomatic HIV disease is common and spans the gamut of disorders from transient sadness to full-blown, debilitating major depression. The most commonly seen reactions are those which do not qualify for a diagnosis of major depression but are briefer in duration and lack the most severe problems of appetite changes, weight loss, insomnia, suicidal thinking and loss of interest in usually enjoyable activities. These reactions are characterized by sadness and are most often related to the acute existential crises raised by acute death anxiety, the development of new medical problems, social isolation, and the multiple losses that are so common among people with HIV disease. Supportive treatment is again the treatment of choice, and helping patients to feel that someone is particularly interested in their problems and well-being is essential. Treatment of those with major depressive syndromes is discussed below, and those with significant suicidal ideation are discussed elsewhere in this volume.

Central Nervous System HIV Infection and the AIDS Dementia Complex

It is now well known that infection with HIV results in infection of the brain and central nervous system with the virus, and a progressive dementing disorder, the AIDS Dementia Complex (ADC), can occur as a result. It is also increasingly appreciated that ADC is a significant cause of disability in those with AIDS, especially among those in advanced stages of the disease.

In recognition of this fact, the Centers for Disease Control amended the surveillance definition of AIDS to include the diagnosis of ADC as one of the signal complications of AIDS in August 1987. People with AIDS are additionally prone to other causes of neurological disease, including other viral and non-viral infections, neoplasms, and stroke. This section will focus on the AIDS Dementia Complex while noting that these other at times partially treatable causes of mental status changes may occur and should always be considered when difficulties in thinking are seen in people with AIDS.

ADC is a clinical diagnosis with a variable course. It is a frightening prospect shown to include symptoms in three different areas: cognitive, behavioral and motor symptoms. These are summarized in Table 1(4).

Table 1. Neuropsychological Symptoms in the AIDS Dementia Complex

	EARLY	LATE
Cognitive	Poor Concentration	Global Dementia
	Slowed Mental Processing	
	Impaired Initiation (amotivation)	
	Forgetfulness	
Motor	Slowed Movements of Eyes and Limbs	Incontinence
	Abnormal Reflexes	Generalized Muscle Weakness
	Ataxia (abnormal gait)	
Behavioral	Apathy and Social Withdrawal	Mutism
	Personality Changes	Agitated Psychosis

Early cognitive symptoms of ADC include difficulties with concentration and memory and a general slowing of mental function. The successful completion of daily tasks may become difficult, and friends or family members may report the patient "is not himself" or "isn't as quick or as witty as he used to be." At times, personality changes may predominate, and the person who has always been neat and tidy may become careless and sloppy; the person who has always been kind and understanding may become irritable and quick to criticize. Common behavioral symptoms include social withdrawal and a generalized apathy. In addition, early motor problems can include difficulty with balance, clumsiness, and leg weakness.

The late stages of ADC include global dementia, often with limited ability or willingness to speak (mutism), multiple neurologic abnormalities, including bowel and bladder incontinence, and an overall vegetative state requiring total bed care. The level of consciousness is usually preserved, though the patient simply lies in bed, stares vacantly, and has little social involvement with his caretakers.

Natural History and Epidemiology

The exact epidemiology and natural history of ADC has not been defined due, in part, to a lack of clear definitions of what constitutes cognitive impairment. In addition, comparing findings between studies has not always been possible because differing criteria were used by investigators in describing subjects' level of impairment, and the much needed longitudinal studies that will document the frequency and quality of these problems have only been under way for a few years (9). However, a system for staging individuals with cognitive impairment has been suggested and is gaining wider use (Table 2) (5).

Symptoms of cognitive impairment have been seen in otherwise asymptomatic seropositive people; and rarely, ADC has been reported in otherwise medically healthy but seropositive individuals. However, cognitive impairment is usually not seen in asymptomatic individuals. Nonetheless, the possibility of developing problems is the cause of a great deal of worry for those infected with HIV.

Occasionally, (5-10%) patients will develop these symptoms before the development of any opportunistic disease (6,7). Once clinically apparent neuropsychiatric symptoms emerge, however, a progressive decline in intellectual function is to be expected, although individual patients may experience a waxing and waning of symptoms in which patients may seem fairly sharp one day and grossly confused the next. In one study, 25 percent of patients with mild or equivocal findings of ADC progressed to clinically apparent symptoms within 33 weeks, while 50 percent of these same patients progressed to clinically apparent disease within 59 weeks (8). Nonetheless, the precise time course is uncertain, and some

Table 2. Clinical Staging of the AIDS Dementia Complex

Stage 0 (Normal)	Normal mental and motor function
Stage 0.5 (Equivocal/ Subclinical)	Absent, minimal or equivocal symptoms without impairment of work or capacity to perform activities of daily living (ADL). Mild neurologic signs (slowed eye or extremity movements) may be present. Gait and strength are normal.
Stage 1 (Mild)	Able to perform all but the more demanding aspects of work or ADL but with clear evidence of intellectual or motor impairment. Can walk with assistance.
Stage 2 (Moderate)	Able to perform basic activities of self-care but cannot work or maintain the more demanding aspects of daily life. Ambulatory, but may require a single prop.
Stage 3 (Severe)	Major intellectual incapacity (cannot follow news or personal events, cannot sustain complex conversation, considerable slowing of all output, walker or personal support needed, usually with slowing and clumsiness of arms as well)
Stage 4 (End Stage)	Nearly vegetative. Intellectual and social comprehension and output are at a rudimentary level. Nearly or absolutely mute. May have no strength in arms or legs with inability to control bowels and bladder.

patients have experienced at least temporary improvement in their symptoms.

While the extent and degree of the ADC remains unclear, researchers estimate that following an AIDS diagnosis, approximately one-third of patients will develop moderate to severe dementia and one-quarter will have subclinical or mild dementia that can be documented only by careful neuropsychological assessment. As many as two-thirds of patients may develop some signs of dementia by late in their disease. These estimates need confirmation by systematic, longitudinal studies.

Clinical Assessment and Diagnosis

When a patient develops mental status or personality changes, the clinician must remember that neurological complications such as these may arise from treatable opportunistic infections such as toxoplasmosis or cryptococcal meningitis, in addition to those resulting from nontreatable brain infections such as the AIDS Dementia Complex (ADC). Other treatable disorders also need to be considered and ruled out, such as metabolic disorders, psychiatric disorders such as depression, recreational drug use, side effects of medication, and nutritional deficiencies.

The individual suspected of having neurological complications related to AIDS should always receive a complete medical and neuropsychiatric evaluation. This should include a neurological exam, neuroradiological procedures, and neuropsychological testing. Standard laboratory bloodwork should be carried out, including CBC, urinalysis, serum chemistry, thyroid panel, syphilis serology, serum cryptococcal antigen, and B-12 level.

Computerized tomographic (CT) scans and Magnetic Resonance Imaging (MRI) are also recommended. The CT scans of individuals suffering from ADC may show cortical atrophy frequently accompanied by ventricular enlargement. The MRI is now thought to be more sensitive than the CT scan in identifying white matter abnormalities associated with ADC. However, it is important to keep in mind that during the early stages of ADC, both CT scans and MRI will often appear normal.

Cerebral spinal fluid analysis generally shows non-specific findings; however, it may indicate a treatable opportunistic infection. The electroencephalogram (EEG) may exhibit mild slowing early in the course, but it is otherwise non-specific. Its sensitivity in detecting early ADC has not yet been determined. Finally, a neuropsychological evaluation is often the most useful diagnostic tool in differentiating between functional psychiatric disorders and neurological impairment.

The diagnosis of ADC, then, is a diagnosis of exclusion. All other possible causes of mental status change must be ruled out before the diagnosis can be made. In addition, the practitioner is asked to exercise professional judgment in making the diagnosis, as the criteria are partially subjective and require:

> Clinical findings of disabling cognitive and/or motor dysfunction interfering with occupation or activities of daily living (10).

In children with HIV disease, a similar problem resulting from HIV infection of the nervous system can also occur, and again the criteria require that all other possible causes of neurological damage be excluded before the diagnosis is made. The criteria for children include:

> The loss of behavioral milestones progressing over weeks to months, in the absence of a concurrent illness or condition other than HIV infection that could explain the findings (10).

In both adults and children, additional diagnostic criteria include a positive HIV antibody test, a negative analysis of the cerebrospinal fluid, and a negative CT scan or MRI scan, or findings consistent with atrophy of the brain.

Neuropsychological Assessment

Neuropsychological tests have distinct advantages over traditional clinical interviews or mental status exams. The neuropsychological test battery is administered in a standardized fashion and integrated with a normative data base. Additionally, the patient's cognitive abilities can be quantified in a manner that allows for accurate retest comparisons over time and helps in the planning of patient care.

A neuropsychological evaluation should include a clinical interview, which includes a history of the present illness and past medical and psychiatric history. The neuropsychological battery should include measures of fine motor speed, verbal fluency and language comprehension, attention and concentration, memory, problem-solving skills, and visual-spatial constructional skills.

Measures of mood state and psychiatric symptoms should also be included. Neuropsychological testing involves considerable patient time (generally one to four hours) and requires patient cooperation. Because HIV-infected individuals are usually frightened by the prospect of testing, fatigue easily and do not have the stamina for extensive neuropsychological testing, a limited, brief, and focused testing approach should be utilized. A recommended test battery is included in Table 3 (9).

When working with people with HIV disease, special attention should be given to regularly performing a thorough mental status exam. Assessing orientation, attention, memory, language abilities, and judgment should be a part of any evaluation. It is important to keep in mind, however, that the brief screening exams in common use (for example, Mini-Mental Status Exam) often fail to detect early and subtle deficits associated with ADC (10).

Perhaps one of the most common requests of mental health professionals is to differentiate the early symptoms of ADC from functional depression. This can be a tremendously difficult task, and most often formal neuropsychological testing is required.

Several clinical points may, nonetheless, be helpful. First, the mental health practitioner should realize that apathy is not depression. Patients who are apathetic may be lethargic and indifferent, but they usually do not reach out emotionally or communicate

---

Table 3. Neuropsychological Measures

- Buschke Selective Reminding Test
- Wechsler Memory Scale (Russell Revision) - Immediate & 30' Delay Memory
- TRAIL Making Test
- Controlled Word Association Test
- Finger Tapping Test
- Strength of Grip
- Shipley Institute of Living Scale
- Digit Symbol (WAIS-R)
- Digit Span (WAIS-R)
- Item 99 (LNNB)
- Short Category Test (Wetzel-Boll Revision)

---

emotional or affective pain. The interviewer is encouraged to pay attention to how the patient makes him or her feel when they are together. Being with depressed patients usually makes the interviewer feel sadness or distress. Apathetic dementing patients, in contrast, leave the interviewer feeling emotionally flat. Verify your impressions with friends or family members if possible. Similarly, assess suicidal ideation. The patient who is depressed is more likely to have distressing suicidal rumination than the patient who is dementing.

Second, be sure to take a psychiatric history. Patients with a history of affective disease are much more likely to have a recurrence of major depression than those without a positive history, even in the face of a life-threatening illness. Also, patients with a family history of depression are at greater risk.

Third, the passage of time will be helpful in verifying your conclusions. If the cognitive dimensions continue to predominate and progress, the diagnosis of ADC becomes more likely.

Fourth, keep in mind that dementia and depression can and often do co-exist. If the usual signs and symptoms of depression are evident, the patient should be referred for psychiatric evaluation and deserves a trial of antidepressants. Some researchers have also used psychostimulants in these patients, and preliminary data suggests cognitive and affective improvement in early ADC patients without addiction or drug seeking. The use of low-anticholinergic antidepressants like desipramine or trazodone are recommended in low doses. Usual anti-anxiety agents, such as the benzodiazepines, should be avoided, as they may confound the already compromised cognitive capacities of the patient with ADC.

Finally, while there is currently no treatment for ADC, AZT has shown at least temporary improvement in the symptoms of ADC in both children and adults; others receiving the drug have been stabilized with little deterioration in cognitive abilities. Others have received no benefit. Larger studies are currently under way to assess more reliably the effectiveness of AZT in AIDS patients with dementia. At present, however, a trial of AZT is clearly warranted in any patient who develops ADC.

Conclusion

Mental health professionals must be aware of the potential for people with AIDS to develop neuropsychiatric problems and must have some understanding of their diagnosis and management. Practitioners working with this group of patients should be quick to contact patients' physicians whenever a question of mental status change arises. In addition, practitioners should establish a working relationship with an AIDS-knowledgeable psychiatrist.

■

References

1. Tross S: Psychological Impact of AIDS Spectrum Disorders in New York City. Paper presentation at the American Psychological Association Annual Meeting, Washington, DC, August, 1986
2. McKusick L, Horstman W, Coates TJ: AIDS and sexual behavior reported by gay men in San Francisco. Am Journal of Public Health 1985; 75:493-496
3. Ostrow DG, Emmons CA, O'Brien K, et al: Magnitude and Predictors of Behavioral Risk Reduction in a Cohort of Homosexual Men. Paper presentation, International Conference on AIDS, Paris, France, June 23-25, 1986
4. Navia BA, Jordan BD, Price RW: The AIDS dementia complex: I. Clinical features. Ann Neurol 1986b; 10:517-524
5. Price RW, Brew BJ: The AIDS dementia complex. J Infect Dis 1988; 158:1079-1083
6. Janssen R, Stehr-Green J, Starcher T: Epidemiology of HIV Encephalopathy in the United States. Paper presentation, Fifth International Conference on AIDS, Montreal, Canada, 1989, Abstract, p. 50
7. Abos J, Graus F, Alom J, et al: Incidence of the AIDS Dementia Complex as the first Manifestation of AIDS: A Prospective Study. Poster presentation, Fifth International Conference on AIDS, Montreal Canada, 1989, Abstract, p. 448
8. Sidtis JJ, Thaler H, Brew BJ, et al: The Interval Between Equivocal and Definite Neurological Signs and Symptoms in the AIDS Dementia Complex (ADC). Poster presentation, Fifth International Conference on AIDS, Montreal, Canada, 1989, Abstract, p. 215
9. Dilley JW, Boccellari A, Davis A, et al: Relationship Among Neuropsychological, Psychiatric and Immune Variables in HIV Positive Gay Men. Paper presentation, American Psychiatric Association Annual Meeting, San Francisco, 1989
10. Revision of the CDC Surveillance Case Definition for AIDS. MMWR, Vol 36, No. 15, Center for Infectious Diseases, Centers for Disease Control, Aug 14, 1987.

11. Dilley JW, Boccellari A, Davis A, et al: The Use of the Mini-Mental Status Exam as a Cognitive Screen in Patients with AIDS. Poster presentation, Fifth International Conference on AIDS, Montreal, Canada, 1989, Abstract, p. 384

Editor's Notes

Page 138. Three issues of importance should be addressed here. First, after much investigation over the past few years, it remains true that, while a rare case of cognitive deficit may occur in a person with asymptomatic HIV infection (see Stern et al below), these difficulties are much more likely to occur in those with advanced HIV disease (see McArthur et al below). Second, the official name of AIDS Dementia Complex has been changed: "HIV-1 Associated Dementia" refers to impairment severe enough to affect social or occupational functioning; "HIV-1 Associated minor cognitive/motor disorder" refers to those with subtle or mild cognitive impairment (see Working Group below). Third, the large scale development of HIV-related cognitive impairment has not materialized as was predicted in 1989 (see Portegeis et al below).

Updated References

Stern Y, Marder K, Bell K, et al: Multidisciplinary baseline assessment of homosexual men with and without human immunodeficiency virus infection, III: neurologic and neuropsychological findings. Arch Gen Psychiatry 1991; 48:139-142

McArthur JC, Cohen BA, Selnes OA, et al: Low prevalence of neurological and neuropsychological abnormalities in otherwise healthy HIV-1 infected individuals: results from the Multicenter AIDS Cohort Study. Ann Neurol 1989; 26:601-611

Working Group of the American Academy of Neurology AIDS Task Force: Nomenclature and research case definitions for neurologic manifestations of human immunodeficiency virus-type 1 (HIV-1) infection. Neurology 1991; 41:778-785

Portegies P, de Gans J, Lange JM, et al: Declining incidence of AIDS dementia complex after introduction of zidovudine treatment. Br Med J 1989; 299:819-821

■

James W. Dilley, MD, is Director of the UCSF AIDS Health Project and Assistant Clinical Professor of Psychiatry, University of California San Francisco School of Medicine in San Francisco. Alicia Boccellari, PhD, is the Director of the Neuropsychology Service at San Francisco General Hospital and Assistant Clinical Professor of Psychology, University of California San Francisco School of Medicine in San Francisco.

HIV Disease and Suicide

Peter B. Goldblum, PhD, MPH and Jeffrey Moulton, PhD

Suicide among people with HIV disease thrusts upon every-one involved serious philosophical, legal, and ethical dilemmas. Health professionals often find that these profound questions of life, death, and choice disrupt their sense of professional obliga-tion and force a review of moral responsibilities and legal restrictions.

The issue of suicide is especially complex among those with HIV disease because of the profound and progressive nature of the illness, the seeming unchangeability of the condition, and the often painful and disfiguring deterioration that occurs. These factors may place thousands of people—from those with evidence of HIV infection to those with AIDS—at particularly high risk for despair and hopelessness and thus, at eventual risk for suicide. As the incidence of AIDS has risen, health care professionals have become involved with increasing numbers of clients concerned about suicide.

Definitions and Distinctions

HIV-related suicide behavior is a specifically defined term which delimits the problem. Suicide behavior includes suicidal thoughts, suicide attempts, and completed suicides. Suicide at-tempts range from efforts by those with a high intention to kill themselves to those whose aim is something other than self-destruction—for example, a cry for help. The term "HIV related" refers to a whole range of individuals: those diagnosed with HIV disease, those experiencing grief related to AIDS, those with concerns about their antibody status, and generally anyone concerned about contracting the disease.

Rational suicide has been defined by Siegel (1) as a suicide in which a) the individual possesses a realistic assessment of his situation, b) the mental processes leading to the decision to commit suicide are unimpaired by psychological illness or severe emotional distress, and c) the motivational basis of the decision would be understandable to the majority of uninvolved observers from one's community or social group. For example, individuals may seek consultation about how to end their lives when pain and deterioration have increased beyond the point that they feel they can endure. Rarely, however, do real life cases fall neatly into the categories of rational or irrational suicide.

The Extent of the Problem

Establishing the extent of HIV-related suicide behavior is difficult. There has been increased speculation that suicide among persons with HIV-related concerns is on the rise as a result of several highly publicized HIV-related suicides. It is clear that some persons along the continuum of HIV disease have taken their lives. Over a six-week period in 1987, seven asymptomatic people in the Miami area committed suicide after receiving a positive result on the HIV antibody test (2). Social service agencies have reported that many of their AIDS clients express concerns about suicide; for example, the San Francisco Suicide Prevention Center receives 60 to 100 AIDS-related telephone calls per month.

Early empirical evidence related to the prevalence of suicidal behaviors among persons with HIV-related concerns leaves many questions unanswered. Two recent studies, one conducted in New York City (3) and the other at Lackland Air Force Medical Center (4), suggest that, at least in these two locations, the incidence of suicidal behaviors among persons along the continuum of HIV infection is significantly higher than for the population at large. Researchers, however, conclude that in San Francisco the incidence of completed suicide is not increasing (5).

In order to make sense of these apparently contradictory findings, we must further refine our question and ask: Which persons (personal/community characteristics) and which AIDS concerns place a person at increased risk for what kind of suicidal behavior (suicidal ideation, attempt, or completed)?

Each of the studies above looked at somewhat different variables or used slightly different methods of analysis, which makes direct comparisons impossible. The studies in San Francisco and New York investigated completed suicides among persons diagnosed with AIDS, while the Air Force examined suicide attempts among persons who had received a positive HIV antibody test result. Using medical examiner's reports cross-matched with the AIDS registry of the NYC Department of Public Health, the New York study found twelve documented cases of completed suicide among persons diagnosed with AIDS in 1985, yielding a relative risk 66.15 times that of the general population. All twelve cases were men; nine (75%) were gay or bisexual.

Employing a comparable case-finding procedure, researchers in San Francisco found only three documented cases of suicide among persons with AIDS in 1985, which comprised less than one percent of the AIDS deaths in that year. Furthermore, they documented only thirteen suicide deaths from 1981 to 1986, and no apparent increasing trend was found. All identified suicide deaths were gay or bisexual men. The researchers did not compute the relative risk to the general population.

To make matters even more confusing, it is likely that in both the San Francisco and New York studies, some individuals who committed suicide near the end of life were not included in the study results. These individuals often completed suicide with the knowledge of friends and were pronounced dead without a coroner's report of suicide as the cause of death. Some actual suicides, then, are likely to be reported by sympathetic physicians as "death due to complications of AIDS." Additionally, some suicides occur and may not be reported when a physician is not present at the time of death and the body is sent to the funeral home without examination. Thus, the figures reported in both of these studies are likely low.

The Air Force research team studied suicidal behavior among recruits. They had unique access to all members of the Air Force who were identified as seropositive through that branch of the military's mandatory testing program. Of the 650 seropositive patients evaluated between June 1, 1986, and December 15, 1987, psychiatric consultations were requested for 150 individuals and 147 were followed over time. In this group, six men attempted suicide. This translates into an alarming suicide attempt rate of 4,535 per 100,000. Among the most consistent factors in the patients who attempted suicide were perceived social isolation (p=.002) and lack of available social supports (p=.015). All six described their social isolation as being externally imposed (p=.002). One man identified as seropositive, yet not evaluated nor interviewed by psychiatrists, completed suicide.

While in some ways comparing these studies is like comparing apples and oranges, several tentative conclusions may be drawn: the suicide rate among persons with HIV concerns varies from one location to another, and an important factor in the prediction of the rate of suicide behavior in a specific environment is the individual's level of perceived support. Finally, from the Air Force study, we receive an important warning: Given the increased rate of suicide attempts in this population, "careful and thoughtful consideration should be given to potential consequences of implementing mandatory testing programs, especially with regard to confidentiality."

Clinical Challenges

To provide competent clinical services to people with HIV-related suicide behaviors, the clinician must be aware of basic suicide interventions and be adept in applying them to the more specific HIV issues involved. The following discussion highlights clinical insights (6) derived from working with people who experience the full range of HIV concerns.

Assessing Risk Factors for Suicide in Life-Threatening Diseases

To assess the suicide potential of a person with HIV-related concerns, the first step is to consider standard risk factors: depression, recent loss, substance abuse, age, sex, current stressors, prior suicidal behavior, current plan, resources, and adequacy of the client's support system. Risk factors identified in patients with other life-threatening diseases may be helpful in alerting health providers to the risk among people with HIV disease.

Faberow (7) found distinctive psychosocial differences between terminally ill cancer patients who committed suicide and a control group of terminally ill cancer patients who did not commit suicide but who died from their disease. Characteristics of those who committed suicide are summarized below:

1. emotional stress over and above the physiological aspects of the disease;

2. exhaustion of physical and emotional resources (including a feeling of lack of family and hospital support);

3. prior suicide attempts;

4. significantly more complaints of pain and discomfort;

5. near-death physical condition; and

6. alcoholism or drug abuse.

Specific Risk Factors for People with HIV-Related Concerns

To date there have been no formal studies to determine factors that specifically place a person with HIV-related concerns at risk for suicide. However, the following represent possible risk factors gleaned from clinical insight in working with a predominantly gay male population:

1. multiple losses related to HIV disease—either deaths or illnesses of friends or lovers; or other losses, such as employment or housing;

2. intimate involvement with another person who has died of AIDS (this past experience often has a decided impact on people as they enter the final stages of their own illness);

3. different stages of the disease may pose different risks of suicide and personal needs may change as the illness progresses;

   - *The recently diagnosed stage.* The person may have a lack of information related to the course and nature of the disease and may not understand the resources that are available. The situation is compounded if the person does not have financial resources or a strong emotional support network. People may use varying types of defenses in coping with the news of their diagnoses, some of which may be more helpful than others; and given the nature of psychological defenses, they may vacillate between intrusive thoughts and feelings and psychological numbing.

   - *The midstage.* At this stage a person's defenses may begin to break down, and thoughts of death and suffering may intrude into consciousness.

■ *The final stage.* At this stage, clients confront increased issues of dependency, pain, and loss of control of bodily functions.

4. great anxiety for people at a midpoint with HIV symptoms who are uncertain of their health status and their future, find their life planning disrupted, experience a loss of physical stamina, and enjoy little of the special "status" given to those with AIDS;

5. recent notification of a positive result from the HIV antibody test, prompting confusion about the meaning of the test result and its implications for future health status;

6. discrimination, insults, or injury related to the fear of AIDS or homophobia;

7. personal histories of losses related to homophobia (family history of rejection, history of employment or legal problems related to being gay);

8. a prevailing attitude that "the world is a dangerous place to be gay" and subsequent suspiciousness and anger toward non-gays;

9. remaining in "the closet," that is, taking part in homosexual behavior but avoiding identification with the gay community and thus often experiencing guilt and personal conflict;

10. an unsettled sexual identity, especially experienced by adolescents who feel that they may be gay;

11. lack of a social and financial support system that is adequate for coping with the AIDS epidemic (this may occur especially for those gay people who recently moved to a large urban area as a haven from discrimination in other parts of the country).

Personality Factors

Personality factors play an important role in how people cope with the full range of HIV concerns. Siegel and Tuckel (8) suggest that a person's psychological makeup is more important than any particular disease in effecting the suicidal or non-suicidal outcome for a person coping with terminal illness.

People with severe personality problems may be blocked in their access to services due to their manipulative behavior and to the management problems they present.

Jerome Motto (9) proposed a classification scheme of two distinct categories of people at risk for committing suicide. These categories may be useful in assessing suicide potential in persons with HIV-related concerns. The two models are a) those who are "stable and experience a forced change" and b) those who are chronically "alienated." The first group commit suicide after a significant loss or threatened loss. These individuals have a "high" rating for overall stability of prior life patterns. The "alienated" group, on the other hand, experiences suicidal ideas extending over years or a lifetime. They experience chronically low self-esteem, feel different from others, and nurture the thought of death as a promise that will someday be fulfilled, thus relieving them of the need to exist in a world in which they feel estranged. These people may commit suicide without an apparent significant loss.

Clinical Interventions

Clinical interventions for those who have HIV-related suicide behavior begin with a good clinical assessment of individual client needs. The practitioner should consider the following clinical issues and strategies:

1. Develop a good working alliance, and strive to understand and work through any blocks to the alliance. If these impediments cannot be overcome, the client should be referred to another mental health provider.

2. Discuss suicidal thoughts early. Given the progressive, deteriorating nature of the latter stages of HIV disease, suicidal clients may plan their suicide many weeks in advance for "when the time comes." The final act may follow a change in health status, which may "trigger" the suicide.

3. Allow clients to make choices and to take an active role in their treatment. People with AIDS may think of suicide as a means of having a measure of control over their lives. Concern about control may be exacerbated when facing the prospects of severe pain, loss of bodily functions, and mental status changes such as confusion and disorientation.

4. Emphasize the importance of perceived hopelessness in suicidal potential (10). Cognitive approaches to depression and hopelessness are often useful tools. Efforts to help clients

derive a measure of hope in the crisis are important. Clients often reach this goal by developing relationships with other AIDS patients who have been able to gain some personal meaning while coping with the disease.

5. Provide clinical assistance to support networks (partners, friends, and family). People with HIV disease moving into the final stage of the illness may commit suicide as an altruistic act to protect loved ones from protracted suffering. In sharing openly the wants and needs of others in the support system, clients may be reassured that their loved ones' needs are being addressed.

6. Encourage expression of feelings. Suicidal thoughts may be an expression of anger directed at people in the immediate support system or in the larger system. The opportunity to take corrective action where appropriate should not be overlooked.

7. Validate the grief that accompanies the loss of physical attractiveness and changes in body image that are common in AIDS. These concerns must be taken seriously and the mourning of these losses validated.

8. Allow clients to express negative thoughts and feelings about themselves or others and then discuss how they want to relate to them. Issues of blame and guilt are very complicated for people with HIV-related concerns. Issues of internalized homophobia are particularly important in determining how gay people cope with HIV.

Countertransference

Emotional issues surrounding HIV may cloud clinicians' judgment. Clinicians unfamiliar with working with medically ill clients may feel overwhelmed by the pertinent medical information and terminology. Clinicians may also be affected by several countertransference responses. These include the following:

1. Clinicians should recognize their own reactions and biases when working with people who have suicidal thoughts related to HIV.

2. Clinicians must face their own death anxiety. Uncertainty regarding the course of the illness may be unsettling to clinicians as well as to clients.

3. Clinicians must balance overreacting (taking unnecessarily restrictive actions to protect clients from themselves) and underreacting (not taking appropriate measures to protect clients). Several factors may influence this balance: a) experience—the less one deals with suicide, the more frightening it is; b) clouded judgment due to the emotional nature of death, suicide, AIDS, homosexuality, or substance abuse; c) lack of clear procedures—when clinicians have clear procedures and understand their legal responsibilities, they can focus on assessing client needs and determining appropriate actions rather than trying to devise procedures on the spot.

4. Clients with long histories of unsuccessful involvement in the mental health system (especially those with severe personality disorders) may prompt clinician reactions that can cloud their judgment in assessing these clients' suicide risk.

By clarifying personal reactions, the health care provider will be better prepared to assess a client's suicide risk and to design an appropriate intervention strategy.

Responsibility of the Clinician

The basic premise of this discussion has been that a clinician must understand and balance a person's right to competent professional mental health care with the right to die with dignity. With this in mind, the first responsibility for clinicians who counsel people considering suicide is to understand as clearly as possible what has led to their clients' suicidal thinking. The clinician must identify whether the person's thinking is clouded. By helping clients clarify their thoughts and feelings, options other than suicide may be developed. In any case, the distressed individual has an opportunity to review the situation with a compassionate person. For people who continue to consider suicide after carefully examining the issues, the clinician must consider taking more active measures such as the use of psychotropic medication or involuntary hospitalization.

The law in the United States clearly disallows clinicians from aiding and abetting a person to commit suicide. Individual states address this issue differently. For example, in California the Welfare and Institutions Code provides specific conditions under which the health care provider is required to intervene to prevent suicide, i.e., if a person is judged to be a danger to self due to "mental disorder or defect." Under these circumstances the clinician must admit the person for psychiatric hospitalization—even if this is against the person's wishes.

Difficult questions arise throughout the counseling process with suicidal clients. Some of the difficulty lies in the realm of clinical judgment: "Are the individuals truly a danger to themselves?" Vagueness in psychological theory and practice may also make decisions difficult: "What is meant by mental disorder or defect?" "Is suicidal thinking by itself an indication of psychological illness?" Other questions are more philosophical and ethical in nature: "Are there situations in which clinicians can agree with their clients that they are better off dead?" In other words, are there rational suicides? If so, what is the clinician's responsibility—a passive stance of noninterference or a more active stance of assisting? What are the limits of this assistance?

The Legal Dimension

Health professionals should consider three legal concerns to determine their clinical responsibilities toward clients who are considering suicide: a) malpractice, b) aiding and abetting, and c) the need to hospitalize or detain people on an involuntary basis.

Malpractice

In a thorough review of legal decisions related to suicide, Bursztajn et al. (11) concluded that in terms of malpractice, the courts have taken a realistic view of the uncertainties inherent in clinical science. To avoid liability, the practitioner does not have to be proven "right" by the outcome. But clinicians have been found liable for defective clinical reasoning: for example, for the failure to recognize the risk of suicide, for underestimating the seriousness of the risk, and for not taking the precautions needed to counter it. Three standards are commonly used to evaluate negligence: a) community standard, b) maximization of benefits relative to costs, and c) the reasonable and prudent practitioner.

Community standard means that clinicians have exercised due care if they have done what others in the relevant professional community would do in a similar circumstance. *Maximization of benefits to costs* is a way of understanding the complexity of decisions on the part of the clinician in order to prevent a client from committing suicide. The decision to hospitalize a client (voluntarily or involuntarily), to place a client under close observation or physical restraint in the hospital, or to discharge a patient are all complex decisions requiring the clinician to balance a host of possible costs and benefits. What is known as the "Learned Hand Rule" holds that negligent behavior represents the failure to invest resources up to a level that is equal to the anticipated savings in damages. The courts do recognize, however, that no amount of precautions can give absolute assurance that the patient will not commit suicide. The assumption is that the clinician's job is to prevent suicide. The question is ultimately "Could a *reasonable and prudent practitioner* have been expected to foresee the likelihood of a completed suicide or suicide attempt or taken greater precautions to prevent it?"

Aiding and Abetting

Although it is not illegal to commit suicide, most state laws clearly forbid aiding and abetting. Any such action is considered a felony. This applies to everyone, not only to health professionals. Such illegal activities might include providing the actual means for committing suicide or actively encouraging a client to undertake a suicide. Furthermore, health care providers cannot tell patients how to commit suicide. However, informing someone about the Hemlock Society, by itself, would probably not constitute aiding and abetting. The courts would probably look on this in light of other actions taken by the practitioner.

Decision to Hospitalize

When deciding whether to hospitalize or detain people on an involuntary basis, the clinician once again must balance overreacting and underreacting. Paramount issues related to balancing legal responsibility involve protection of the client from self-harm and the rights of clients not to be incarcerated unjustifiably.

A legal requirement for the clinician working with a suicidal client is that of *informed consent*. Informed consent is the discussion of treatment options with the client, such as antidepressant medication and hospitalization, including a discussion of the possible negative side effects of each.

Clinicians must be especially careful to maintain *confidentiality* when dealing with people who have HIV-related concerns. The possible damage to a person is considerable given the hysteria and possible reprisals connected with AIDS. This issue is made more difficult when people are assessed to be imminently a danger to themselves. At such a point, their safety supersedes their rights of confidentiality.

The following conclusions of Bursztajn et al. (11) are relevant to these issues:

1. Clinicians should feel reassured by recent court decisions which demonstrate a congruence between clinical and legal standards. Courts have not tended to be overzealous in their expectations that mental health providers can always prevent suicides; rather, they expect clinicians to use good clinical judgment in dealing with suicidal clients.

2. Clinicians need to understand legal standards of negligence and informed consent.

3. Clinicians are best safeguarded from malpractice suits by careful documentation of both objective and subjective information.

4. Clinicians need to review treatment options with clients and document consultation in cases where action on the part of the clinician can be misconstrued.

Summary

Issues of suicide are always difficult for the health care worker. The controversial social and political nature of HIV disease only compounds these difficulties. Yet this complex issue is one that is likely to confront practitioners in increasing frequency as the number of people affected by HIV continues to increase. An understanding of the clinical, ethical, and legal concerns involved can help alleviate some of the uncertainty and distress for health care providers, who must cope with this emotionally charged issue.

■

References

1. Siegel K: Psychosocial aspects of rational suicide. Am J Psychotherapy 1986, 15:405-418

2. Pierce C: Underscore urgency of HIV counseling. Clinical Psychiatry News, October 1987, p. 1

3. Marzuk PM, Tierney H, Tardiff K, et al: Increased risk of suicide in persons with AIDS. JAMA 1988; 9:1333-1337

4. Thomason JL, Rundell JR, Boswell RN: Factors associated with suicide attempts in a mandatory human immunodeficiency virus screening program. Editor Rundell, Wilford Hall USAF Medical Center, Lackland AFB, Texas, 1988 (Reprints available: James R. Rundell, M.D.; Chief, Consultation Psychiatry; SGHMSL/Department of Psychiatry; Wilford Hall USAF Medical Center; Lackland AFB, TX 78236-5300)

5. Engelman JE, Hessol NA, Lifson AR, et al: Suicide patterns and AIDS in San Francisco. Paper presented at Fourth International Conference on AIDS, Stockholm, 1988

6. Working group of mental health specialists convened by the UCSF AIDS Health Project to discuss the dual problems of AIDS and suicide behavior, April 1986, San Francisco, CA

7. Farberow NL, Schneidman ES, Leonard CV, et al: Suicide among patients with malignant neoplasms, in Psychology of Suicide. Edited by Schneidman ES, Farberow NL, Litman RE. New York, Science House, 1970

8. Siegel K, Tuckel P: Rational suicide and terminally ill cancer patients. Omega 1984-85; 15:263-269

9. Motto JA: Estimation of suicide risk by the use of clinical models. Suicide and Life-Threatening Behavior 1977; 7:236-245

10. Beck AT, Steer RA, Kovacs M, et al: Hopelessness and eventual suicide: a 10-year prospective study of patients hospitalized with suicidal ideation. Am J Psychiatry May 1985; 142:559-563

11. Bursztajn H, Gutheil TG, Hamm RM, et al: Subjective data and suicide assessment in the light of recent legal developments. Int'l J Law and Psychiatry 1983; 6:331-350

Updated References

Schneider SG, Taylor SE, Kemeny ME, et al: AIDS-related factors predictive of suicidal ideation of low and high intent among gay/bisexual men. Suicide and Life-Threatening Behavior 1991; 21(4):313-326

■

Peter B. Goldblum, PhD, MPH is the former Deputy Director of the UCSF AIDS Health Project, a faculty member of the Pacific Graduate School of Psychology, Palo Alto, California, and co-author of Strategies for Survival: A Gay Man's Health Manual for the Age of AIDS. *Jeffrey Moulton, PhD is Program Evaluator, UCSF AIDS Health Project and Director of Psychological Services, HIV Evaluation & Treatment Unit, Letterman Army Medical Center.*

AIDS Anxiety Syndromes

Charles R. Tartaglia, MD

The threat of exposure to HIV and the fear it inspires have forced many at-risk individuals to adopt a variety of coping mechanisms. These coping mechanisms range from outright denial to differing levels of confrontation with risk, including significant adaptations of life-style. If these coping efforts are successful, fear subsides to a level of reasonable caution or may vanish altogether. If they are unsuccessful, however, fear may proceed unchecked, at times progressing to irrational levels, prompting actions which can be destructive and debilitating.

Among this group of AIDS-anxious individuals are those who respond to their fears by turning to the medical establishment, seeking evaluation, treatment, and emotional solace from physicians. For a variety of reasons, these physicians may refer such persons to mental health professionals, who must be prepared to deal with the issue of AIDS anxiety.

The observations about this group and suggestions for working with them outlined below have been developed over five years of experience in evaluating and treating a number of such patients. While representing a varied though far from comprehensive cross-section of AIDS-anxious individuals, this group consisted primarily of homosexual or bisexual men. Their concerns spanned the spectrum of the disease, from pre-antibody testing to terminal care of those with AIDS. Less prominently represented have been heterosexuals and intravenous drug users.

Interventions employed with these patients have included brief counseling and crisis management, ongoing individual psychotherapy over a few weeks to several years, and medication management.

This experience with several dozen patients seen in individual psychotherapy provides the basis for a number of observations about the issues and psychodynamics of AIDS-anxious individuals and some thoughts about the conduct of therapy with such patients. There is always a risk of error in generalizing from the particular; therefore, broad extrapolation from the groups examined must be undertaken with caution.

Symptoms of AIDS Anxiety

Descriptions of the symptoms of AIDS anxiety can be readily found in the psychological and psychiatric literature and typically include panic attacks, phobic symptoms, generalized anxiety, morbid obsessions, anger, depression, persistent hypochondria, self-absorption, and despair.

Virtually all individuals with this syndrome have experienced serious disruptions in various aspects of daily life beyond those attributable to any physical disease. Some have had problems at work, including poor concentration, poor performance, withdrawal from co-workers, and frequent, occasionally protracted absences. Others have suffered severe disruption of their social activities and avoid their friends and acquaintances. Most have spent some period of time withdrawn from the outside world, although they may exhibit a morbid interest in media reports about AIDS.

Frequently these patients have guarded their anxiety from all but their physicians, and while the physicians generally try to support the patient, their efforts are often unsuccessful or in some instances have even intensified the patients' anxiety. At times, these patients have avoided visits to the doctor because of a fear of what might be discovered.

The severest symptoms have tended to occur early in the course of events—sometimes before seroconversion, most often upon testing HIV-antibody positive or being diagnosed with HIV-related disease.

AIDS Anxiety Among Gay and Bisexual Men

Gay and bisexual men represent the largest group affected by HIV and the one most frequently encountered in our treatment experience with AIDS anxiety. The situation of this group of patients can be best understood as a confluence of several sets of factors: the character of AIDS itself, certain behavioral characteristics of the gay community, and the psychological characteristics of individuals with AIDS anxiety.

For this discussion, AIDS can be characterized as a fatal sexually transmitted disease whose incubation period can be as long as 15 years. It is a disease that has incited more fear and social and moral stigmatization than any disorder in recent memory.

Relevant factors about the gay patients we have treated for AIDS anxiety include a common phenomenon of multiple sexual partners, a frequent history of sexual practices closely associated with transmission of HIV, and most importantly, the prevalence of the virus in the gay community. In an earlier descriptive study, insight into the individual psychological characteristics of AIDS-anxious gay and bisexual men were reported (5). In this study a tendency toward obsessionality, a pattern of chronic dysthymia (mood fluctuation) associated with prominent dependency needs, and a strong pressure to "take action" to relieve anxiety were noted. For example, patients would frequently and repeatedly seek reassurance from physicians, even when the reassurance did little or nothing to allay their anxieties. In addition, there was a strong tendency for some of these patients to identify themselves first and foremost in terms of their sexual orientation.

AIDS, as a sexually transmitted and fatal disease, establishes a real link between sexual behavior and risk. This fact, coupled with the uncertainty as to whether, when, and in what ways the disease will manifest itself, provides a basis not only for rational fear but also for a patient's sense of responsibility for his or her HIV infection. These fears of death and disability legitimately occupy time and attention but do not seem to adequately account for the distress and social dysfunction observed among AIDS-anxious individuals. Other issues contribute to the phenomenon of AIDS anxiety.

Psychological Issues in AIDS Anxiety

One important issue contributing to AIDS anxiety is the significance of the role of sexual orientation in the definition of self. In the best adapted individuals, it might be expected that sexual orientation is experienced as one facet of a multifaceted whole. For a number of AIDS-anxious patients, however, homosexuality seems to be the single most important feature of their personality. While no one explanation suffices to explain this phenomenon, repetitive encounters with homophobia and considerable reliance for support on the gay community provided powerful societal reinforcement of such a self-view. With regard to AIDS anxiety, however, this emphasis on sexual orientation and sexual behavior at a time when aspects of that behavior may be life threatening serves as a constant and relentless reminder of risk, and a spur to associated fear and anxiety.

Moreover, many AIDS-anxious patients are ambivalent about their homosexuality and experience feelings of guilt and shame about their sexual orientation. In some cases, these feelings have not been acknowledged prior to the development of AIDS anxiety. Attendant to this may be an expectation and fear of punishment reinforced by the social censure to which gay people are subjected. Finally, these patients may feel simultaneously angry and resentful toward other gay men as potential sources of infection. In addition, feelings of concern and regret over past sexual activity, and later, shame and guilt for the possible harm to others in the gay community for which they may be responsible are frequently expressed.

Shame and guilt about sexuality, with which the sense of self is so closely equated in this group, contributes to a serious loss of self-esteem and often results in social withdrawal. This, in turn, permits an escalation of existing feelings of depression, obsessionality, and hypochondria that typically characterize AIDS-anxious individuals. Social withdrawal also removes patients from their sphere of activity and diminishes their capacity to take constructive action to meet their own needs. The resulting frustration further inflames existing anger—at themselves for their own helplessness and at others for their failure to be constructively helpful. Finally, the recognition of these feelings increases anticipation of punishment for that anger.

Treatment of AIDS Anxiety in Gay and Bisexual Patients

Treatment approaches should be designed to meet the dual goals of building rapport and addressing issues specific to the patient's distress and dysfunction. The form of psychotherapy most often recommended can be best categorized as "supportive": that is, working toward the restoration of function and preexisting comfort, rather than toward personality growth or change. This approach also implies a focus on here-and-now matters, with little emphasis on linking current issues with the experiences from earlier years which have helped to shape them.

Particularly at the outset of treatment, the distrust, depression, and apprehension demonstrated by AIDS-anxious patients require active engagement. Specific questioning, encouragement, communicating interest and attentiveness, and acknowledging expressed or implied feelings are helpful interventions.

Ruminations about disease and symptoms often require interruption in order to obtain a reasonable history. To counter this tendency, it is fruitful to ask about the time of onset of symptoms and their meaning to the patient in relation to life events occurring concurrently. Often there is initial resistance to discussing these matters. In the end, gentle persistence and demonstration to patients that the origin of their anxiety is broader than the real threat of AIDS may be successful in stimulating their curiosity about themselves and their situations. In addition, the implication that a patient's psychological symptoms have a beginning may stir the hope that they might also have an end.

In this regard, it is helpful to explore why the patient is feeling anxious and asking for help at this particular point in time. One patient seeking help for debilitating symptoms of AIDS anxiety discovered that a mid-life crisis was at the crux of his anxiety. This crisis, however, began at a time when media attention was focused on the AIDS epidemic. This confluence of events encouraged his age-related anxiety to center on his vulnerability to AIDS and served to distract him from the more relevant concern about his age.

A second important element in working with AIDS-anxious individuals is the conscientious maintenance of therapist neutrality, particularly regarding sexual orientation and behavior. This recommendation differs from a number of therapists who stress the importance of actively reassuring patients that their sexual behavior is natural, healthy, and desirable. Such an advocacy position, which is intended to diminish guilt over sexual orientation, in many instances actually discourages the patients' expression of negative feelings and judgments about being gay without helping to resolve or accept them. Indeed, given the frequency with which this ambivalence is encountered and the intensity of the negative feelings expressed, this neutrality may well have been the decisive factor in allowing patients to acknowledge and speak of such conflicted issues.

Moreover, refraining from suggestions about what patients should and should not do, and adhering to a policy of accepting with concern and interest whatever patients might offer, seems to correspond to a fairly rapid development of the capacities to better accept themselves, to think about their situation, and to re-establish their more durable and adaptive coping styles. Last, but not least, neutrality and acceptance without judgment, either positive or negative, seems pivotal to the patients' capacity to trust the therapist. The development of this trust seems to be a significant ingredient in their willingness to begin to trust others in their social and work environments. Eventually, this trusting attitude leads in turn to a breakdown of social isolation and renewed access to usual sources of support.

A third important element is the therapist's effort to become acquainted with the patient as fully as time and circumstances permit. The exploration helps patients become more aware of the varied dimensions of their personalities and to expand the excessively narrow self-definition (self = gay only) to a broader one (self = gay plus other aspects). In some, this entails leading patients to rediscover dimensions of their personality that were recognized prior to the development of AIDS anxiety but which had become obscured by a focus on sexual behavior and concern about health matters. To others, it meant a new awareness of self. To the extent that this succeeds, patients are able to appreciate themselves more fully and to recover a measure of self-esteem.

In addition to the psychotherapeutic elements just described, medication may have a significant, though most often adjunctive, place in the treatment of AIDS-anxious patients. Polycyclic antidepressants are clearly indicated in the presence of major depression which may accompany AIDS anxiety. More recently, Ritalin has proven safe and effective in managing clinically depressed patients. When panic attacks present as a feature of AIDS anxiety, low doses of Imipramine, for example, may be of use, as may various anti-anxiety agents. These "anxiolytic" agents, largely benzodiazepine-type medications, also have a limited role in the symptomatic relief of debilitating anxiety, and sleeping medication may be occasionally indicated for severe and unremitting insomnia. Therefore, when panic disorder, severe anxiety, or depression are noted, referral to a psychiatrist for a medication consultation is strongly advised.

AIDS Anxiety Among Intravenous Drug Abusers

The drug-abusing person with AIDS anxiety, though barely represented in our treatment group, warrants at least a brief comment. Members of this sizable and very significant group, in our experience, do not seem to find their way as readily into medical referral channels, and the few who have been referred have been much more resistant then other AIDS-anxious patients to seeing a mental health professional. Those who continue their drug usage have tended to drop out of medical follow-up as well. Those who have been withdrawn from drugs and continue their medical follow-up for HIV infection have almost exclusively sought help with both drug dependency and AIDS anxiety from self-help groups such as Narcotics Anonymous and various supervised peer support groups. They have shown little or no sustained interest in the sort of individual approaches described above.

Effects of AIDS Diagnosis on Anxiety

When faced with a diagnosis of AIDS, there may be a decrease in manifest anxiety in some patients. Some individuals even express a sense of relief that their situation has been clarified and much of the uncertainty removed. In virtually all patients, the issues relating to AIDS anxiety recede from prominence. In their place reality-based issues emerge with increasing urgency, accompanied by affects appropriate to these new issues. Accordingly these patients are no longer properly thought of as "AIDS-anxious." Even where the issues typical of AIDS anxiety continue to partially influence the emotional state of these patients, they are less accessible to psychotherapeutic intervention, and the focus of the work shifts to the reality-based concerns and problems. Physical discomfort and disability, including encephalopathic changes, become issues for, as well as impediments to, psychological treatment. Internal pressure to attend to unfinished business, often including reconciliation with estranged loved ones, becomes powerful and may involve the therapist as facilitator, consultant, and mediator. The lessons learned in assisting patients with other fatal illnesses, such as cancer, are invaluable, and therapists with clients dealing with an AIDS diagnosis would do well to acquaint themselves with the rich literature on the subject.

Despite shifts in the issues patients face after diagnosis, multiple problems remain, including maintaining self-esteem, retaining a clear sense of identity, finding purpose and meaning in day-to-day activities, holding on to important relationships until the end, and preserving a sense of control. A therapist's assistance is often required to help the patient cope with these issues.

Awareness of these issues permits the therapist to more clearly identify a series of goals for this stage of treatment. Therapists ought, for example, to be diligent in assessment and aggressive in helping to bring the full therapeutic arsenal to bear on the physical symptoms which accompany AIDS. Advocating for follow-up visits with the patient's medical provider is sometimes necessary. In addition, therapists need to be attentive, supportive, and reliable in their efforts to assist patients' needs to maintain as much self-reliance as they can manage.

Patients with life-threatening diagnoses are subject to a powerful regressive force which will tend, at times, to make them regard themselves as childlike and often to behave accordingly. They are, of course, not children and ought not to be treated as such. To do so would inadvertently reinforce their growing sense of helplessness and undermine their adult sense of identity and self-esteem. On the contrary, the therapist must be alert to whatever remaining capacities the patient has, and support and reinforce them at every opportunity.

The presence of psychological regression allows certain behaviors on the therapist's part to assume a greater than usual significance. Touching a patient, for example, by way of a handshake or a pat on the shoulder, can be extremely important in communicating in a concrete way the therapist's connection with the patient. For persons with AIDS who often feel contaminated, unclean, and untouchable, physical contact can be a powerful antidote and a reinforcement that they are accepted and valued. But the therapist must touch patients respectfully, in accordance with the patients' preferences, and must avoid gestures which might be deemed patronizing or infantilizing.

As in the earlier stages of treatment, therapists need to become acquainted with the patient's personal history that describes and defines who that person has been and, notwithstanding the limitations imposed by illness, may still strive to be. Such information allows the therapist to better understand how to reinforce patients' senses of personal identity and spare them the ignominy of being simply AIDS patients or dying patients.

Conclusion

As the AIDS epidemic worsens, AIDS-anxious patients will likely become more common and will be increasingly seen by mental health practitioners. These patients are frequently challenging and often demand considerable effort. Therapists can be successful in helping to bring relief to these patients through an active engagement of their patients. Through understanding the meaning of symptoms (such as the fear of death or disability) and recognizing patients' psychological characteristics and past coping styles, therapists will be able to provide meaningful support appropriate in all stages of work with AIDS-anxious patients.

■

References

1. Morin SF, Charles KA, Maylon AK: The psychological impact of AIDS on gay men. Am Psychol 1984; 30:1288-1293

2. Nurnberg HG, Prudic J, Fiori M, et al: Psychopathology complicating acquired immunodeficiency syndrome. Am J Psychiatry 1984; 141:95-96

3. Holland JC, Tross S: The psychosocial and neuropsychiatric sequelae of the acquired immunodeficiency syndrome and related disorders. Ann Intern Med 1985; 103:760-764

4. Folstein M: AIDS anxiety in the "worried well," in Psychiatric Implications of Acquired Immune Deficiency Syndrome. Edited by Nichols SE, Ostrow DG. Washington, American Psychiatric Press, 1984

5. Filson CR, Tartaglia CR, et al: Psychological characteristics of individuals with AIDS-related concerns. Paper presented at the First International Conference on the Acquired Immune Deficiency Syndrome, Atlanta, 1985

6. Nichols SE: Psychosocial reactions of persons with acquired immunodeficiency syndrome. Ann Intern Med 1985; 103:765-767

7. Perry SW, Markowitz J: Psychiatric interventions for AIDS-spectrum disorders. Hosp Comm Psychiatry 1986; 37:1001-1006

8. Tartaglia CR: Psychological aspects of hospice care: research areas. Hospice J 1987; 3:75-84

■

Charles R. Tartaglia, MD, is an Assistant Professor of Psychiatry and formerly the Director of Consultation-Liaison Service at Georgetown University Medical Center. He is presently the Director of Student Health Psychiatry, Georgetown University, and a consultant to the AIDS Clinic at Georgetown University Medical Center.

Treatment of People with AIDS on an Inpatient Psychiatric Unit

Jay W. Baer, MD; Joanne M. Hall, RN, MA; Kris Holm, RN; and Susan Lewitter Koehler, RN, MS

As the incidence of illness related to HIV increases, more of those affected are requiring inpatient psychiatric care. This article describes 18 months' experience with 36 patients with AIDS and symptomatic HIV infection who were treated on a locked psychiatric inpatient unit. The special issues raised in the care of these patients are discussed below: staff reactions to caring for patients with a terminal illness, the complexity of psychiatric diagnosis and treatment in infected patients, and the ethical concerns raised by working with this patient group.

The special needs of people with AIDS and those infected with HIV, combined with the demands of patients, some of whom are psychotic, on acute inpatient psychiatric wards create a unique and challenging set of problems. People with AIDS can change clinically, quickly and repeatedly; they require significant medical management, may engender fear in other patients and staff, are frequently the sufferers of multiple stigmas, and are dying.

Clinical Issues and Staff Responses

The presence of HIV-infected patients on inpatient psychiatric units requires specific adaptations by each mental health discipline. Researchers have reported increased staff anxiety in response to the hospitalization of psychiatric patients with AIDS or related problems and predicted that such anxiety would become a common, troublesome phenomenon (1-3). In addition, the gradual adaptation of staff to working with AIDS patients on psychiatric units has also been described (4). Experience with treating people with AIDS, staff education, and ongoing staff support helped improve staff coping and also contributed to the ability of other patients on the ward to tolerate the presence of

AIDS patients. In addition, structural changes in the treatment milieu are often necessary. These issues are addressed separately below; many are illustrated with case vignettes.

Staff Reactions

The need for staff to attend to a myriad of physical problems, the long patient stays, and the need to work with patients who are dying all intensify the quality of staff-patient relationships. This is illustrated by the case of Mr. A.

> Mr. A was admitted to the unit in a floridly manic state after recovering from his first bout of *Pneumocystis carinii* pneumonia. Although some of his manic symptoms receded, signs of AIDS encephalopathy appeared and steadily worsened. He remained on the ward for many months and grew dependent on nursing staff for toileting, eating, bathing, and ambulation. The nurses became particularly fond of him. One day Mr. A developed a high fever and weakened dramatically. He became unusually lucid and poignantly thanked staff members for the care he had received. The next day, Mr. A's fever broke and he returned to his former mental and physical condition.

Most staff members were significantly troubled by working with terminally ill patients and dreaded the possibility of dealing with a patient death. (Actually, none of these 36 patients died on the unit.) In fact, several reported they had chosen psychiatry as a specialty in part to avoid such involvement. Staff tended to empathize and identify with these patients, who are largely young, middle-class gay men, since they had much more in common with them than they did with the usual patients with chronic mental illness cared for on the ward.

Additionally, patients with HIV-related dementia were the most challenging to care for on inpatient psychiatric units. These patients needed ongoing physical care and frequently suffered fluctuating cognitive abilities. They gradually lost the ability to care for themselves, became unable to control their bladder or bowels, and sometimes developed such disfiguring symptoms as Kaposi's sarcoma or profound emaciation, all of which intensified a sense of isolation. Touch, often proscribed in psychiatric staff-patient relationships, was an essential part of the daily medical care of these patients. All staff members had to learn how to "shift gears," to attend to the needs of patients with AIDS.

Continuing staff support must be available in a variety of settings, including general meetings, small groups, and individual supervision sessions. These should consist of didactic sessions (e.g., updates on AIDS treatments) and opportunities for ventilation and morale maintenance. It is also important to apply the concept of respite care, developed for families caring for chronically ill individuals, to the staff (e.g., giving the primary nurse for a particularly difficult patient an occasional day off from caring for that patient).

Milieu Management

Like many inpatient psychiatric settings, our unit was designed to emphasize communal living space and milieu therapy. The regular appearance of AIDS and HIV-infected patients led to several modifications in the ward program, as the following case illustrates.

> Mr. B manifested rapidly progressive AIDS dementia and became incontinent of urine and feces. On several occasions, he urinated in the dayroom in an area where patients smoke and watch television. Patients expressed open hostility toward him, complaining that he was pampered by nursing staff, and feared that they would contract AIDS even after the soiled areas were properly cleaned.

> The immediate problem was solved when staff supplied Mr. B with adult diapers and limited his appearances in communal areas. Longer-term solutions included purchasing furniture that could be easily cleaned and providing ongoing patient education to reinforce lessons about the modes of transmission of HIV.

Patients' Responses

The other psychiatric patients on the ward had a variety of responses to the medically ill AIDS patients. Many expressed fears of "catching AIDS." Others were concerned that AIDS patients might strike out in angry retaliation for having become ill or for suffering discrimination. Many also had great difficulty understanding that people their age could become demented; they saw these patients as individuals who constantly tested limits and who were unfairly absolved from responsibility by the staff. Several, like the patient described below, incorporated AIDS patients into their delusions.

Mr. C, a young schizophrenic patient admitted for catatonic behavior, was gradually improving when he suddenly retreated to his bed for a week. Through a blanket pulled over his head, he confessed that he had "caused" the illness of one of the recently admitted AIDS patients. Gradually, he was able to respond to staff's efforts to educate him about AIDS and he rejoined the patient community.

Educational Interventions

To address the educational and emotional needs of patients like Mr. C, a weekly health group was added to the ward program. The groups were led by staff physicians and nurses, and focused primarily on HIV-related illness. Patients were taught about modes of transmission, the risks of intravenous drug use, common symptoms of AIDS, and safer sex practices. A written summary of this information was used in the group as a teaching tool and was given to patients for later reference. The group provided a regular forum for discussing HIV disease whether or not AIDS patients were present. The staff respected the privacy of AIDS patients and did not reveal their identities; however, many chose to talk openly of their illness and served as informal group leaders.

The unit's patient orientation booklet, which all patients received on admission, was amended to include a description of the AIDS program, so that all new patients knew that care of AIDS patients was a significant part of the ward's routine.

AIDS patients also were encouraged to join the group activities administered by the occupational therapist, though at times, fatigue or confusion limited their participation. Cooking, grooming, and pet-assisted therapy groups were very successful activities for these patients. The functional level of the individual patient determined which groups were the most appropriate.

Those AIDS patients with significant cognitive impairment were often unable to respond to the usual limit setting used to promote change in behavior on the unit. Failing memory and increasing impulsiveness made behavior modification techniques minimally effective. Demented AIDS patients frequently used the telephone inappropriately: they badgered friends, ordered unaffordable products, and called public officials to report grandiose revelations. Establishing routines for toileting, meals, and recreation helped demented patients by minimizing new stimuli and allowed staff to efficiently help patients with more of their daily functions.

Despite progressive encephalopathy, most patients had painful glimpses of their own physical and mental decline. Patients were helped to express anger about their loss of control and helped to resign themselves to their need for increased assistance. Most patients searched for a meaningful explanation for their illness. Some consulted clergy in this process, while others were drawn to less traditional spiritual formats, such as guided visualization or meditating while listening to music. Although all of our AIDS patients were gay and bisexual men, few spoke of guilt about their homosexual lifestyles.

Infection Control

The unit followed the hospital's infection control guidelines which proscribe direct handling of patients' body fluids. HIV-infected patients who had an active, undiagnosed cough or who were unable to dispose of excretions hygienically were housed in private rooms, while others had roommates.

Occasionally, our AIDS patients were assaultive and required seclusion and restraint. Whenever staff felt there was significant risk of contact with bodily secretions, they wore protective coverings. This practice was later adopted for seclusion of all patients, since the HIV status of the patient requiring seclusion was usually not known.

Diagnostic Dilemmas

Numerous pitfalls occur in the diagnosis of AIDS patients with psychiatric disorders. The case of Mr. D is a good example.

Mr. D had been treated for AIDS for three years. He had a history of mixed personality disorder with narcissistic and borderline features that made him notorious to providers in the local AIDS service delivery system. He had made several suicide gestures, abused street drugs and alcohol, and was prone to rage attacks whenever he felt criticized. He came to the AIDS outpatient clinic complaining of suicidal thoughts and was referred to our unit for treatment of "depression." It soon became apparent that Mr. D was markedly demented, as evidenced by his severe cognitive deficits, incontinence, and disinhibited behaviors.

The diagnostic process in AIDS-related illness is a complicated one (5-10). Although a majority of our patients had one predominant problem, many evidenced mixed psychopathology that included conditions or behaviors already present before the onset of AIDS or HIV infection. In addition to these pre-existing conditions, the stress of adapting to terminal illness and the insult to the brain from HIV infection complicated the clinical picture. In these patients, it was the rule that mental states continually evolved; Mr. D had been well known to providers for years but was simply no longer himself at the time of admission.

Medication Complications and Limitations

Psychoactive medication can be extremely useful in AIDS patients who exhibit psychotic behavior or severe agitation. However, because mental status changes may occur rapidly in these patients, careful monitoring is needed. The patients' response to a particular medication can also change rapidly and is illustrated by the case of Mr. E.

> Mr E was admitted to the psychiatric ward from the medical service after his behavior had become unmanageable: he struck out at staff, was sexually aggressive toward other patients, and attempted to start a fire. Diagnoses of organic affective disorder and AIDS encephalopathy were made. Haloperidol in doses of 10 mg daily quickly calmed him and stopped his violent, impulsive behaviors. After several days of treatment, however, he developed severe side effects that were not responsive to standard treatment. He was transferred back to the medical service when his difficulty swallowing resulted in aspiration pneumonia. His extrapyramidal symptoms and, interestingly, his conduct improved after Haloperidol treatment was discontinued.

Although many patients receive neuroleptics without unusual complications, demented patients are especially susceptible to side effects and toxicity. Unlike the chronic schizophrenic patient, those with progressive neurological impairment due to HIV may not require ongoing psychoactive medication, and if started on such therapy, should receive low dosages. Our experience with lithium, antidepressants, and benzodiazepine medications was limited. However, we observed several demented patients treated with lorazepam who developed adverse reactions, including visual hallucinations and worsened cognitive deficits.

Ethical Issues

Staff working with AIDS patients must grapple with a variety of ethical issues. The case of Mr. F illustrates a common example.

> Mr. F had been sick with AIDS for more than a year, suffering two bouts of *Pneumocystis carinii* pneumonia, a disseminated mycobacterium infection, and painful peripheral neuropathy. His family, with whom he lived, was unable to manage his medical problems. After resolving his business affairs, Mr. F attempted suicide by carbon monoxide inhalation and was involuntarily admitted to the psychiatry service. Witnessing his debility and discomfort, staff debated the morality of preventing him from killing himself. During the first few days of his hospitalization, Mr. F expressed ambivalent feelings about suicide and then progressed to consistently deny suicidal intent. One week after discharge, he died of recurrent *Pneumocystis carinii* pneumonia, for which he had declined treatment.

Although suicidal behavior has been described in terminal illnesses before the advent of AIDS, it may be more prevalent in this context because of complicating factors attending the illness, such as social stigma and loss of supports, including the deaths of one's friends and peer group. Staff did not seem distressed by the involuntary treatment of suicidal patients early in the course of their illness, but different feelings emerged when patients who were in an advanced state of illness were admitted for suicidal ideation.

All suicidal patients left the hospital with some hope for their immediate future, but for many the commitment to life required daily renewal. Undoubtedly, for some whose commitment waned after an additional opportunistic infection or some other emotional or physical blow, the decision to actively end suffering was made. While the frequency of such occurrences is unknown, an undocumented but well-known phenomenon is the AIDS patient's planned goodbye party. The evening begins with a final visit with loved ones and ends in the patient's suicide. The common themes among the suicidal patients were the wish to exert control and to end suffering. It is important to note that at the same time, there were widely varying individual reasons for becoming suicidal (for example, pain, shame, loss, fear, or some combination of these) that needed to be explored and were often amenable to intervention.

Other ethical issues surround the use of the HIV antibody test in the inpatient setting; these have been described earlier (11) and include the individual's right to privacy as well as the health professionals' responsibility to warn others of danger. Antibody testing was not a routine procedure on our unit; instead, patients were educated and informed of antibody test sites in the community where they could receive additional counseling and anonymous testing.

Needs of Friends and Family

Ward visitation policies were often altered to allow visitors more time with AIDS patients. This flexibility was justified by the family's need to make use of precious time. Although we adapted this policy, we also tried to balance visitation by our commitment to keep the patients involved in the activities of the patient community as much as possible.

Families often struggled with unresolved issues concerning the patients' sexuality and life-styles while confronting the issues of contagion, social stigma, and grief that accompany AIDS. They gained significant relief by ventilating their concerns, receiving current medical information, and receiving assistance with the exhausting work of caring for their loved ones, particularly those who were demented. Family members frequently required and received referrals for their own mental health treatment.

Disposition Planning

The 36 AIDS and ARC patients who were part of this 18-month experience remained in the hospital for a mean of 15.8 days (30.7 days for the subgroup of demented patients). All of these patients required some form of continued care after discharge from the hospital. An example is Mr. G.

> Mr. G was admitted to our unit after an overdose of sleeping pills and was found to have moderate to severe AIDS dementia. His family was unable to provide the 24-hour care he required. His insurance carrier was convinced to pay for home attendant care, a benefit not included in his original policy, rather than continuing to pay for acute care in the hospital. Mr. G died at home seven weeks after discharge.

In some cities, like San Francisco, we are fortunate to have a number of agencies that assist patients with housing, psychological support, transportation, and finances. Nonetheless, the placement of the AIDS patient with ongoing behavioral and cognitive deficits remains difficult. This is due, in part, to the health care system's strict stratification into medical and psychiatric settings and, in part, to institutions' massive resistance to dealing with AIDS.

Discussion

The presence of a person with AIDS or symptomatic HIV infection on the inpatient psychiatric milieu requires adaptation by members of each mental health discipline. Psychiatrists must master a complex diagnostic process and exercise caution and flexibility in their use of medications. Nurses must cope with patients who have physical limitations and who are often unable to retain information or respond to behavior modification techniques. Occupational therapists must tailor their interventions to patients' levels of energy and cognitive ability. Disposition workers face limited community resources. Members of all disciplines must cope with a significant cognitive and emotional strain: keeping up to date in a burgeoning field of knowledge; tolerating legal, ethical, and scientific ambiguity; and working with patients who are dying despite their best efforts.

Education and support are essential components of milieu management in the face of the AIDS epidemic. Our efforts in these areas proved to be very helpful to staff. The acute inpatient setting, however, will always have staff and patients who will be severely stressed by the presence of AIDS patients. Staff who were uncomfortable with the advent of the AIDS program in this institution were given the opportunity to transfer. However, it is unclear how long health care workers will continue to be able to choose settings in which they will not encounter people with AIDS.

At times, it is difficult for AIDS patients to participate in the larger therapeutic milieu; this is particularly true for demented patients and those in a more advanced state of illness who begin to withdraw from life. Staff need to make decisions on how much to involve these patients in the milieu on a case-by-case basis.

Epidemiologists predict that the AIDS epidemic is only beginning. It behooves mental health practitioners, then, to develop resources to grapple with this growing medical and psychiatric problem. From our experience, such resources must include an adequate subacute care system, neuropsychiatric diagnostic tools, prospective studies of the benefits and side effects of psychoactive medications and of agents that may stop or slow the neurological progression of disease, teaching tools to help in preventing AIDS, and behavioral management techniques tailored to the patient with progressive AIDS dementia.

This article has been adapted from a previously published article that appeared in Hospital and Community Psychiatry, December 1987, Vol. 38, No. 12.

■

References

1. Polan HJ, Hellerstein D, Amchin J: Impact of AIDS-related cases on an inpatient therapeutic milieu. Hosp Community Psychiatry 1985; 36:173-176

2. Cummings MA, Rapaport M, Cummings KL: A psychiatric staff response to acquired immune deficiency syndrome (letter). Am J Psychiatry 1986; 143:682

3. Rosse RB: Reactions of psychiatric staff to an AIDS patient (letter). Am J Psychiatry 1985; 142:523

4. Amchin J, Polan HJ: A longitudinal account of staff adaptation to AIDS patients on a psychiatric unit. Hosp Community Psychiatry 1986; 37:1235-1238

5. Dilley JW, Ochitill HN, Perl M, et al: Findings in psychiatric consultations with patients with acquired immune deficiency syndrome. Am J Psychiatry 1985; 142:82-85

6. Hoffman RS: Neuropsychiatric complications of AIDS. Psychosomatics 1984; 25:393-395, 399-400

7. Nurnberg HF, Prudic J, Fiori M, et al: Psychopathology complicating acquired immune deficiency syndrome (AIDS). Am J Psychiatry 1984; 141:95-96

8. Perry S, Jacobsen P: Neuropsychiatric manifestations of AIDS-spectrum disorders. Hosp Community Psychiatry 1986; 37:135-142

9. Kermani E, Drob S, Alpert M: Organic brain syndrome in three cases of acquired immune deficiency syndrome. Comprehensive Psychiatry 1984; 25:294-297

10. Wolcott DL, Fawzy FI, Pasnau RO: Acquired immune deficiency syndrome (AIDS) and consultation-liaison psychiatry. Gen Hosp Psychiatry 1985; 7:280-293

11. Binder RL: AIDS antibody tests on inpatient psychiatric units. Am J Psychiatry 1987; 144:176-181

Updated References

Cohen MA: Biopsychosocial approach to the human immunodeficiency virus epidemic: a clinician's primer. Gen Hosp Psychiatry 1990; 12:98-123

Commission on AIDS: AIDS policy: guidelines for inpatient psychiatric units. Am J Psychiatry 1992; 149(5):722

Ochitill H, Dilley J, Kohlwes J: Psychotropic drug prescribing for hospitalized patients with acquired immunodeficiency syndrome. Am J Med 1991; 90:601-605

Hriso E, Kuhn T, Masdeu JC et al: Extrapyramidal symptoms due to dopamine-blocking agents in patients with AIDS encephalopathy. Am J Psychiatry 1991; 148(11):1558-1561

■

Jay W. Baer, MD, is an Assistant Professor of Psychiatry, Tufts University, School of Medicine, Boston, Massachusetts. Joanne M. Hall, RN, MA, is a Doctoral Student in Nursing, Department of Community Mental Health and Administrative Nursing, University of California, San Francisco. Kris Holm, RN, is a Psychiatric Nurse at Highland Hospital, Oakland, California. Susan Lewitter Koehler, RN, MS, is a Clinical Nurse Specialist, Department of Psychiatry, San Francisco General Hospital, and Assistant Clinical Professor, University of California San Francisco School of Nursing, San Francisco, California.

Caring for Patients with AIDS Dementia

Alicia Boccellari, PhD and James W. Dilley, MD

Awareness of the AIDS Dementia Complex has led to frequent requests for information from providers, family, and friends of the person known to have HIV-related cognitive changes. These requests center around questions of how best to work with these patients and how best to be helpful in improving their lives.

The kinds of cognitive impairments seen in individuals with the AIDS Dementia Complex (ADC) require different kinds of interventions. The specific intervention indicated depends on several factors, most important of which are the severity of symptoms and the stage of the disorder. Although ADC can be varied in its appearance and course, there are essentially two stages of the complex that need to be considered. Each stage requires a different intervention strategy.

Stage One: Early to Midstage AIDS Dementia Complex

In early stages of impairment, the individual with ADC will demonstrate mild difficulty with the ability to pay attention, to concentrate, and to remember details. Family and friends may describe a sense that the patient has "changed" in ways that are subtle but important. They may feel that the patient is less interested in those things which used to be of great interest, or they may comment that the patient is no longer as talkative or as "sharp" as before. At the same time, patients themselves will often report similar observations: they may complain of thinking more slowly and of having difficulty in organizing and carrying out complex tasks. In addition, they may report balance and coordination problems. Behavioral changes frequently noted are general apathy, a tendency toward social withdrawal, and an overall slowness of speech and movement.

While the individual during Stage One may have noticeable signs and symptoms of ADC, some capacity to get along in the world is maintained. Specifically, the individual remains fully oriented (aware of the day, the date, and time of day) while being prone to brief periods of disorientation and confusion. The patient continues to walk (with some motor slowing or decreased coordination) and typically retains the ability to speak clearly and without difficulty. Occasionally, slurring of speech may be a problem.

During this stage, the individual with ADC can participate actively in treatment and management decisions, and providers should encourage them to do so. The intervention strategy most appropriate at this stage of impairment is one which helps the patient learn to adapt to changing abilities by learning to compensate for any deficiencies. This model, discussed in greater detail below, is referred to as the Adaptation and Compensation Model.

Stage Two: Mid- to Late-Stage AIDS Dementia Complex

As the disease progresses and cognitive skills continue to decline, the ability to make reasonable judgments becomes increasingly impaired. Frequent periods of disorientation can occur. Individuals with mid- to late-stage ADC are easily recognized as impaired by non-professional people, since the nature of the impairment is severe and involves virtually every aspect of the individual's ability to cope with daily life. These patients develop severe attention deficits and are unable to follow conversations. Concentration becomes increasingly difficult, making reading a problem. Obvious memory problems are apparent as they are unaware of previous conversations or as they forget appointments or other important information. Individuals who progress to this stage usually cannot live independently. They may have difficulty performing even routine tasks, such as finding a phone number in the telephone book or driving a car safely. These patients may progress eventually to a degree of disability that leaves them unable to get out of bed. They can become virtually mute and unable to respond to questions or attempts at conversation.

By this time, the ability to participate in self-care is obviously impaired, and the patient requires help with cooking, dressing, and other basic tasks. Once this degree of disability is reached, the individual has lost the means to learn how to adapt creatively to the disability. The intervention strategy that is now most appropriate is one referred to as Environmental Engineering.

Stage One: Adaptation and Compensation Model

This approach acknowledges that during Stage One, individuals are still able to interact with others, are still reasonably intact, and are able to care for themselves (although they may not be as "quick" or as "sharp" as they once were). The main thrust of this approach is to encourage and reinforce the individual's remaining cognitive and emotional strengths.

Education is the most important strategy during this phase. Patients and caretakers, including family, friends and lovers, need to be educated about the physical, cognitive, and behavioral changes that may occur with ADC.

Counselors should be aware that patients and their families may misunderstand the term "dementia," which has different meanings to different people. For some, the term implies images of insanity and violent, out-of-control behavior; for others, the image is one of the frail and helpless elderly person. Asking patients and their caregivers to discuss their concepts of dementia and their fears about it can help to clarify any misconceptions or myths about the condition.

Educating caregivers about ADC is often a difficult process because the exact natural history and course of ADC remains ill defined. In fact, ADC appears to take a variable course from person to person. Counselors can, nonetheless, inform people about certain aspects of ADC, such as some of the expected symptoms.

Encouraging and Reinforcing Compensatory Mechanisms

While significant variations in the course of ADC can occur, it is essentially a progressive dementing illness. Nevertheless, strategies can be used during the early stages to help individuals compensate for their cognitive problems and to encourage them to stay active and involved in the world. The following suggestions may prove helpful.

1. Encourage the patient to keep a written record of appointments and important dates.

2. Encourage patients to slow down, undertaking one task at a time. Individuals with dementing illnesses often employ an

impulsive problem-solving style; they become frustrated or overwhelmed easily by multiple or simultaneous demands.

3. Suggest that patients keep mentally active in ways that are not stressful. Playing games such as Scrabble, cards, checkers, crossword puzzles, jigsaw puzzles, and video games encourages and reinforces concentration abilities and keeps many patients stimulated and involved. A balance needs to be achieved, however, between games that are stimulating and challenging and those that are frustrating and overly difficult.

4. Encourage patients to get plenty of rest and to schedule appointments in the early part of the day. Fatigue usually causes a worsening of cognitive problems.

5. Encourage patients to verbally monitor their behavior. For example, problem solving out loud helps improve the patients' ability to concentrate and focus upon the task at hand.

6. Help patients be realistic about stressful situations and encourage them to avoid or minimize exposure to stressful environments. For example, the patient should consider shopping or dining out during off hours when there is less stimulation.

7. Suggest that patients employ stress reduction and relaxation techniques to reinforce their coping skills.

8. Encourage patients to avoid tasks that were once easily accomplished but are now difficult. For example, balancing a checkbook may become difficult, and helping the patient find resources or friends who can assist with such tasks can be an important intervention.

9. Encourage patients to exercise regularly. Daily walks may help to relieve tension, reduce stress, and keep the patient involved in the world. Some evidence indicates that motor skills may be retained longer if they are used regularly (1).

10. Encourage patients to manage their own medications for as long as possible. This can be facilitated through the use of an automated pill box that can be set to beep when it is time to take the next dose. These devices are available in many drug stores.

Psychotherapy Issues

Educating the patient with ADC is often best accomplished within the context of supportive psychotherapy or counseling. In this setting, the therapist needs to shift from a traditional non-directive role to that of an active interaction with the patient in which the therapist actively encourages and supports the patients' attempts to manage their cognitive problems. Therapists should remember that individuals with Stage One ADC are frequently depressed and anxious. Depression and anxiety can worsen the underlying cognitive deterioration, making it even more difficult for patients to compensate for their intellectual losses. Active intervention through psychotherapy can improve not only the patient's emotional state, but can also reinforce and enhance the patient's attempts to compensate for his or her losses. The use of antidepressant and anti-anxiety medications may also be helpful; these will be discussed below.

In addition to individual psychotherapy, it is often helpful to provide couples therapy or group therapy to the person with ADC and to caregivers. During group therapy, lovers, friends and family involved with the ADC patient can discuss the ways in which the patient's disabilities have changed the interaction between the patient and loved ones. These role changes may include "assuming the role of parent to one's spouse (or lover) or resuming the parental role with an adult child who had once gained independence. These role changes require switching well-established habits that have evolved over years of interaction and involve complex, often subtle, and quite subliminal, virtually automatic, behaviors (1)." These role changes often upset the balance of power within a relationship. The individual with ADC may feel a loss of control and loss of position within the family system, resulting in feelings of helplessness, worthlessness, anger, and resentment. Caregivers in turn may feel burdened and overwhelmed by the increasing responsibility placed on them; they also may experience feelings of helplessness, depression, anger, or loss. Couples or group therapy can help to clarify the nature and implications of these role changes and can give the patient and caregiver a better understanding of how to cope with them when they occur.

Two extremes in relating to the ADC patient may occur. One extreme is that of denial, in which both the patient and the caregivers downplay the seriousness of the emerging symptoms. For example, the following statement is frequently heard: "He's always been like that; this is nothing new." Therapists should remember that for the ADC patient, denial may be due to either the psychological mechanism in which the patient literally does not want to consider the reality of what may be happening, or it may be related to an "organic denial." Organic denial can be the by-product of a dementing illness, in which individuals may lose the ability to appreciate fully the impact of their behavior on them-selves or on other people because of their brain dysfunction.

Caregivers, especially family and friends, may also experience psychological denial because the reality of the illness is too painful to face. This form of denial risks colluding with the patient, and it can result in endangering the patient and others if, for example, difficulties with driving a car or forgetting to snub out lighted cigarettes are ignored.

On the other hand, the other extreme may occur, and care-givers may act as if the patient with ADC cannot do *anything* inde-pendently. There may be a tendency to take over and take charge of the patient's life before it is indicated. This situation often results in the patient's feeling out of control and increasingly hopeless and powerless.

In fact, during early stages of ADC, individual and group therapy should focus on what the patient can still do, and the patient should be actively included in all decision making. Fam-ily, friends, and therapists should help the individual establish daily and short-term goals that are both realistic and achievable. An important goal during this stage, therefore, is to help the patient maintain a sense of responsibility and self-esteem.

In later stages of the illness, the therapist's role changes to one of helping the patient and the family adjust to changes caused by advancing disability. The therapist is in a position to help care-givers understand how to change the environment, not the pa-tient. This is a dramatically different approach from that usually employed by mental health professionals.

Legal Issues

Upon receiving a diagnosis of ADC, patients should be en-couraged to arrange for estate planning through an attorney if they have not already done so. This process needs to be completed early, while the patient is still competent and "of sound mind."

There have been many examples of the wills of HIV-infected individuals being contested afterwards on the grounds that the individual was mentally incompetent due to ADC. Neuropsychological testing conducted at the time of the writing of the will or videotaping the execution of the will can provide proof of the patient's judgment and state of mind should questions about the validity of the will be raised at a later date.

Stage Two ADC: Environmental Engineering

ADC is a progressive dementing illness without a cure, although recent evidence suggests that the antiviral AZT may help improve cognitive function in these patients. In the early stages of ADC, there is clearly more sense of hope and autonomy. The patient is able to interact and be an active participant in treatment planning. For the individual with Stage Two ADC, however, life becomes a struggle to survive and maintain a sense of one's personal identity. In this second stage, interaction among therapists, physicians, caregivers, and nursing professionals is essential to successful management, and environmental engineering becomes increasingly important.

Environmental engineering acknowledges that people in the mid to late stage of a dementing illness lose their ability to be mentally flexible, to adapt and adjust to changes, and to deal with novel situations. Since individuals with advanced ADC may no longer be able to change, control, or monitor their behavior, caregivers need to provide an external structure to help make the world less confusing.

Environmental engineering refers to structuring a patient's world to minimize the impact of their lost abilities. As the patient loses the capacity to deal with changing circumstances, an emphasis on routine becomes necessary. The more structure in the environment, the easier it is for dementing patients to understand and process the world around them. The following guidelines may help in the management of these patients.

Orientation: Patients should be given frequent reality and orienting cues as to the year, month, date, time, and place. Calendars and clocks should be kept in view; occasionally, digital clocks are easier for the dementing patient to read. An orientation blackboard that includes the day's date and the patient's daily schedule is often helpful, as are night lights, particularly for those who become more disoriented in the dark.

Structured Environment: Familiarity is a key feature in helping keep patients oriented and less afraid. Familiar objects and photographs should be placed in the patient's room, particularly if the patient is hospitalized or being cared for away from home. Furniture, personal objects, and utensils of daily living should be kept in the same place at all times.

If the patient is being cared for at home by a home health aide or visiting nurse, every attempt should be made to have the same staff member assigned to the patient.

For the patient who gets lost easily, large, clear signs labeling rooms is often helpful. Current photographs of the patient may help locate patients should they wander away from home. The patients themselves should always carry identification cards with names, addresses, and telephone numbers of their caregivers included.

Communication: Information should be presented slowly and one step at a time. Patients do not always understand what is being said to them. Asking patients to repeat instructions ensures that they have understood. If the patient can still read, encourage the recording of appointments, important information, and telephone numbers.

Long-term remote memory is often intact in individuals with ADC, whereas memory for recent events can be quite impaired. Encouraging the patient to talk about familiar places, interests, and past experiences can be comforting and reassuring while it enables the patient to feel competent. Avoid frustrating patients by asking them to discuss topics they no longer remember.

Assess Level of Stimulation Needed: Too much or too little stimulation may lead to a worsening of confusion, agitation, and fearfulness. The patient's living space should be kept uncluttered. While friends and family should be encouraged to visit regularly, the number of people visiting at one time should be kept to a minimum. If the patient is bedridden, physical therapy (e.g., passive range of motion) or massage can provide needed tactile stimulation as well as a sense of psychological support.

Emotional and Personality Changes: The patient's cognitive problems and personality changes are often misunderstood by those around them. For example, the distractibility often seen in these patients may be attributed to anxiety, disinterest, or lack of attention. The patient who appears stubborn in the face of ordinary requests may be demonstrating the mental inflexibility seen with dementing illnesses. The patient who is easily upset, has labile moods, and who is difficult to be with may be exhibiting behavioral changes common with ADC. Therefore, caregivers should recognize that many of the behaviors being manifested may not be deliberate, and the patient may have little ability to control them.

Patients with significant dementia are particularly prone to developing "catastrophic anxiety." The term catastrophic anxiety describes the emotional behavior of the brain-damaged individual who experiences panic, and it is often accompanied by irritability, emotional lability, angry outbursts, and inappropriately severe reactions to minor environmental stimuli. These symptoms are particularly heightened when the patient is feeling overly stimulated or faced with tasks that can no longer be accomplished.

The following may help decrease catastrophic reactions (2):

1. Notice what stimuli in the environment seem to trigger the reaction. For some individuals, it may be too much noise; for others it may be too many people or being asked too many questions at once.

2. Simplify tasks for the patient by breaking them into smaller components. For example, instead of asking the patient to get dressed in the morning, it might be more helpful for the patient's clothes to be laid out for him. This reduces the need for the patient to choose clothes for the day.

3. Don't rush the patient; allow for a personal pace. Expect the patient to perform tasks slowly.

4. Remove the patient from stressful situations and offer calm reassurance if the patient becomes upset.

5. Avoid the temptation to argue or reason with the patient during the outburst. Attempts at reasoning may result in a worsening of the situation.

Occasionally, patients with ADC may develop an organic psychosis (3), particularly an "organic manic" episode characterized by confusion, agitation, hyperactivity, grandiosity, and delusional thinking. Generally, such a patient will require the use of antipsychotic medications (to be described below) and may need to be hospitalized for psychiatric care.

Need for Continued Clinical Assessment

Practitioners should regularly assess whether patients are able to care for themselves and live independently. Special attention should focus on the patients' ability to shop, prepare meals, drive a car, pay bills, keep medical appointments, and take medications reliably.

ADC patients should be monitored for sudden changes in mental status. Sudden changes need not be attributed immediately to a worsening of ADC; other causes of acute mental status changes should be excluded first. Patients with ADC are susceptible to increasing disorientation from medication side effects, nutritional deficiencies, and dehydration; all these respond to medical intervention and should be treated accordingly.

Medication for Individuals with ADC

Antidepressant medications can be helpful in treating the ADC patient who is depressed. In choosing antidepressant medications, those lowest in anticholinergic properties should be used to minimize the possibility of an anticholinergic psychosis. Sedatives should be avoided unless a patient has a depression with marked anxiety or agitation. Experience at San Francisco General Hospital suggests that dosages should be built up gradually over seven to ten days to minimize side effects (4). Preferred medications include Nortryptyline and Desipramine.

Occasionally, the individual with ADC may develop an organic psychosis accompanied by agitation and hyperactivity. Patients with ADC appear to be particularly sensitive to side effects caused by antipsychotic medications, especially in developing extrapyramidal syndromes—for example, muscle stiffness, weakness, or inability to sit still. These side effects have occurred particularly with Haloperidol and the use of mid-range potency antipsychotic medications, such as Perphenazine, Trifluoperazine, or Thiothixene. These drugs, if needed, should be given along with low dose anti-parkinsonian agents given prophylactically (4).

If patients fail to respond to the above regimen, the introduction of benzodiazepine derivatives, such as Alprazolam, is recommended. First order benzodiazepines, such as Valium, tend to increase confusion and cause a worsening of cognitive deficits and balance problems and should be used cautiously (4). Some researchers report that the use of psychostimulants, such as methylphenidente (Ritalin) and dextroamphetamine (Dexedrine), given in low doses to individuals with moderate cognitive deficits due to ADC, may result in improvements in both cognitive impairments and in apathy and depression (5). Continued longitudinal research on the efficacy of psychostimulants in the treatment of ADC is needed.

Research is also under way to determine the role that Azidothymidine (AZT) may play in diminishing neurological symptoms. Preliminary studies suggest that AZT may result in an improvement in tests of attention, fine-motor coordination, and memory, within two to sixteen weeks of treatment (6,7). Similar improvements have been seen with the use of the AZT analogue, ddI, a drug that is gaining importance as an anti-viral treatment in those with HIV disease. Additional research in this area is needed as well.

Regardless of the medications used with ADC patients, caregivers should appreciate that dementing individuals are particularly sensitive to medications, and monitor them closely for side effects.

The Needs of Caregivers

Caring for the individual with AIDS who develops dementia can be an overwhelming and burdensome experience. Family members face a terminal illness with increasing physical debilitation, as well as deteriorating cognitive abilities, personality changes, and increasing financial responsibilities. They may also, for the first time, encounter other stressors, including AIDS phobia, knowledge of their loved one's homosexuality or a history of drug use, or other life-style behaviors that had been unknown. Additionally, caregivers may feel that their need to settle unresolved issues or to complete their "final goodbyes" is thwarted by the patient's dementia. Thus, they may be left with a sense of unfinished business or guilt over unresolved interpersonal issues.

For many individuals with ADC, their sole source of support comes from lovers or friends who are also HIV infected. These caregivers must not only confront the stress of caring for a loved one who is ill, but must also do so while feeling ill and weak themselves. Additionally, these caregivers are frequently reminded of their own issues of death and dying, fears of dementia, and fear of physical pain and suffering through their caregiving role.

The needs of the caregiver can be extensive. Supportive psychotherapy, peer support groups, and psychoeducational groups on ADC may provide some benefit. Caregivers need to talk about their emotional reactions to their role. Feelings of abandonment, anger, resentment, despair, and inadequacy often emerge, accompanied by a deep sense of guilt and isolation. Discussing these feelings in a supportive group setting helps to minimize the pain and validate the experience.

Negative or ambivalent feelings towards the patient, such as anger and resentment, can be particularly difficult for the caregiver to admit. Yet recognizing and accepting these feelings can result in a decrease in tension and feelings of guilt.

Caregivers should recognize warning signs that might indicate their own need for assistance in times of severe stress. These warning signs include increased feelings of isolation, social withdrawal, frequent crying spells, increase in irritability, sleep disturbance, a reliance on tranquilizers and alcohol (2), and total devotion to the care of the loved one to the exclusion of all other activities.

Respite programs that allow the caregiver "time out" from their caregiving role are also essential. Perhaps most important is the message that *caregivers also need help and support, and that they need not be alone.*

Conclusion

HIV-related cognitive impairment and the AIDS Dementia Complex are frightening possibilities for those who are infected and those who care about them. Suggestions for managing the complications of AIDS dementia have been offered, and a framework for considering these issues has been described. Finally, issues for caregivers in working with this population have been discussed, and while this work can be difficult and emotionally stressful, the informed caregiver who establishes a thoughtful treatment plan can find the care of these patients rewarding and meaningful.

■

References

1. Lezak M: Living with the characterologically altered brain injured patient. J Clin Psychiatry 1978; 39:592-598

2. Mace N, Rabins P: The 36-Hour Day. Baltimore, John Hopkins University Press, 1981

3. Boccellari A, Dilley JW, Shore M: Neuropsychiatric aspects of AIDS dementia complex: a report on a clinical series. Neurotoxicology 1988; 9:381-390

4. Baer J, Dilley JW, Boccellari A, et al: Altered mental states: treatment issues, in San Francisco General Hospital AIDS Knowledgebase. Edited by Cohen PT, Sande MA, Volberding P, et al. New York, Lantham, 1987

5. Fernandez F, Adams F, Levy JK, et al: Cognitive impairment in AIDS related complex and its response to psychostimulants. Psychosomatics 1988; 29:38-46

6. Yarchoan R, Thomas R, Grafman J, et al: Long term administration of 3' - azido - 2', 3' - dideoxythymidine to patients with AIDS-related neurological disease. Ann Neurology 1988 (Supplement); 23:92-94

7. Schmitt FA, Bigley JW, McKinnis R, et al: Neuropsychological outcome of Zidovudine (AZT): treatment of patients with AIDS and AIDS Related Complex. N Eng J Med 1988; 319(24):1573-1578

■

Alicia Boccellari, PhD, is the Director of the Neuropsychology Service at San Francisco General Hospital and Assistant Clinical Professor of Psychology, University of California San Francisco School of Medicine in San Francisco. James W. Dilley, MD, is Director of the UCSF AIDS Health Project and Assistant Clinical Professor of Psychiatry, University of California San Francisco School of Medicine in San Francisco.

Educating Chronic Psychiatric Patients About AIDS

Amanda M. Houston-Hamilton, DMH; Noel A. Day and Paul Purnell

AIDS education programs have focused largely on the general public and have been slow to reflect the needs of many special populations, especially those considered hard to reach, such as drug users out of treatment, partners of infected persons, and "closeted" men who have sex with men. It is not surprising that the mentally ill and developmentally disabled have received little if any attention in the prevention effort thus far. Health education has never been a priority for staff of psychiatric facilities, who have little training in prevention and even less time in the face of the service needs of their large caseloads. Beyond these obstacles, the omission of primary AIDS intervention is encouraged by the common belief, even among those of us who serve them, that the mentally ill are incapable of assimilating such information or engaging in self-care. Furthermore, the sexuality of the mentally ill provokes discomfort and avoidance, evidenced by the encouragement of routine sterilizations in the all too recent past.

Yet the chronically mentally ill are also at risk of exposure to HIV since, like most adults, they are sexual beings. In addition, some may be regular victims of the sexual abuses of others, or still others may, by virtue of identity, display polymorphous sexual behaviors. Some psychiatric patients are also known to use illicit drugs which precipitate, compound, or medicate their psychotic symptoms. Finally, HIV-infected adults, heterosexual and homosexual, are appearing on psychiatric wards, and their presence suggests a need not only for primary and secondary prevention, but to allay anxious disruptions in the ward milieu.

Adolescents hospitalized in psychiatric facilities may, in fact, have a higher risk of HIV infection than other teens, since sexual and drug-taking behaviors are higher. At the same time, the number of adolescents on psychiatric wards is increasing (1).

AIDS prevention programs must reach beyond transmitting knowledge and educational messages to general audiences. The task at hand is to personalize HIV interventions and focus attention on changing the attitudes and, more importantly, behaviors of vulnerable individuals. Education techniques can be developed to address the ethnically, cognitively, and diagnostically diverse mentally ill population as well.

This article will describe a successful training program for HIV prevention designed for psychiatric outpatients of a large urban hospital called "Riverview" in this chapter. Approximately 1300 patients with diagnoses ranging from psychoses, including schizophrenias and bipolar illness, to character disorders and alcoholism, were educated over a period of six weeks. Most were relatively well functioning, attentive, alert, and many were articulate and eager for information. A few were intellectually limited, preoccupied with internal stimulation, or heavily medicated. In other words, they represented the full complement of the psychiatric outpatient population in such settings. (See Editor's Notes, page 208.)

Concerns and Constraints

The first consideration in any program design relates to the characteristics of the audience. Age, gender, culture, and educational level are all factors to be considered; however, when planning AIDS prevention for the mentally ill, educators must also consider the cognitive and emotional development, diagnosis, and historic significance of the material presented.

The key to the success of such efforts is the early participation of staff whose experience of the patients helps determine the patient characteristics, needs, and thereby, scope of the intervention. Furthermore, their "buy-in" to the activity is essential to its implementation. If they have not had the opportunity to feel a part of the process and have their questions answered, the program will lose its effectiveness. Both administrative and provider staff will have concerns or apprehensions, which can be incorporated into the design. At the same time, unrealistic fears or resistances must be addressed before the patient program can proceed. Indeed, needs assessment discussions with staff are the beginning of the patient education effort. Long after the workshops are over, mental health staff will be the ongoing source of clarification and personalization of the material shared. Their anxieties about the subject, as well as their assumptions about the population's capacities for change, will affect the impact of the intervention.

The issues raised by Riverview staff largely focused upon the anticipated limitations of their patients. They wished the trainers to 1) avoid any emotional disruption caused by images or colors; 2) create unambiguous, direct, but minimally stimulating sexual information; use simple, accessible terms, free of jargon and scientific concepts; 3) overcome perceptual difficulties caused by medication side effects or other health problems; 4) schedule a time of day when patients would most easily be available and attentive; 5) agree on consistent messages; and 6) consider the magical or concrete thinking of some patients (i.e., if we say bleach kills the AIDS virus, why not drink it?). In fact, many of their psychiatric patients were well educated and able to assimilate sophisticated information; nevertheless, such factors were of concern to staff and had to be reviewed carefully.

Attitudes or policies of the institution can be constraints. For instance, the delivery of drug transmission information was surprisingly controversial at Riverview despite the high rate of drug use in this urban community. Although remarkably open to safer sex messages, the administration strongly felt references to possible drug use by patients were inappropriate and could not be included. Such concerns must be viewed in the context of the information considered critical to stopping infection. The basic prevention message is shaped by the needs of the audience and the sponsor, but the program design must maintain a fundamental integrity. Rather than lose this essential aspect of AIDS education, we designed content which encourages the audience to "help a friend who uses" with this information.

The "AIDSSAFE" Program

Staff concerns became part of the training goals. The identification of clear goals and objectives is neglected too frequently in program development. Even if not directly providing the education, staff must be clear about the purpose of the AIDS education activity and the specific effect it will have on their patients and on their own roles.

The Riverview program, later known as "AIDSSAFE," was designed to achieve several goals:

1. To increase patients' awareness of HIV disease as a public health problem with personal relevance;

2. To provide accurate information about the ways in which AIDS is and *is not* transmitted, and methods for preventing exposure to HIV;

3. To elicit and correct myths and misconceptions about AIDS, HIV transmission, risk factors, and prevention while decreasing irrational fears and anxieties about AIDS which might affect the institutional treatment setting;

4. To emphasize that AIDS is preventable but not curable, and to distinguish between prevention and cure;

5. To assist patients in assessing their personal risk based on behaviors related to drug use and sexual practices; and

6. To motivate participation in ongoing risk reduction counseling with their therapists or physicians.

With these criteria in mind, a training was designed which would meet several objectives:

■ be limited to 60 minutes, so that all outpatients could be reached;

■ consist of small groups to facilitate interaction;

■ focus on transmission, not epidemiology, in the short time available so that patients would learn how to avoid infection even if they did not entirely understand the nature of HIV;

■ be technically accurate but would, if necessary, sacrifice pure scientific accuracy for the sake of comprehensibility (e.g., using terms like "catching AIDS," and "AIDS virus");

■ minimize the dependence on written text or formal presentation;

■ remain interactive, encouraging communication between participants and between trainer and audience;

■ address any paranoia about the purpose of the workshop by quickly orienting the participants and soliciting their ideas about reasons for their presence;

■ use numerous devices for message reinforcement;

- develop cartoon visuals which are graphic, but not disturbing or arousing;
- include trainers who not only have considerable experience as AIDS educators, but reflect the ethnic, cultural, and linguistic characteristics of the audience;
- use a rotating two-person training team in each session, including one trainer who is a mental health practitioner; and
- refer any clinical issues which emerge to counseling staff, and generally encourage continued discussions with staff on personal risk, use of and access to safer sex items, such as condoms and foams, and skill-building practice.

As a result, the two daily AIDS education sessions were organized around seven critical components:

1. **Introduction of trainers and group members.** Group members were given name tags as they entered and, if necessary, were offered help in writing their names. Trainers also wore name tags and wrote their name on a flip chart. Each participant was then greeted by name and welcomed to the session.

2. **Identification and clarification of trainee expectations.** To assure that participants did not have either unrealistic expectations or irrational fears about the purposes, process, or length of the training session, they were asked to describe what they had been told about the session, what they expected to happen, and how long they thought they would be there. The trainers then corrected any misconceptions, underscored appropriate expectations, and informed trainees that they had permission to leave the session at any time they became uncomfortable with the discussion.

3. **Audiovisual presentation.** An eight-minute slide-tape presentation on AIDS developed especially for this audience was presented. A cartoon format was selected for the slide-tape to allow for the presentation of explicit information about HIV transmission without being stimulative or suggestive. The presentation showed people of all races, ages, and body shapes, and was narrated by both male and female voices.

4. **Question and answer period.** Trainers invited questions from participants in order to identify any areas of confusion or questions generated by the slide-tape presentation. As much

as possible, trainers involved the participants in answering these questions for other group members (2).

5. **"Where Do You Stand" exercises.** These exercises addressed a series of questions or statements, such as "I am afraid that I will catch AIDS," and "I know how to protect myself against AIDS." Participants were asked to stand at either "Agree" or "Disagree" positions, or anywhere in between, that coincided with their personal response. Each was then asked to explain why they had taken that position. Then, with the trainers' assistance, other participants commented on these reasons, corrected misconceptions, and reinforced ideas and positions that were correct.

6. **AIDS risk assessment questionnaires.** Questionnaires designed to pinpoint personal risk behaviors were distributed to trainees, and assistance was provided in completing and scoring them. They provided estimates of each trainee's "range of risk" and highlighted risk areas for further risk reduction counseling with counselors.

7. **Reinforcement.** a) Trainers used wall charts or slides to reiterate and reinforce key points from the session; b) trainees were referred to their therapists or physicians for further risk reduction counseling, condoms, or prescriptions for viricidal foams and jellies; c) handouts were distributed to repeat the main prevention messages and allow trainees to share information with partners or clarify personal issues with staff; and d) the hospital also gave each trainee a "diploma" certifying that they had completed the training.

Outcomes

Although no formal evaluation was conducted, responses from both staff and patients were highly positive. It was clear from audience questions, as well as the "Where Do You Stand" exercise, that they understood the information presented and were able to relate it to others and translate it into desired behaviors in their own lives. The patients cooperated to clarify each other's concerns, referring frequently to statements made by the trainers or appearing in the slides. They were especially interested in the risk assessment instruments, and many requested extra copies for sexual partners, family, or friends. (The staff were also given copies to enable them to review the answers with their clients.)

Many more staff chose to attend the sessions than anticipated. Although originally welcomed by members of the groups, the presence of more than one or two proved disruptive to the process. Not only did the patients seem less open to express their thoughts, but the staff occasionally dominated the question and answer period.

Recruitment of the audience is, perhaps, the most challenging part of an outpatient effort. In contrast to an inpatient, day treatment, or board-and-care setting, an ambulatory unit may have little control over patient time and availability. Although twenty patients were scheduled for each session, groups consisted of ten to eighteen individuals.

Appropriate scheduling of the education is also important. The timing of the sessions affects compliance as well as the attentiveness of the audience, especially for those on certain medications. Workshops were scheduled to reach as many as possible and to fit into regular ongoing outpatient therapy appointments. Those patients with the strongest transference to the institution, or therapists who are supportive advocates for the activity, appeared to have the best attendance.

Several trainings were successfully conducted with special subpopulations. Deaf patients in day treatment were educated with the help of translators who were given materials in advance to assure their comfort with the use of unfamiliar terms. Other day treatment patients, as well, were responsive to training; however, some clinical skill was occasionally needed to address appropriately or incorporate a patient's loose associations or delusions into the group interaction. Often, however, these comments were moments of great charm, as when one women struggled (literally) to get a sexual word out of her mouth and a second, seemingly preoccupied with her own singing, looked up from the back and offered "fornicate." The grateful first lady thanked the second and continued her question.

Less beneficial were activities directed at those in temporary, involuntary holds on the locked units. Technically outpatients, they were typically disoriented, either heavily medicated or not stabilized, and acting out. In contrast, those patients voluntarily placed on the short-term wards responded exceptionally well. Several used the opportunity to discuss their own AIDS or symptomatic HIV disease diagnosis to the trainer in order to find support and clarity. These sessions served not only to prevent infection, but secondarily to mitigate the stress to patients and staff uncertain of the communicability of the infection. Trainers were able not only to talk about the disease, but also to model appropriate physical interactions with such persons.

Conclusions

Clinical research suggests the superiority of cognitive-behavioral therapies with the chronically mentally ill and demonstrates the need for models which engage the patient in active participation in the intervention. Many studies point to greater treatment success with structured, directive protocols than with open-ended, individualized talking therapies (2,3,4,). AIDSSAFE reflects this theoretical research as well as staff concern and intuition about patient education needs. We believe that parallels can be drawn between therapeutic and health education principles. The program was designed to minimize the presentation style of most AIDS education activities(5,6). Instead the group was engaged, at many levels, in their own learning. The use of multiple communication media (auditory, visual, and physical movement), repetition, group interaction, handouts, and enlistment of participants themselves as respondents to other member's questions are examples of the message reinforcement necessary for this population.

Ideally, staff should be trained in prevention of HIV transmission before the patient program begins. Their continued discussions with their clients is a critical part of the further personalization of the message. Training should focus on building specific skills in risk-reduction counseling which supports positive client attitudes, and problem solving, as well as how to have safer sex and access to condoms.

Thus, patients must be given education which empowers them in their social relations outside the safety of the hospital or clinic. This principle of empowerment or enabling has been noted as a critical element of therapy with many disenfranchised populations, but it is also essential for educating mentally ill persons with little experience of their ability to direct their life and choices (7,8).

A critical part of AIDS education to the mentally ill must encourage the strengthening of self-efficacy or the sense of personal capacity for change. Certainly self-esteem, competence, and autonomy are not achieved in a health education session; nevertheless, this principle must be a guiding force in program design and implementation. Everything in the intervention must reinforce a sense of competence. If AIDS education is to be useful with this population, providers will have to resist their burn-out and cynicism to support their clients' power. Only then will the client be able to follow through with these potentially life-saving behaviors.

Program design should reflect careful analysis of the particular group targeted. Most institutions do not have the resources or the time to create separate sessions which divide patients by vulnerabilities, ethnicities, or level of skills. AIDS educators most likely will have to accommodate a range of backgrounds and experiences and be prepared to respond to the needs of the patients as they emerge. Thus, any program must include trainers with mental health experience as well as a solid grounding in AIDS information. Trainers with extensive backgrounds in AIDS education must resist the temptation to lapse into discussions of etiology of the disease and virology and instead focus on the most important transmission issues and specific prevention concerns of the group.

In summary, AIDS education can and must be offered to the chronically mentally ill. People with HIV disease are already patients in psychiatric facilities. Mental health professionals have become aware of their roles in providing supportive counseling for HIV-infected clients and their families, friends or lovers. As the epidemic widens, there is a growing need for their participation in primary education to a population largely ignored by AIDS education efforts. The chronically mentally ill as well as the developmentally disabled have special clinical needs which require the skills and sensitivity mental health providers can bring.

■

Bibliography

1. DiClemente RJ, Ponton LE, Hartley D, et al: Prevalence of high-risk sexual and drug-related behaviors among psychiatrically hospitalized adolescents: preliminary results. Bethesda, MD, National Institute of Menal Health Monograph (in press)

2. Rubin A: Community-based care of the mentally ill: a research review. Social Work 1984; 9:165-177
3. Test MA: Effective community treatment of the chronically mentally ill: what is necessary? J Social Issues 1981; 37:71
4. Videka-Sherman L: Meta-analysis of research on social work practice in mental health, part 1. Social Work 1988; 33(4):325-337
5. Harder P, Wexler S, Houston-Hamilton A, et al: Evaluation of California AIDS Community Education Program. San Francisco, URSA Institute, July 1987
6. Jang M, Moore M, Houston-Hamilton A, et al: Second Year Evaluation of California AIDS Community Education Program. San Francisco, URSA Institute, August 1988
7. Solomon B: Empowerment: social work in oppressed communities. J Social Work Practice, May 1987, pp 79-91
8. Pinder Hughes E, Pittman A: A socio-cultural treatment model: empowerment of worker and client, in The Socio-Cultural Dimensions of Mental Health. Edited by Day MW, Vantage Press, New York, 1985 pp 82-111

Editor's Notes

Page 199. Significant numbers of the chronically mentally ill report AIDS risk behaviors (see Kelly et al below), and the HIV infection rate among psychiatric inpatients is many times that of the general population (see Cournos et al below). Additionally, AIDS prevention can be successfully achieved with this group of patients (see Ponton et al below).

Updated References

Kelly JA, Murphy DA, Bahr R, et al: AIDS/HIV risk behavior among the chronic mentally ill. Amer J Psychiatry 1992; 149(7):886-889

Cournos F, Empfield M, Horwat E, et al: HIV seroprevalence among patients admitted to two psychiatric hospitals. Amer J Psychiatry 1991; 148 (9):1225-1230

Ponton LE, DiClemente RJ, McKenna S: An AIDS education and prevention program for hospitalized adolescents. Journal of the Amer Acad Child Adol Psychiatry 1991; 30(5):729-734

■

Amanda M. Houston-Hamilton, DMH (Doctor of Mental Health), is Senior Research Associate, Polaris Research and Development; Clinical Director, Center for AIDS Prevention and Education of Polaris/URSA Institute; and Associate Clinical Professor of Psychiatry, University of California San Francisco. Noel A. Day is the President and Founder of Polaris, a social and public research and consulting firm based in San Francisco and Washington, D. C. Paul Purnell is a Senior Associate of Polaris.

VI
Legal and Ethical Issues for the Mental Health Professional

Ethical Dilemmas in HIV Disease: A Conceptual Framework

Cheri Pies, MSW, MPH

Ethics, values, morals. The esoteric nature of these terms often means that people shy away from discussing them. Many feel that an understanding of such terms is best left to lawyers, theologians and philosophers. Others fear that they can't really understand these words anyway and thus have little use for them. Not surprisingly, however, mental health practitioners regularly find themselves in the middle of controversies which require skills in addressing ethically challenging situations. For those practitioners involved in the care of people with HIV disease, ethical questions are particularly common, and the need to untangle ethical dilemmas can occur on a daily basis.

What if HIV-infected clients are exposing others to infection through needle sharing or sexual activity? How should one counsel an HIV-positive woman who is planning to become pregnant? And what do we tell the IV drug user who wants to begin treatment, but each program has a waiting list of at least three months? These dilemmas raise key questions which are central to the discussion of ethics, values and morals. And at the same time, other pressing questions highlight the broader nature of these dilemmas (1). What duties do HIV-positive individuals have? Is there adequate justification for restricting the liberties of competent adults? What restraints, if any, should HIV-infected individuals voluntarily place on themselves? There are no simple and straightforward answers to these questions. However, an understanding of ethical principles and theories may offer some direction in identifying how to think about them.

Most people may be aware of ethical principles but only vaguely aware that taken together they form an ethical system. A great deal of what mental health practitioners do on a daily basis is applied ethics—that is, the application of general ethical theories, principles and rules to problems of therapeutic practice, health care delivery and biological research (2). This chapter offers a brief overview of several ethical principles and describes selected ethical systems. In addition, several examples of ethically challenging situations are included to encourage the reader to explore the process of thinking through these situations. The increasing complexity of the dilemmas created by the AIDS epidemic will no doubt require further decision making. Furthermore, frequent and thoughtful conversations with colleagues, those with whom you agree and those with whom you disagree, are essential tools in broadening one's understanding of applied ethics.

As a beginning, take a few moments to identify the values and moral reasoning necessary to sort out the following situations. Try to clarify what you think about these situations. What comes to mind initially? How would you address the situation and on what principles, values, assumptions do you base your actions?

A suicidal patient on a 72-hour hold has shown signs of dementia. The patient reluctantly agrees to HIV antibody testing but clearly states he does not want the results. The patient's test result is positive and he is about to be released back into the community.

A local hospital has just received funding for a research protocol for antiviral trials with HIV-infected infants and children. The protocol includes the use of placebos. One of your clients asks your opinion about placing her child in the study.

A colleague known to be HIV infected begins to show signs of neurological manifestations. He doesn't acknowledge these problems and insists on continuing his private psychotherapy work with individual clients.

Basic Terms

The term "ethics" is used to describe a set of beliefs and practices concerned with rights and duties (2). Ethics is the study of rational processes for determining the best course of action in the face of conflicting choices. Values play a key role in an individual's decision-making process and are pivotal in the development of one's ethical framework. Values are often developed at an early age and are influenced by one's religious upbringing, class background, parenting, and geographic roots. The development of values and moral commitment is also thought to be influenced by gender (3).

Psychological conditioning as men and women appears to condition one's personal approach to moral dilemmas (3). As boys and girls learn how to view the world, a different emphasis is placed on duty and consequences as a result of gender and social conditioning. This social conditioning is thought to contribute significantly to the different ways in which men and women approach and resolve moral conflicts.

Observations of boys and girls playing games of soccer and facing situations of potential conflict during the games illustrate particular themes. Boys appear to resolve the problems posed during the game by relying upon the rules of the game. Girls, on the other hand, may redesign the game or end the game in order to preserve the relationships of those involved. These themes appear to continue into adulthood. Men frame moral problems in terms of conflicting rights and abstract justice, also described as rules. Following the stated "rule" is held in high esteem. And women frame moral problems in terms of conflicting personal responsibilities to preserve relationships. Maintaining the integrity of a personal relationship in the face of conflict is of primary importance.

What is central to this discussion is the idea that men and women may in fact approach ethical dilemmas from different perspectives. As psychological development influences other aspects of human behavior, so, too, does it influence our approaches to resolving moral conflict.

Ethical Dilemmas

An ethical dilemma is precipitated by the existence of a real choice between two equally desirable or undesirable courses of action (4). Ethical dilemmas are frequently philosophical in nature and rely upon the use of values, moral reasoning and ethical principles to reach a resolution. Although medical, legal, religious and financial criteria are often part of the decision-making process, knowledge of ethical theories and an ability to articulate one's values and moral prerequisites are critical.

Ethical systems clarify theoretical and general levels for ethical reasoning. Ethical systems are sometimes described as consequence oriented or duty oriented (4). The consequence-oriented systems focus on the outcome of actions or the consequences.

Utilitarianism is one form of consequence-oriented theory. The use of this system seeks the most happiness or the greatest good for the greatest number of people.

A second, commonly used ethical system is the duty-oriented system. In this system, it is the act that is considered to be right or wrong, rather than the outcome alone. Rules and principles are the primary guide in determining rightness or wrongness. The decision-making process is guided by rules, such as "thou shalt not kill."

These ethical systems are not mutually exclusive. A person may take a consequence-oriented position on one issue and a duty-oriented position on another. People are rarely solely utilitarian or duty oriented in their process of untangling the web of ethical dilemmas. In fact, some situations pose a convergence of these two schools of ethical thought. A case in point is that of therapist-client confidentiality. The "rule" that confidentiality be maintained between therapist and client is widely held. However, in those circumstances where harmful consequences may result or a principle of a higher social good is desired, confidentiality may be broken. Based on this established "rule," how does one behave if there is a threat of morally corrupt consequences? Certainly there are degrees that one must consider. These degrees are best understood with an explanation of ethical principles.

Ethical Principles

Ethical principles are general, fundamental truths, laws and doctrines which are used in resolving particular dilemmas. Six ethical principles are briefly described here. They include autonomy, veracity, nonmaleficence, beneficence, confidentiality and justice. These principles have many common applications in the field of mental health and are also frequently employed in medicine, law and human relations.

Autonomy

Autonomy is a form of personal liberty in which an individual determines his or her own course of action in accordance with a plan chosen by him or herself (4). It has been suggested that autonomy includes the freedom to decide, the freedom to act, and acknowledgement and respect for others' autonomy. The concept of informed consent is derived from the principle of autonomy and urges that we respect others and their strides toward self-determination. This principle gives individuals the freedom to act on their own behalf given that the individual is so situated as to be able to act on and implement free choices.

Consenting to HIV antibody testing is one example of how autonomy is addressed. In some states, an individual is required to sign an informed consent prior to taking the HIV antibody test. And it is also expected that the individual will receive thorough and informative counseling and information concerning the pros and cons of the test before being asked to sign this informed consent. In this way, it is hoped that individuals who are agreeing to take the test have at least a basic understanding of the possible implications of taking the test.

Veracity

The principle of veracity calls upon one's moral obligation to tell the truth. In the case of a therapist-client relationship, telling the truth is the obligation of both individuals. The principle of veracity is closely aligned with that of autonomy. That is, we respect one's ability to make reasonable decisions when given all the information and when told the truth. Some practitioners employ the practice of "benevolent deception" (5). For example, some think it may be in a patient's best interests not to know the whole story of a terminal illness. Or a client may indicate not wanting to know the whole truth, preferring to leave the decision making regarding treatment, care, and talking with other family members up to the practitioner. Veracity requires that we tell the truth to the best of our knowledge and ability.

The testing of various antiviral treatments provides one example of the principle of veracity. Because most of these treatments are experimental, it is uncertain if they will work, how they will work, and what side effects an individual will experience. With this in mind, all study participants must be made fully aware of the limitations of knowledge about this drug therapy. At the same time, those utilizing alternative treatments must receive as much truthful information as possible about these treatments. Often in an effort to promote the use of a particular therapy, whether it be experimental or alternative, vital information is omitted for fear of discouraging participation or utilization.

Nonmaleficence

Perhaps the most familiar principle is that of nonmaleficence, frequently known as "do no harm." It is the principle derived from the Hippocratic oath which supports and promotes the noninfliction of harm. It frequently requires that we ask ourselves "What is the most humane treatment?" One is also asked to consider which treatments are morally obligatory and which are morally and/or medically optional.

What are the responsibilities of the mental health worker to warn a client's partner that the client is HIV infected? How do we promote the noninfliction of harm in a situation in which another individual is knowingly putting others at risk of infection? To whom would the harm be done if the mental health worker informed a partner?

Beneficence

Beneficence is closely linked with the principle of nonmaleficence. While nonmaleficence is concerned with doing no harm, simply stated, beneficence is concerned with promoting good health and welfare. Beneficence requires that we analyze the costs and benefits of particular treatments, drugs, and the like to determine whether the benefits outweigh the costs.

Take the drug treatment protocol mentioned in one of the earlier examples. This research protocol involving infants and children may include the use of placebos. Can the long-term benefits of such a study outweigh the short-term effects such treatment may have on infants and children? Will such a study contribute significantly to the health and welfare of others, and at what expense? It is here that one must analyze the benefits and costs of treatment and decide whether the way in which a particular protocol is designed will truly be of benefit and to whom and in what time period.

Confidentiality

The principle of confidentiality establishes a social contract between client and therapist. It seems simple and straightforward, promoting the rights of others to private information. It implies that the secrets of another will be respected and maintained. Its simplicity is misleading, however, as the art of balancing a client's rights to confidentiality against the rights of others (and often society) can sometimes lead to complex and challenging situations.

When a client is knowingly putting others at risk of infection and refusing to notify these others of their risk, how should the mental health worker proceed? Can the principle of nonmaleficence take precedence over that of confidentiality? Do we acknowledge the autonomy of clients, informing them that such behavior is unacceptable and that others will be informed if the client will not inform them? Ideally, it would be hoped that we could create a moral climate in which it is taken for granted that partners will not expose each other to HIV infection (6). Until that is achieved, mental health practitioners must grapple with the desire to maintain confidentiality and that of balancing the rights of all individuals to a healthy and risk-free existence.

Justice

The principle of justice urges the fair and equitable distribution of resources, treatment, and economic goods. It addresses the issue of equality, suggesting that cases which are alike in context and nature be treated equally while cases which are different be treated differently.

Since the beginning of the AIDS epidemic, questions of justice have proliferated. Familiar to most are those concerning the adequate distribution of monies to support basic research, treatment trials, education, and prevention programs. Other concerns raised by the justice principle are evident in the management of health insurance. Where is the justice in terminating or denying health insurance to someone who is HIV positive or has low T-4 count? How can an insurance company refuse to pay for a prophylactic treatment of an HIV-infected individual on the grounds that the treatment will prolong the person's life? Is this a just response in a society that funds the implantation of artificial hearts at an astronomical cost?

Decision-Making Models

Although there is no magic formula or five-step recipe for quick resolutions to difficult moral problems, there are a variety of ethical decision-making models which can provide guidance to those struggling with ethical dilemmas (2,7,8,9). Each model is slightly different, thus offering the reader an opportunity to explore various approaches. Perhaps the most basic model suggests that the first task is to define the problem. Gather any additional information you need to make a judgment. Clarify who will be affected by this decision. Here is where you are also identifying the relevant moral issues, your own values and those of your client (s).

Determine if there is a decision to be made and whose decision it is. Weigh the various alternatives by looking at the short-range consequences, the long-range consequences and identifying any risks created by this alternative. Take time to explore the ethical justifications for each alternative as well.

Although it is often not easy, we must select the most ethical and acceptable decision based on the possible alternatives. It is always useful to compare the actual outcome with the desired outcome. We learn from our decisions in that they give us guidance of what to expect in the future.

Conclusion

These are complex times, and there are no simple solutions to the difficult dilemmas facing mental health practitioners or others involved in the care of those with HIV disease. In this chapter, ethical principles have been described and systems of ethical decision making have been outlined. Applying ethical principles to clinical work requires practice. And, in addition to practice, it demands that we talk with others about how and why we choose to make certain decisions.

■

References

1. Pierce C, VanDeVeer D: AIDS Ethics and Public Policy. Belmont CA, Wadsworth Publishing, 1988

2. Francoeur RT: Biomedical Ethics: A Guide to Decision Making. New York, J. Wiley and Sons, 1983

3. Gilligan C: In a Different Voice. Cambridge MA, Harvard University Press, 1982

4. Beauchamp TL, Childress JF: Principles of Biomedical Ethics. New York, Oxford University Press, 1983

5. Bunting SM, Webb AA: An ethical model for decision making. Nurse Practitioner 1988; 13(12)

6. Bell NK: AIDS and women: remaining ethical issues. AIDS Education and Prevention 1989; 1(1):22-30

7. Thompson JE, Thompson HO: Bioethical Decision Making for Nurses. Norwalk CT, Appleton-Century-Crofts, 1985

8. Aroskar MA: Anatomy of an ethical dilemma: the theory. Am J of Nursing 1980; 80:658-660

9. Murphy MA, Murphy J: Making ethical decisions systematically. Nursing May '76; pp 13-14

■

Cheri Pies, MSW, DrPH, is a private consultant with an emphasis in reproductive ethics, public health, and health education practice. She has worked extensively in the past as an AIDS prevention trainer and educator and as a consultant to a variety of AIDS agencies, media projects, and research studies.

■

The Duty to Protect: Confidentiality and HIV

Howard V. Zonana, MD

The same persistent fears and irrational beliefs that once overshadowed syphilis, bubonic plague, cholera, and leprosy prior to effective treatments now hamper attempts to deal with AIDS and HIV disease. People who contract diseases like AIDS that are sexually transmitted are especially prone to the additional judgment that their fate results from moral laxity or turpitude that deserves punishment. Even into this century these fears of contagion have led to efforts to quarantine and isolate those deemed to be at risk for transmitting these diseases (1,2).

The treatment of people who are HIV positive again brings these fears and beliefs into focus. The related public issues are complicated by attempts both to prevent the spread of the infection and to protect the individual's right to medical treatment without discrimination and stigmatization. Mental health professionals increasingly confront these issues as HIV-infected individuals present themselves in a variety of counseling and treatment settings. This chapter focuses on one of the more common ethical concerns of practicing mental health practitioners: the issues of confidentiality, HIV antibody screening and testing, and the duty to warn.

General Principles of Confidentiality

Prior to the 19th century, when physicians were subpoenaed to testify in court, there were no barriers that prevented disclosures of information revealed in the course of the physician/patient relationship. Such a testimonial privilege grants the right to maintain confidentiality when confronted with a subpoena in court or other judicial proceedings. This "privilege" afforded to attorneys and clergy did not apply to the medical profession.

Gradually states began to protect information disclosed to physicians by enacting statutes creating a privilege. This now means that without permission, statutory exception or waiver, the physician cannot testify in court about such communications (i.e., the privilege belongs to the patient). During the past 30 years this privilege has been extended to psychologists in many states and other psychotherapists in a smaller number of jurisdictions.

On the other hand, mental health professionals have generally felt that information obtained from clients, if treatment was to be successful, must be regarded as confidential. It should be protected not only in court proceedings, but more broadly. Beginning around 1961, statutes governing the confidentiality and release of information derived in medical and psychotherapeutic settings began to be enacted. These codified and set limits upon the ethical codes, such as the Hippocratic Oath, which professionals had relied upon for guidance. Now most states deem communications between a psychiatrist and patient legally confidential, although there are many exceptions that permit disclosure without patient consent.

For nonmedical psychotherapists, however, the scope of confidentiality duties is generally defined by discipline: i.e., psychologists, social workers, nurses, rape counselors. Some states have confidentiality and/or privilege statutes which apply specifically to a particular discipline, and where these exist the therapist can be confident in approaching issues of confidentiality. However, for some professional groups the only guidelines may be ethical principles promulgated by the specific professional organization. While these may provide some help, it is also important to note that these guidelines may not have legal standing in courts of law.

Where confidentiality statutes exist, they usually involve any communication between the therapist and client. This includes both verbal and written communications, including letters, notes, or memos to the chart. This protection of confidentiality generally means information may not be shared with others without the patient's specific written informed consent. The scope of this duty and exceptions to it which allow disclosures without patient consent are defined generally by state statute. Exceptions vary somewhat from state to state, but exceptions to these rules are generally made when disclosures have to do with emergency treatment, imminent dangerousness, child abuse, or the need for hospitalization. If a client enters his or her mental condition in a lawsuit, the opposing side generally will be afforded access to all prior mental health records.

However, because it is true that all communications between patients and treating clinicians are not strictly confidential, the limits of confidentiality should be explicitly discussed with the client in the initial treatment or evaluation period.

Operating within the framework of the general principles of confidentiality discussed above, the American Psychiatric Association has developed guidelines for treating HIV-positive patients in a variety of settings. The guideline for the initial evaluation period states:

> Physicians have an ethical obligation to recognize the rights to privacy, to confidentiality, and to informed consent of all patients. During the initial clinical evaluation, the physician should usually make clear the general limits of confidentiality. If the physician has reason to suspect the patient is infected with HIV or is engaging in behavior that is known to transmit HIV disease, the physician should notify the patient of the specific limits of confidentiality. Further, if the physician intends to inquire specifically about a patient's HIV status, the physician should, in such instances, notify the patient about the limits of confidentiality in advance of asking such questions. (3)

These principles may be useful to all mental health professionals. As with any set of guidelines, some circumstances will occasionally arise when a patient will make a statement before the limits can be made clear. Such circumstances may require consultation with colleagues and/or an attorney, as well as a full discussion with the patient before resolving any conflicts about disclosures.

Screening and Testing for Antibodies to HIV

Mandatory testing of individuals for HIV antibodies remains restricted to specific groups under specific circumstances. Screening for the presence of the HIV antibody currently occurs in the armed services and the U.S. foreign service, in processing U.S. immigrants, in federal prisons, and in blood, semen and organ donors. In addition, some states and some insurance carriers require testing of prisoners or convicted prostitutes, or to obtain marriage licenses or health insurance.

All states require reporting of individuals diagnosed with AIDS, but only a handful require reporting of those testing HIV positive without other symptomatology. Many states offer anonymous testing sites. These testing sites are probably the only way to ensure anonymous testing results.

For the purposes of our discussion, the issue of testing is closely tied to the issue of disclosure. This issue is most often problematic in two ways: the first in making decisions about charting HIV-related information, and the second in warning third parties at possible risk. The issue of warning third parties is discussed separately below.

In terms of charting, each state will likely have specific recommendations regarding the handling of HIV test results. When the testing is performed in a hospital or clinic setting, the findings will usually be recorded in the medical record and will be disclosed when valid requests for the record occur. Although some physicians have suggested that HIV testing be treated like routine blood tests, most hospitals require specific written informed consent before HIV testing and before disclosing the results to others outside the hospital setting. However, several recent reports revealed that some hospitals were testing patients without their knowledge and consent (4,5,6). In inpatient mental health settings, the distinction between testing for the purpose of staff awareness and individual patient need is blurred. Testing merely for staff awareness is not felt to be justified because of potential negative social consequences to the patient. It may also lead to more carelessness with infected patients who have not yet developed antibodies, as well as creating difficulties in disclosing positive results to patients who did not even know they were tested.

Initially, many hospitals did not place HIV test results in the medical record. Currently this practice has changed and medical records now contain test results. Generally the record (inpatient or outpatient) should contain only information that is necessary for the clinical care of the patient. Thus discharge summaries may or may not contain HIV information depending upon the purpose of the disclosure. Some state statutes have not allowed disclosure of HIV antibody status to other health care facilities without specific patient consent.

Much has been written about the need for careful counseling and sensitivity in the initial disclosure to individuals that they are

HIV positive. Since this disclosure has been interpreted by many as an immediate death sentence, it is not surprising that there have been a number of suicides and suicide attempts within a short period of time after a patient learns of positive results. In fact, many have elected not to find out test results when blood had been collected for other purposes on an earlier occasion (7). Depression as a reaction to disclosure or anytime in the course of the disease is not uncommon.

When the mental health professional is working with an out-patient who is HIV positive, there is good reason to review any sexual or drug-related practices which may place others at risk for exposure. There is evidence that counseling, if it is to be effective, should be more than a one-time event. Clients may become quite angry by the suggestion that high-risk behaviors must be stopped or modified. Some mental disorders may make control of impulses difficult, and at times, clients may overtly threaten to knowingly engage in high-risk activities. The decision to seek voluntary or involuntary hospitalization in these circumstances is a difficult, clinical decision. These clients may require emergency certification or petitions to courts, under a standard of danger to others. Contingency planning with the client may make this choice less likely if other resources are available. Greater flexibility in appointments, inclusion of family or friends, or judicious use of medication may be viable alternatives. While many patient fears about disclosure of their HIV infection are warranted, some may not be. Careful exploration regarding the reality of such fears may make voluntary disclosure an opportunity for support rather than further stigmatization.

Protecting Third Parties and the Duty To Warn

Especially troublesome to mental health care professionals has been the duty to warn third parties who may be at risk of HIV infection by their patient's actions. Is there a "Tarasoff" or other legal duty to protect potential victims from infection? This dilemma balances the duty to an individual patient against the duty to society or other individuals who may be harmed by the patient.

While a clear answer is not yet available, the Centers for Disease Control (CDC) recommends that if persons who are HIV infected "are unwilling to notify their partners or if it cannot be assured that their partners will seek counseling, physicians or health department personnel should use confidential procedures to assure that partners are notified"(8). Unfortunately this guideline does not specify how or what "confidential procedures" the drafters had in mind, nor does it comment on the general situation when an HIV-infected individual is reasonably believed to be engaging in high-risk sexual activity with unidentifiable parties. The guideline also does not address whether notification is necessary when the HIV-infected person consistently practices safe or low-risk behavior in all sexual encounters.

A California law now permits disclosure of this information by a physician to a person *believed to be* a spouse or needle-sharing partner, if attempts to obtain the patient's voluntary consent have failed. There is, however, no legal duty to make such a disclosure. The statute affords protection from liability if the physician decides to disclose or remain silent (9). Similar laws have been adopted in other states (10,11,12). The trend clearly is moving to permitting disclosures, especially to "spouses" and others in immediate danger.

The APA guideline is in accord with this trend and states:

> In situations where a physician has received convincing clinical information...that the patient is infected with HIV, the physician should advise and work with the patient either to obtain agreement to terminate behavior that places other persons at risk of infection or to notify identifiable individuals who may be at continuing risk of exposure. If a patient refuses to agree to change behavior or to notify the persons at risk, or the physician has good reason to believe that the patient has failed to or is unable to comply with this agreement, it is ethically permissible for the physician to notify an identifiable person whom the physician believes to be in danger of contracting the virus.

The American Medical Association (AMA) guidelines are similar, with the exception that they recommend that if persuasion fails, the first step is to notify the authorities (presumably the Department of Health), and only if the authorities take no action should the physician notify and counsel the endangered third party (13). The President's Commission on AIDS and the CDC also recommend disclosures to individuals who may be unknowingly in immediate danger of being exposed to the HIV (8,14).

The danger of approving guidelines allowing disclosures to third parties without a patient's consent is that professionals will use this permission in a reflex manner and not give sufficient thought to alternatives. There are examples where disclosures are made before the patient is given any opportunity to deal with the situation directly or where there is no risk. Disclosures to third parties without patient consent is a major decision and, in the absence of an emergency, should usually be made after consultation with other knowledgeable colleagues.

In inpatient mental health facilities, the need to protect other patients from harm is a substantial obligation. Especially in large state mental hospitals, this has become a great concern, as the strict control of sexual behavior between patients is exceedingly difficult. Hospitals have tried different approaches, from making condoms available to all patients to the use of seclusion and restraints for patients who refuse to comply with the ban on sexual activity. No clear, workable and successful method has emerged, but disclosure of a patient's HIV status to other patients should not be a substitute for adequate clinical care (15). When other mental disorders such as schizophrenia or bipolar disease are also present, clinical management can become more complicated, and civil commitment may become necessary. Some hospital representatives have suggested that such patients should not be released without court approval if they have histories of discontinuing medication and engaging in behavior that places others at risk.

Another area where confidentiality questions arise surrounds the organic AIDS dementia complex that may be seen in HIV disease. Studies have indicated that dementia may occur in both HIV-positive and symptomatic patients before the development of full-blown AIDS. While the exact incidence is actively under study, some controversial studies have suggested the occurrence of mild cognitive impairment in nonsymptomatic HIV-positive individuals (16). Mental health clinicians will often be in a position of identifying and testing for such symptoms. They will also be in positions of counseling when impairments are of a degree that continued work in certain professions may be hazardous. For example, health care professionals themselves may become impaired, and reporting statutes may require disclosures if patients are unwilling to stop working. Generally, counseling should be sufficient, and other aspects of the illness usually intrude before the dementia becomes the determining factor.

Conclusion

Confidentiality remains an integral and time-honored feature of the therapist-client relationship. The emergence of HIV has brought many new challenges to this issue, and as long as HIV-infected individuals are stigmatized, discriminated against and refused treatment, the confidentiality of such data will remain a dilemma. Furthermore, the more rapid the spread of HIV disease and the growing availability of useful treatments, the greater the demands will be for mandatory testing and disclosures. In this article, the impact of this disease on confidentiality has been discussed and a summary of the thinking of major professional organizations presented. Patients who are HIV infected present a number of unique and complicated issues to the practicing mental health professional. The appropriate balancing of ethical principles in their care is a major challenge.

■

References

1. Brandt AM: No Magic Bullet: A Social History of Venereal Disease in the United States Since 1880. New York, Oxford University Press, 1987, pp 87-96

2. Annual Report of the U.S. Interdepartmental Social Hygiene Board, Washington, D.C., Government Printing Office, 1920

3. AIDS policy: confidentiality and disclosure. APA Policy Statement, Amer J Psychiatry 1988; 145(4):541-542

4. Keith H, Maki M, Crossley K: Analysis of the use of HIV antibody testing in a Minnesota hospital. J Am Med Assoc 1988; 259:229-232

5. Dallas hospital secretly tested patients for AIDS. The Washington Post, February 7, 1988; p A6

6. AIDS testing without consent reported. The New York Times, January 9, 1988; p 7

7. Lyter DW, Valdiserri RO, Kingsley LA, et al: The HIV antibody test: why gay and bisexual men want or do not want to know their results. Public Health Reports 1987 (Sept-Oct); 102(5):468-474

8. Centers for Disease Control: Public health service guidelines for counseling and antibody testing to prevent HIV infection and AIDS. Morbidity and Mortality Weekly Reports (MMWR), August 14, 1987; 36:509-515

9. California Senate Bill No. 2788, 1988

10. New York Bill No. S-9265-A, 1988. Allows physicians to disclose HIV test results to the spouse, sexual partner, or needle-sharing partner of a person who tests positive, if they believe that the contact is in danger of infection and will not be warned by the infected person. Under the new law, physicians are granted immunity from liability for warning the contacts of infected persons, for failing to warn contacts, and for disclosing HIV information to authorized persons. (Effective February 1, 1989)

11. Connecticut Public Act No. 89-246, 1989

12. West Virginia House Bill No. 303-XXX. (Effective September 1, 1988)

13. Wilkerson I: AMA urges breach of privacy to warn potential AIDS victims. The New York Times, July 1, 1988; pp A1 and A11

14. The Presidential Commission: The Final Report of the Presidential Commission on the Human Immunodeficiency Virus Epidemic. James D. Watkins, Chairman. Washington, D.C., Government Printing Office, 1988

15. Zonana HV, Norko M, Stier D: The AIDS patient on the psychiatric unit: ethical and legal issues. Psychiatric Annals, October 1988; 10:587-593

16. Grant I, Atkinson JH, Hesselink JR, et al: Human immunodeficiency virus-associated neurobehavioural disorder. J Royal College of Physicians of London, July 1988; 22(3):149-157

Editor's Notes

Because of the thorny legal and ethical issues raised by the HIV epidemic, the AIDS Health Project has published a book specifically addressing AIDS law for mental health professionals. The book uses a case history approach and addresses dilemmas from both legal and clinical perspectives. While the book is based on California law, it is a comprehensive resource for practitioners throughout the country, and it comes with regular updates highlighting changes that have occurred since the book's publication.

AIDS Law for Mental Health Professionals by Gary Wood, JD, Robert Marks, and James W. Dilley, MD can be obtained from your local bookstore—it is distributed to the trade by Celestial Arts in Berkeley, California—or by writing the UCSF AIDS Health Project at Box 0884, San Francisco, CA 94143-0884.

■

Howard V. Zonana, MD, is Associate Professor of Clinical Psychiatry and Director of the Law and Psychiatry Division at Yale University School of Medicine, New Haven, Connecticut.

VII
Special Populations

- **Ethnic Minorities, HIV Disease and the Growing Underclass**
  Mindy Thompson Fullilove, MD

- **HIV Disease: Issues for Women**
  Nancy Stoller Shaw, PhD

- **Youth and HIV: No Immunity**
  Janet Shalwitz, MD and Ken Dunnigan, MD, MPH

- **Double Jeopardy: Hemophilia and HIV Disease**
  Donna DiMarzo, MSW, MPH

- **The AIDS Bereaved: Counseling Strategies**
  Amy Weiss, MS, MFCC

- **HIV, Stress and the Health Care Professional**
  Mary L. S. Vachon, RN, PhD and Jeanne Dennis, MSW

- **Too Many Casualties: HIV Disease in Gay Men**
  Michael Helquist

Ethnic Minorities, HIV Disease and the Growing Underclass

Mindy Thompson Fullilove, MD

AIDS and Minorities

AIDS has affected disproportionately Blacks and Latins in the United States. Though Blacks in the U.S. are 12% of the population, they represent 26% of the people with AIDS. Latins, who are 7% of the U.S. population, represent 14% of the people with AIDS (1). To explain the excessive impact of AIDS on minority communities, researchers have suggested the presence of large numbers of intravenous drug users in Black and Latin communities (2). Others have wondered (though rarely in print) if, perhaps, levels of sexual activity among minorities are much greater than they are among Whites. Each suggestion bears examination.

Sharing needles is an extremely efficient way to transmit the AIDS virus from one person to another, but the virus must be present in the needle-sharing group before it can be spread (3). Currently, the virus has entered some needle-sharing groups, but not all, a fact which seems to be related to several factors, including the complex ways in which needle users choose shooting partners. For example, many drug users have a regular "spot" to which they go for drugs. Often these "sharing locations" are organized by race—Blacks tend to share with Blacks and Whites tend to share with Whites—but also, within specific groups, there are ties of friendship and family relationship that bond the group. Some needle groups are rigid and closed, and members never share outside their own group; these groups are sometimes called "endogamous." Other groups, sometimes labeled "exogamous," are not as rigid and allow members to move in and out.

Drug groups, whether exogamous or endogamous, are sensitive to changes in the environment. An examination of the changes in New York's South Bronx in the late '70s and early '80s (4) indicated that people living in those communities suffered a "forced migration" when an epidemic of fires destroyed block after block of low-income housing. Many of the people living in those neighborhoods were addicts. It is likely that when the addicts moved, they were forced to re-establish their needle-sharing groups, thus spreading the virus throughout the Bronx, which currently has one of the highest rates of HIV infection anywhere in the nation.

Despite the importance of the issue, there is more talk and speculation about minority sexuality than there is hard evidence. Perhaps what is most clear is that there is a common belief in the fantasy that Blacks and Latins have an exotic and different sexuality that distinguishes them from Whites (5).

Researchers from the Multicultural Inquiry and Research on AIDS (MIRA) group in San Francisco reviewed the literature on the sexuality of Blacks and Whites (6) and talked to black adults and teens in order to learn about their sex lives. While there is a great deal more to learn—for example, little is known about the sexuality of Latin and Asian cultures—the following observations appear solid (7):

1. Black teenagers initiate sexual intercourse at earlier ages than White teenagers. This is especially true for black boys, half of whom become sexually active by about age 13. Sexually active teens, especially when young and inexperienced, are at high risk for sexually transmitted disease.

2. Blacks are less likely to use contraception, including condoms, and are less knowledgeable about contraception than their white peers.

3. Where other things are equal—that is, where there is economic stability and social integration—black adults and white adults will attempt to create stable, loving relationships in which to raise children and grow old companionably. In general, minority heterosexuals, not in contact with the drug-using networks, are at no more risk for AIDS than white heterosexuals isolated from drug-using networks.

4. Minority homosexuals experience many of the same pressures as white homosexuals, as they work through "coming out" as gay or lesbian. But for minorities, there is a dual oppression to

be faced: one from the minority heterosexual community which is extremely rejecting of homosexuality, and the other from the white gay community which can be as racist as other white communities. Among minority men who identify as "gay," there are close-knit networks that provide social and economic support.

What we have proposed, in this brief synopsis of an extremely complex body of information, is that the term "race," as applied to AIDS statistics, does not stand for biology, or culture, or social class so much as it stands for "network." When we look at AIDS statistics, we are looking primarily at intimate groups, groups that love each other, that share with each other, and that take care of each other.

This article will not focus so much on the past, however, as it will make suggestions about the future of the AIDS epidemic. Changes in the environment and economy as they have affected Black communities in the past decade will be presented and the impact of these changes on substance users will be suggested. Further, the effect of heterosexism on the minority community's response to the AIDS epidemic will be discussed, and finally, the effects of changing economic conditions and social denial on the future of the AIDS epidemic for minority substance users and minority gay men will be described.

Changing Environment and Economy

Illiteracy and semiliteracy rates are high in the black population, a fact that is linked to the current economic situation of the community. As the U.S. economy has shifted away from unskilled labor in basic industry toward highly skilled labor in service industries, literacy has become the key to getting and keeping a job. Miller noted, "Although the cause-and-effect relations are extremely complex, it has long been recognized that semiliteracy, poverty, and racial discrimination are inextricably connected (8)."

In the past, Blacks have competed for unskilled jobs, but these have largely disappeared from the modern marketplace. Positions in the "information economy" increasingly dominate the job market, but Blacks are poorly prepared to compete for them. This has created a mismatch between human and economic resources which has serious consequences for the economy of black communities. Black men have been particularly hard hit, with unemployment rates in that group reaching as high as 43% of all those of working age.

The growth of black male unemployment has had a devastating impact on men, women and children. In an excellent description of the link between economic and family structures, Bowser wrote, "As the community declines, the family is a key institution which will reflect it. As the nuclear family has become the normative structure for participation in advanced industrial society, Blacks have had to devise or maintain alternative social units in order to survive on the edge of advanced industrial society. The alarming rise in divorce, separations, female-headed households and children born into single-parent households indicates community decline" (9).

Family structure has important implications for education. Early reports examining the relationship between single-parent families and child development suggest that such children are at risk for behavioral and academic difficulties. However, some studies suggest otherwise. One study of teenage mothers and their children followed over a number of years found a range of outcomes and that "children of children" were not necessarily doomed to a life of failure, particularly if the mother had high educational aspirations and was able to complete school (10). However, for those children whose mothers continued to be single parents, and particularly for those with limited income (including those on welfare), repeating a grade in school and having other difficulties in behavior were more common. Thus education, family structure, and economic class are closely linked in present-day America.

Overall, in the past decade, black communities have faced increased economic instability, accompanied by the growth of a largely male underclass whose economic survival depends on criminal and semi-criminal activities. Family instability alone would lead to changing sexual mores and behaviors, but the added factor of the growth of a new economic class, with a distinctly different relationship to the means of production, may increase the rate of change in sexual behaviors toward more permissive, less protective norms. Young men in the underclass have been drawn into employment in the vast crack-dealing networks that have flourished in inner-city communities around the country. When asked, "Do you think there's a future in selling crack?" many will reply, "No." Unfortunately, there are few other alternatives upon which to draw.

Implications for Substance-Using Networks

While many AIDS cases in the past have been related to intravenous drug use, data now suggest that a narrow focus on needles and needle use alone will not control the spread of the epidemic. In interviews with black teen crack users, we found that 42% reported a history of sexually transmitted disease (STD) (11). The STD rate was even higher among teens who reported combining sex and drugs. In this "sex and drugs" group, 52% had had a sexually transmitted disease. Overall the teen crack users reported large numbers of sexual partners and little use of condoms. Finally, about 10% of the teens had used needles to inject heroin, cocaine, or amphetamines. Thus, there were two vectors for HIV infection to be carried from the intravenous drug-using community to the crack-using community: sexual activity and needle sharing.

Yet, rather than simply adding crack users to the list of AIDS "risk" groups, it is probably more helpful to see all substance users as at risk. This is so because drugs and alcohol interfere with protective decision making and because mind-altering substances are interchangeable. Many heroin users have become alcoholics; more recently they have switched to crack. For people who like to get high, any drug will do. Drug availability and drug use are context driven. Many unhappy soldiers in Vietnam used heroin but gave it up on returning home. Black teens, typically less likely than white teens to use drugs, have been swept into the crack epidemic in a dramatic fashion (12). As long as society condones getting high and suffering people see drug use as a means of escape, problems with addiction will continue though the name of the current favorite substance will periodically change. Hence, only broadly based prevention efforts will be useful in the long run.

Minority Gay Men, Social Denial and Heterosexism

Gay men are seen by many as ideal consumers; relative to those supporting children, they have a large amount of disposable income and are willing to spend it. One of the questions that our research group has grappled with is: To what extent does this status of relative economic privilege (assuming it really exists) also encompass black gay men? It is our early impression that some black gay men—especially those who have consolidated and are comfortable with a gay identity—are, like their white counterparts, relatively well-to-do.

This is not to say that all gay men are wealthy; rather, I wish to suggest that in understanding the gay community and its minority subsections, we need to develop a complete understanding of the socioeconomic conditions in which homosexual men live. Also, while these observations may be true of "gay-identified" men—that is, a relatively small subset of all the men who have sex with men—this may not be true of men who, though they have sexual encounters with other men, do not see themselves as homosexual.

The issue of identity is important here, in part because it defines the networks in which people will function. Because of their network attachments and supports, gay-identified minority men are most likely to receive and to attend to AIDS prevention messages. Minority men who have same-sex activity, but who do not have a gay identity, may be at a different level of risk. On the one hand, their more isolated sexual encounters may not take place within networks that have high rates of infection. On the other hand, they may be less likely to use safe sex practices.

As gay communities—minority and white—are struggling with the AIDS epidemic, they have been fortified by the existence of strong and politically astute gay networks. As gay men die from the disease, however, we may see an accelerated shredding of these networks. Just as shredding of networks had an effect on the spread of AIDS among addicts in the South Bronx, we can anticipate that the destruction of gay networks will have deep consequences for the epidemic among gay men. Though the directions of the consequences are as yet unclear, careful attention must be paid to this issue. Possible outcomes might include (but are not limited to): 1) depression and anxiety as people lose multiple members of their social set, 2) increasing unsafe sex arising from feelings of hopelessness, 3) increasing unsafe sex because people cannot maintain the behavior changes they have made in recent years, 4) decreasing ability to cope with the social and political pressures related to the epidemic, or 5) some adaptation of sexual practices as much earlier evidence suggests.

Minority and white gay networks must also be seen in the context of social and cultural rejection of homosexuals (13). Thus, the strength of the network is an important source of support in maintaining a positive sense of one's self in spite of rejection from the larger society. The rejection of homosexuals by our culture—called "heterosexism" in this paper—has been an important factor in determining the slow response to the AIDS epidemic in our country.

Social Denial

Epidemics present a serious danger to the functioning and survival of the social group. The early stages of recognition and identification of an epidemic are characterized by social denial, a group reaction similar in many respects to the individual reaction of denial of a threatening event. Social denial, like its individual counterpart, is an unconscious mechanism of defense that protects against fear and anxiety. But if not rapidly resolved, this denial can endanger the group by inhibiting appropriate responses to the epidemic.

Several factors may impede the resolution of social denial, including geographic or emotional isolation from the threat. "Emotional isolation" refers to the belief that the threat is not a threat to the "group" because those at risk represent a "different" group as defined by age, race, sex, social class, religion or other identifiers.

These issues are also illustrated in the AIDS epidemic which has, almost exclusively, affected racial and sexual minority groups traditionally discriminated against in U.S. society (14). The "out-group" character of the victims of the epidemic has slowed epidemic response and fed hostility. National surveys confirm that the general public feels hostility toward people with AIDS (15). Firebombings, discrimination in housing, employment, and education, and lack of funds for research and treatment have all been part of the social denial in reaction to AIDS.

Heterosexism in the Black Community

During the course of our research on black sexuality (6), we asked black adults and adolescents to describe their experiences with homosexuality and their reactions to it. Heterosexual adults had various reactions to homosexuality. One man said, "Gays are dangerous. They are very, very dangerous." A woman told us, "Homosexuality gags me with a spoon." Others were perhaps more tolerant, including one woman who said, "I think, whatever makes you happy." The most extreme reactions of rejection and hostility were recorded in a group of young male crack dealers: One young man said, "If he's a real nigga, he ain't gon be no faggot." Heterosexual informants saw their emotions rising in reaction to the behavior of homosexuals. The tendency was for the informant to generalize from the behavior of one individual to the group.

Homosexuals, presenting the other side of the story, saw many of these reactions as projections and stereotypes created by heterosexuals. One man described, "There's that whole relationship of fending off women who are convinced that it will take just one piece of p— to change you to a real man." With heterosexual men he noted, "I have to let straight black men know that not one of them has anything they could offer me. . . because the first thing they do is put up their barrier. . . I wouldn't make a pass at them in a million years."

The comments from homosexual informants included many descriptions of rejection by heterosexuals. For gays and lesbians, the process of coming out was protracted, involving recognition of oneself as gay, discovering one's sexuality with a lover, acknowledging one's sexual orientation to intimate friends and family, and for some, acknowledging this sexual orientation publicly. The family was of little help in this process, as family members did not suggest the possibility of homosexual identity until the homosexual person asserted it. For a number of informants, the response from family members was, "Well, we always knew." But for others, the announcement was followed by intense rejection. For all, the isolated search seemed to have been lonely, frightening, and often painful.

Comments on the AIDS epidemic underscored the social denial of some heterosexuals toward the epidemic. These informants generally saw the epidemic as something happening to another group that was not of concern to the black community and further, as something that was taking resources out of the community.

In Summary: Two Epidemics

Minority communities have been hit with two AIDS epidemics: one among intravenous drug users and one among gay men. Given the vast economic changes seen over the past decade, we can anticipate worsening in the conditions that link drug use and sexually transmitted disease. Thus, HIV infection among substance users—in general—will almost certainly expand over the next few years. Minority gay-identified men and other men who have sex with men face a threat not only from the loss of personal networks that will follow in the wake of the AIDS epidemic, but also from the hostility toward homosexuality that exists in American culture.

Much of the material reviewed here supports the contention that there is a link between deepening poverty and increasing disease. More subtle are the linkages between social and economic disintegration and social ostracism. It seems that as things fall apart, the need to blame, to reject, and to distance will increase in many sectors of society. As this "blaming" feeds social denial and slows the response to the epidemic, the cost will be many lives. This is one of the greatest threats that faces minority gay men, minority substance users and minority communities, in general, in the coming period.

What can health workers do? They can envision their role on two levels: first, they need to understand and treat the ills that bring the individual person into treatment. Obviously this will include people with AIDS-related anxiety and dementia, the worried well, and the HIV-infected person who is trying to cope. Second, they need to identify and "treat" the social denial that is holding Blacks, as a society, back from making a rapid, appropriate and just response to this epidemic. The many efforts to address this—the Names Project Quilt, the "Faces of AIDS" Project, Act Up, etc.—all deserve our support. As mental health professionals we may be able to bring new insights to bear on the awful "illness" of social denial.

■

References

1. Selik RM, Castro KG, Pappaioanou M: Distribution of AIDS cases by racial/ethnic groups and exposure category in the U.S., 6/1/81-7/4/88. MMWR, 1988; 37:1-10

2. Bakeman R, Lumb JR, Jackson RE, et al: AIDS risk-group profiles in whites and members of minority groups. New Eng J Med 1986; 315:191-192

3. Haynes KC: Minorities, intravenous drug use, and AIDS: a review. MIRA Newsletter, 1988; 2(4):1-2

4. Wallace R: A synergism of plagues: "planned shrinkage," contagious housing destruction and AIDS in the Bronx. Environmental Research 1988; 47:1-33

5. Gilman S: Difference and Pathology. Ithaca, New York, Cornell U. Press, 1987

6. Weinstein M, Crayton E, Goodjoin R: Black Sexuality: A Bibliography, 2nd Edition. San Francisco, CA, MIRA Publications, 1989

7. Fullilove MT, Weinstein M, Fullilove RE, et al: "Will you still love me tomorrow?": Race/gender issues in the sexual transmission of AIDS. Unpublished manuscript, 1989

8. Miller GA: The challenge of universal literacy. Science 1988; 241:1293-1299

9. Bowser B: Community and economic context of black families: a critical review of the literature, 1909-1985. Amer J Soc Psychiatry 1986; 6:17-26

10. Furstenberg FF Jr, Brooks-Gunn J, Morgan SP: Adolescent mothers and their children in later life. Family Planning Perspective 1987; 19:142-151

11. Fullilove MT, Fullilove R: Intersecting epidemics: black teen crack use and sexually transmitted disease. J Am Med Women's Assoc 1989 (in press)

12. Zabin LS, Hardy JB, Smith EA, et al: Substance use and its relation to sexual activity among inner city adolescents. J Adolescent Health Care 1986; 7:320-331

13. Boswell J: Christianity, Social Tolerance and Homosexuality: Gay People in Western Europe from the Beginning of the Christian Era to the Fourteenth Century. Chicago, University of Chicago Press, 1980

14. Shilts R: And the Band Played On: People, Politics and the AIDS Epidemic. New York, Penguin Books, 1987

15. Blendon RJ, Donelan K: Discrimination against people with AIDS: the public's perspective. New England Journal of Medicine 1988; 319:1022-1026

Updated References

Ellerbrock TV, Lieb S, Harrington PE, et al: Heterosexually transmitted human immunodeficiency virus infection among pregnant women in a rural Florida community. N Engl J Med 1992; 327:1704-1709.

Chiasson MA, Stoneburner RL, Hildebrandt DS, et al: Heterosexual transmission of HIV-1 associated with the use of smokable freebase cocaine (crack). AIDS 1991; 5:1121-6.

Fullilove RE, Fullilove MT, Bowser BP, et al: Risk of sexually transmitted disease among black adolescent crack users in Oakland and San Francisco, Calif. JAMA 1990; 263:851-5.

■

Mindy Thompson Fullilove, MD, is Assistant Clinical Professor of Psychiatry, University of California San Francisco (UCSF) School of Medicine and Director of Multicultural Inquiry and Research on AIDS (MIRA), which is a project of the Bayview-Hunter's Point Foundation and the UCSF Center for AIDS Prevention Studies in San Francisco.

HIV Disease: Issues for Women

Nancy Stoller Shaw, PhD

HIV disease has had an effect on every segment of American society. However, it is increasingly an illness of the poor and of ethnic and sexual minorities. As we move into the nineties, this will be more the case than ever. (See Editor's Notes, page 248.)

Demographics

Thousands of adolescent and adult women in the United States and Puerto Rico have been diagnosed with AIDS and other manifestations of HIV disease. Many more are seropositive without symptoms. Until the epidemic is controlled, a steadily increasing number of women will become infected.

National rates of HIV infection and disease are much higher in the Black and Latin communities than among Whites. Although Blacks constitute about 12% of the U.S. population, black women comprise over 50% of the women with AIDS. Puerto Ricans and Chicanas are similarly overrepresented among seropositive women. The social source of these ethnic differences is a combination of several factors: multigenerational segregation; widespread sale of addicting, mind-altering, and injectable drugs in poor ghetto communities; deteriorating public health services; and grossly inadequate health education for Black and Latin populations.

The majority of seropositive women are intravenous drug users who contracted the virus through contaminated needles. The second most frequent route of infection is heterosexual intercourse. The already infected male partners have most often been IV drug users. Bisexual men, hemophilics, and men with other or undetermined sources of infection comprise the group of other infected partners. Other seropositive women have contracted HIV from blood transfusions. In a small number of cases, the source of transmission has not been determined. Most of these "unknown risk" cases are believed by researchers to be the result of male-to-female transmission in situations where the women did not believe that their partners could have been infected. A few cases are listed as "unknown" because the women died before they could be interviewed. AIDS among lesbians can generally be traced to the same sources of infection as for heterosexual women. Only one case of woman-to-woman transmission has been documented in the United States; that transmission was most probably through blood-to-blood contact (1).

Women with HIV disease were initially concentrated in four states: New York, New Jersey, Florida, and California. As the epidemic has spread, seropositive women have been appearing more and more frequently in every state and in the smaller cities, suburbs, and rural areas of the U.S. By 1988, women already constituted ten percent or more of the reported AIDS cases in five states (New Jersey, Connecticut, Florida, Rhode Island, and New York) and Puerto Rico.

Most women with HIV disease are poor, uneducated women of color. In a pattern similar to that of intravenous drug-using women, they have backgrounds of early family loss and emotionally or physically absent parents (2). Many left home in their early teens and turned to drugs or prostitution for survival. More than half have children under 18. Caring for their children is often the primary emotional focus in their lives. Women with AIDS are predominantly between 13 and 39 years old, making them significantly younger than men with AIDS and indicating that more were infected in their teens than is the case with men. It is common for women with AIDS to express low self-esteem, place their children and their male partners ahead of themselves in terms of importance, and deny their own needs to meet the needs of others (3).

Unlike the men who comprise the majority of HIV patients to date, most seropositive women arrive at medical and mental health systems with low expectations, not only for themselves but also of the system. The system has not served them well in the past and they do not expect much in the present and future.

And although these women are linked by their diagnoses and some background commonalties, they are still divided by race, class, culture, language, and educational background into diverse fragments. Both before and after diagnosis, some of their challenges may be similar: poverty, living in a sexist society, negotiating sexual encounters in an environment in which HIV infection is a possibility. But the forms of these challenges, the contexts in which they occur, and the access to family and/or peer support all vary considerably. Therefore, one set of AIDS prevention techniques and models of care and therapy will be insufficient to serve all of them. A flexible program with appropriate staff and language diversity will be needed.

Counseling Issues

The counseling and mental health needs of women will vary dramatically depending on whether the woman is seronegative, seropositive or symptomatic. An uninfected woman may need to assess and minimize her risk. A seropositive woman will need to adjust to major changes in the meaning of sexual activity and to possible foreshortening of life expectancy. The woman with symptomatic disease will have additional concerns which can include severe economic stress, child custody, physical pain, and imminent death.

Women at Risk of HIV Infection

The mental health practitioner can assist the patient in assessing her own risk of exposure and help her and her sexual partners to protect themselves from future exposure. If the patient is already infected, the counselor needs to be able to teach the client how to avoid infecting a potential sex partner. Mental health workers should be able to talk about sex and the use of condoms in specific terms and in a comfortable, nonjudgmental manner. Given the relative passivity of many women in sexual encounters, the therapist should consider couples counseling, role playing, empowerment strategies, and other innovative approaches to assist the client.

All sexually active women of childbearing age should be made aware of the possibility of perinatal transmission. If a patient is pregnant or considering pregnancy, the practitioner should follow a protocol involving education, HIV counseling and appropriate medical care as well as mental health services (4).

Because intravenous drug use is such a common transmission route for HIV, all mental health providers should be taught to identify early indications of substance abuse. Information about reducing risks for IV drug abusers must be provided to patients in a supportive way. However, long-term treatment and counseling for drug abusers is most appropriately provided by specialists in substance abuse prevention (5).

The Asymptomatic Seropositive

Women with HIV infection often experience heightened anxiety, denial, and a preoccupation with maintaining health. They may also express concerns about HIV transmission; disclosure of antibody status; childbearing and childrearing; access to social and emotional support services; and a feeling of isolation.

Transmission is a special concern to seropositive women for several reasons. The uninfected woman may need to be assertive and creative to lower her risk, but her seropositive counterpart must contend simultaneously with her own responsibility to prevent transmission, her relative powerlessness socially and economically, and the frequent scapegoating of women as "vectors" of heterosexual transmission (6) and as the "causes" of infant infection. These multiple pressures can create significant stress. If she foregoes childbearing and insists on safer sex, she may suffer a loss of status, security and income. Even if she chooses safer sex, she may need to practice new techniques and focus on one or two high-risk activities at a time. Long-term reinforcement of these behavior changes will also be necessary.

Disclosure of antibody status is difficult for both men and women. Women also have unique disclosure problems. Many are highly dependent on public institutions, are on welfare and depend on government funded health care. They are often primary parents, and those who reveal themselves to be seropositive to family, friends, or institutions are sometimes subject to pressure to relinquish care of their children. The confidentiality of their antibody status and their medical records is much less certain, even where promised, than it is for those in the private system. A woman's parenting ability and her longevity may be questioned even when she is asymptomatic. Even when women do not have to fear institutional reprisal or loss of children, they may be rejected or blamed by a lover, a former needle-sharing partner, or their family. Their own economic dependence and their frequent responsibility to care for others will complicate the decision to disclose their status.

Because most women who are seropositive are of childbearing age and many have children, the care of women with HIV and HIV disease almost always requires a family perspective. In the first place, the reproductive role of women and the risk of maternal transmission are ever-present issues for infected women. Clients need counseling concerning pregnancy, the possibility of abortion, breastfeeding, contraception and, if pregnancy is pursued, preparation for uncertainty concerning the infant's status and future. Although the pregnancy should be classified as high risk, the additional complications of confidentiality and medical uncertainty about the course of HIV infections in pregnant women may result in multiple challenges.

The overwhelming majority of children with AIDS have contracted the virus perinatally. In cases where an asymptomatic HIV-positive mother has been identified through a child's diagnosis, further investigation sometimes uncovers additional infections in older children, as well as in male partners. An entire family may be affected. The woman is faced with many problems, ranging from her own ill health and possible death to arrangements for her child (or children). And approximately half of the infected women must contend with an ongoing struggle with needle use. In addition, most of the women are living at poverty levels, are in generally bad health, have a history of inadequate health and nutrition, and are suffering the multiple consequences of racism.

Access to social and emotional support systems can be difficult, especially in smaller cities which have a less developed system of AIDS services. Some services developed for gay men or drug users with HIV can be helpful, but sometimes they are culturally or socially inappropriate.

Connected to this problem is the extreme sense of isolation felt by many women with HIV. Without a support group, and given both the relatively small numbers of women with HIV and a common fear of disclosure, an infected woman may feel she is the "only" person with HIV.

Issues for Women with HIV Disease

For the woman who has physical symptoms of HIV disease, additional concerns emerge. These include physical health and appearance, including changes in body image and chronic infections (such as vaginitis and other gynecological complications); economic stress; child custody planning, including adoption or guardianship after the death of the mother; and emotional issues associated with the death and dying (for herself, her partner, and her child).

A consequence of the changes in gynecological health and of the knowledge that one can transmit HIV sexually is that intimacy is increasingly difficult. They may feel sexually dirty and unloved. They often believe they are no longer feminine. They may withdraw further because of their appearance. They are embarrassed and tired of their frequent gynecological problems. Yet many must attend male-oriented AIDS clinics where they usually see male doctors. At these clinics they may be seen as oddities by the other, predominantly male, patients. Private physicians and women's health clinics on the other hand are often geared to middle-class women with insurance. These women do not feel comfortable there either.

When a woman becomes ill with HIV disease, her role as a primary caregiver to a child or children or to other adults in the household is immediately affected. The family is disrupted. Economic difficulties reverberate throughout the daily life of a woman with HIV disease. Housing can be a significant problem. For example, in 1987, women with AIDS in San Francisco received either General Assistance of $311 a month, or Supplemental Social Security of $560 a month. With these limited funds, they lived in areas with substandard housing and higher crime rates. Safety for themselves and their children became an added stressor.

Many housing and residence programs for people with AIDS do not accept children or partners. In order to get adequate and safe housing, some women have had to separate from their children. If a woman attempts to keep her family together but becomes too ill to care for them, she may still be forced to turn her children over to foster care or give them up for adoption, thus increasing her feelings of guilt, shame, and failure as a woman and as a mother.

Adding to the pain and discomfort of ill health is the increasing necessity to acknowledge the process of dying and one's impending death. And with this acknowledgement comes issues of permanent child guardianship, adoption, and a final farewell to one's children.

The Role of the Therapist

Attention to the special issues of women with HIV should include an awareness of the therapist's own reaction. Especially when the therapist is a woman, countertransference can include fear of contagion, denial, discomfort with sex, sexuality, and sexual behavior change, a sense of combating helplessness and despair, anger and blaming the victim, blurring of ethical and professional boundaries, and fear of professional inadequacy.

Conscious self-management of sexual behavior is a key to preventing AIDS transmission. But discussions of female sexuality can prompt identification and discomfort, especially for a female provider. A client's decisions concerning pregnancy, child-rearing, testing for the HIV antibody or disclosure of HIV status may also challenge a provider's sense of ethics. In these and other situations, mental health providers will need to acknowledge their own concerns in order to identify and correct those factors which may interfere with their work with women clients.

Resources for Women

Because the total number of women infected with the AIDS virus is much smaller than the number of infected men, the resources available for women are limited.

Women need specific AIDS services designed to meet their needs (7). Many AIDS organizations have developed women's support groups and have recognized the need to hire and train staff who are sensitive to women's issues. Because over 70% of all female AIDS cases are Black or Latina women, resources and services (including staffing) should match the ethnic makeup of affected women. Special outreach efforts to women who are economically and socially marginal will also be needed in many communities. Consulting with local ethnically focused health and civic organizations can raise one's awareness of the racial and cultural concerns in relation to AIDS and can be an important step in developing culturally appropriate treatment approaches.

■

References

1. Guinan ME, Hardy A: Epidemiology of AIDS in women in the United States: 1981 through 1986. J Am Med Assoc (April 17) 1987; 257(15): 2039-2042
2. Mondanaro J: Strategies for AIDS prevention: motivating health behavior in drug dependent women. J Psycho Drugs (April-June) 1987; 19(2):143-149
3. Maier C: Women with AIDS and ARC in San Francisco, in Women and AIDS Clinical Resource Guide. Edited by Shaw N. San Francisco, San Francisco AIDS Foundation, 1988
4. Shaw NS: Serving your patients in the age of AIDS. Contemporary OB/GYN (October) 1986; 28(4):141-149
5. Friedman SR, Des Jarlais DC, Sotheran JL, et al: AIDS and self-organization among intravenous drug users. International J Addictions March 1987; 22(3):201-219
6. Alexander P: Summary of Data on Prostitutes and AIDS. San Francisco, National Task Force on Prostitution, 1987
7. Shaw NS (ed): Women with AIDS Clinical Resource Guide. San Francisco, San Francisco AIDS Foundation, 1988

Editor's Notes

Page 241. At the close of 1992, 11.5% of AIDS cases in the U.S. were among women. Women, especially in urban centers in rural southern states, continue to be primarily at risk for HIV through heterosexual contact and injection drug use. While three possible cases of woman-to-woman transmission have been reported, a study of 164 women with AIDS who reported sexual contact only with women revealed other risk factors: 152 reported injection drug use and the remaining 12 had received blood transfusions before March 1985. Thus, HIV education for women having sex with women should focus on injection drug use issues.

Updated References

Ellerbrock TV, Bush TJ, Chamberland ME, et al: Epidemiology of women with AIDS in the United States, 1981 through 1990: a comparison with heterosexual men with AIDS. JAMA 1991; 265:2971-5

Chu SY, Hammett TA, Buehler JW: Update: epidemiology of reported cases of AIDS in women who report sex only with other women, United States, 1980-1991 (Letter). AIDS 1992; 6(5):518-19

■

Nancy Stoller Shaw, PhD, is an Associate Professor, Board of Community Studies, University of California Santa Cruz.

Youth and HIV: No Immunity

Janet Shalwitz, MD and Ken Dunnigan, MD, MPH

The critical role which adolescents may play in the HIV epidemic has become increasingly clear. The relatively small numbers of adolescents aged 13–19 who have been diagnosed with AIDS do not take into account the prevalence of high-risk sexual activities, which is more realistically reflected in the very high rates of teenage pregnancy and sexually transmitted diseases (STDs). It is the purpose of this chapter to draw attention to the need to address adolescents about HIV disease and to suggest strategies for both prevention education and counseling interventions.

The prevalence of HIV among adolescents is largely unknown. This lack of information hampers understanding of the true extent of the problem. To date, there have been few studies of HIV seroprevalence among adolescents, except in a few subpopulations of youth—for example, military recruits and a sample of street youth in New York City. In addition, given the lengthy interval between the time of infection and the onset of HIV-related symptoms, most adolescents with HIV infection will appear healthy. Consequently, the presence of HIV infection remains unknown to the youth and to the youth's health care providers, who may not be motivated to address the possibility of HIV infection. Lastly, while it is possible that HIV may not yet have entered large groups of adolescents, its presence has already been demonstrated in other cohorts. Furthermore, the risk of spreading HIV among adolescents (once it becomes entrenched) is quite high. (See Editor's Notes, page 259.)

High-Risk Activity Among Adolescents

That adolescents represent a potential "powder keg" of HIV infection should be a compelling factor in prevention efforts. Unprotected sexual activity is normative behavior in this population. In a 1983 study, the average age of onset of heterosexual intercourse was found to be 16.2 years for females and 15.7 years for males (1), while in certain communities, the onset of sexual intercourse was found to be as early as 11-12 years of age. Two-thirds of those in the study reported no use or ineffective use of contraceptives, and only 15% of those using contraceptives were using condoms (2). HIV notwithstanding, the consequences of these behavioral norms already pose a staggering problem: in the U.S., more than one million, or one in ten, teenage women become pregnant each year (3,4) and one in seven teenagers are diagnosed with a sexually transmitted disease annually (5). Analysis of the U.S. data on the prevalence of sexually transmitted diseases per sexually active individual reveals that 15-19-year-olds have the highest rates of gonorrhea, syphilis, and hospitalizations for pelvic inflammatory disease than any other age groups (6).

In addition to risk associated with unprotected sexual activity, youth may also be at significant risk because of drug use. Drug use can enhance risk both through the sharing of potentially infected needles and through the sexual disinhibition that can occur when an individual is intoxicated. A 1985 survey of 130 high schools in the U.S. indicated that two-thirds of seniors reported drinking alcohol, 25% reported marijuana use in the last month prior to the survey, and 17% and 1.2% of seniors reported cocaine and heroin use, respectively, at some time in their lives (7). The number who may be injecting these drugs is unknown. However, considering that numerous heavy and/or intravenous drug users drop out of school prior to their senior year, these numbers are likely to be a conservative reflection of adolescent drug use.

There are also some youth, less well studied, for whom the risk of acquiring HIV infection is particularly high and for whom existing services may be least well adapted to identify or treat the problem. These youth include homeless youth and runaways; youth caught up in the drug culture; out-of-school youth; victims of sexual and physical abuse and family violence; youth involved in prostitution; incarcerated youth; and sexual minority youth (gay, bisexual, transsexual, and transvestite).

Adolescents are not a homogeneous population. There is no one set of cultural norms or a common language. Significant variation exists in communication skills, problem-solving abilities, and breadth of experience. All adolescents do, however, share certain common developmental characteristics which account for much of the observed high-risk activity. They are, in general, egocentric, oriented to the present rather than the future, have only a vague sense of personal vulnerability, and are primarily influenced by their peers. They often believe that "clean" and loving persons do not have diseases, and, if they did, they certainly would not transmit the diseases to a loved one. Like many well-educated adults, they have difficulty comprehending the notion of asymptomatic infection. Although studies have revealed that adolescents are aware of the high-risk activities associated with HIV transmission, a very low percentage report actual modification of their sexual behaviors because of concerns of acquiring HIV/AIDS (8).

Finally, the problem of HIV infection among adolescents is compounded by extrinsic realities:

1. Most HIV testing services currently available are not geared to the specific needs of adolescents.

2. Adolescent-specific health care and counseling services are only sporadically available.

3. In spite of the presence of some family life education and some open communication with parents, adolescent sexuality remains a largely taboo subject in American culture.

4. There is virtually no societal support for gay and lesbian adolescents.

5. Many educators, doctors, nurses, coaches, probation officers, youth group leaders, and others who work with youth are uncomfortable talking about sexuality.

6. Traditional approaches to adolescents emphasize controlling unwanted behaviors; there are few examples of approaches which emphasize youth making their own decisions. Nevertheless, adolescence does not lend itself well to attempts at controlling behavior.

Prevention Education and Counseling: Common Strategies

For an educator or a counselor, addressing youth involves at least three common goals: establishing rapport, building trust, and communicating clear, accurate, and appropriate messages. Counseling, as considered here, is based on the belief that behavioral change is best realized as a product of an effective client-counselor relationship which emphasizes personal decision making over social control. That same model also applies to educational interventions; the emphasis rests not with the information itself, rather with the process by which the information is delivered. The following suggestions, then, may prove useful to both educators and counselors alike:

1. **Messages communicated to youth should be developmentally appropriate.** It is unreasonable and ineffective to approach the "concrete" here-and-now thinker with messages emphasizing the future consequences of high-risk activities. Messages will be more successful when they draw attention to immediate outcomes, especially rewards, and when they acknowledge the importance of peer support.

2. **Messages communicated to youth should be brief, explicit, and direct, as well as consistent and repetitive.** Ambiguous and judgmental terminology such as "sexually active," "bodily fluids," and "promiscuous" should be avoided. The opportunity for repeated sessions should also be made available. The experience over the last decade with sex education has glaringly revealed that didactic "one-shot deals" are ineffective in helping adolescents change sexual behaviors, so the opportunity for repeated sessions is essential.

3. **HIV/AIDS information should be presented within the context of broader societal/family life issues which adolescents experience.** HIV education should incorporate values clarification, skills development, and self-empowerment, particularly in the areas of communication, decision making, and assertiveness training. These features should be interwoven throughout a comprehensive family life education scheme which should include human anatomy and physiology; sexual development; cultural values and norms; STDs, HIV infection, and contraception; parenting; violence/abuse; substance use; racism and homophobia; and issues of self-esteem. It is important to communicate the interrelationship of high-risk behaviors and sexually transmitted conditions—for example, pregnancy, sexually transmitted diseases, and HIV

disease. For youth in nontraditional settings, such as those living on the streets, messages regarding HIV should be delivered in a manner which acknowledges that the youth may be experiencing much more pressing needs at the moment, like finding a place to stay or something to eat.

4. **The educator or counselor must be perceived as trustworthy, nonjudgmental, knowledgeable, and interested.** The counselor/educator is encouraged to understand the social norms and values of the identified population, as well as their HIV-related risk factors. Sessions should be linguistically and culturally appropriate to the lifestyle of youth. No assumptions should be made regarding the sexual orientation of the youth involved. Humor can be used to advantage in most any setting. The counselor/educator is also encouraged to reflect upon personal prejudices and values. Youth are highly skilled in stripping off the masks of adults and exposing vulnerability. One should never get caught in a lie; rapport and trust will be lost immediately.

5. **It is important for the educator/counselor to appeal to the emotional as well as the reasoning side of adolescents' personalities.** The involvement of HIV-infected individuals in both educational and counseling interventions may have a more powerful, lasting impact than information alone. Similarly, the educator or counselor is encouraged to examine the possible benefits of disclosing his or her own sexual orientation, history of chemical dependency, or HIV status. Modelling behavior can be a powerful learning technique, and rapport may be facilitated by this level of honest exchange.

6. **The involvement of peers cannot be overstated.** The involvement of peers, including peer counselors, will enhance the effectiveness of both educational and counseling strategies. It is of utmost importance to capitalize on the positive power of peer pressure and support.

7. **Both educators and counselors should receive periodic training on HIV issues, including relevant communication strategies and values clarification.** Individuals need to remain current with respect to the flood of information regarding HIV infection so that accurate knowledge is disseminated. Educators

and counselors alike also need to remain current regarding the changing lifestyles of the youth they serve. It is also important that anyone working with adolescents at risk for HIV be familiar with the range of services available for those youth who may already be infected.

8. **Both educational and counseling interventions should be flexible, creative, and engaging.** The Law of Requisite Variety, a concept employed in family therapy, states that whoever has the widest capacity for communication, or whoever has more flexible behavior options, is in control of the system. Adolescents, with a seemingly endless array of behavioral options, present a challenge to the educator or counselor who needs to be even more creative both to gain attention and to deliver a message. For example, a discussion about how to use a condom may not be effective, while games played with condoms may be. The involvement of a person with HIV may stir emotions, cause some unease, and set the stage for an interactive dialogue which might never occur in a didactic setting. Messages delivered outside the classroom or in a non-traditional setting may give the educator/counselor an edge in gaining the interest of youth. The effective provider should also be able to "shoot from the hip" in most situations.

9. **If the counselor or educator is perceived by the youth to be disapproving or judgmental, rapport has already been lost.** When possible, referral to another counselor or educator is recommended. Adolescents are skilled at recognizing disapproval, and once that occurs, there are few options for mending the relationship.

In summary, for both prevention education and counseling interventions, the common goal is to build effective relationships and thereby empower adolescents to make positive behavioral changes. How this is conducted will depend, of course, upon the specific setting for the interaction.

An educational setting is likely to involve a greater array of planners and providers and may occur in a school, a social service agency, an institutional facility, or a church, to name a few venues. Parents, outreach workers, educators and teens themselves are encouraged to participate in the planning and implementation of prevention education activities and programs. All disciplines will need adequate training, including sensitivity training. It is obvious that every person working with adolescents will not have the time, skills, and opportunities to address carefully and sensitively issues related to HIV. For some youth workers, discussing issues related to sexuality, pregnancy, sexually transmitted diseases, HIV infection, condom use, and the use of illicit drugs may be unacceptable and disquieting. Others will find these activities challenging. Training should be provided for all staff, and those workers who are most comfortable and interested in providing HIV-related counseling and education should be identified. However great the interest, though, it must be remembered that the ability to develop rapport and build trust is the cornerstone of whatever interventions are developed.

Counseling is a personalized process, and whether provided individually or in a group, it is bounded by rules of confidentiality. While many of the principles have already been cited, the counselor has the added advantage of negotiating specific behavioral goals with the client. In doing so, the counselor is encouraged to remain flexible and to accept even the smallest of changes as a sign of progress. If the counselor holds on to expectations which are too high or too unrealistic, the counseling service will be perceived as ineffective and the youth will be perceived as too resistant to change. Success may, in fact, be simply the development of rapport between provider and client; behavioral change may not occur until some time later.

Maintaining Boundaries

Developing rapport with youth requires skill and a constant awareness of one's own feelings regarding the youth and the youth's behaviors. Maintaining appropriate boundaries may be a challenge, and the counselor must identify clearly those feelings in order to maintain boundaries. The counselor may see the adolescent through the eyes of a parent; see the youth as a member of an ethnic minority group which stirs negative feelings; be uncomfortable with homosexuality or, for that matter, any sexuality; be sexually attracted to the youth; have disapproving feelings about some aspect of the youth's lifestyle; or judge his or her own success on whether the youth meets certain behavioral goals. Success in counseling depends upon a counselor's own ability to recognize these feelings, establish appropriate boundaries, and adhere to those boundaries. Adolescents, especially those at highest risk, are likely to have difficulty trusting others, especially those in authority, and will challenge the counselor's ability to build trust without getting enmeshed in the youth's life.

The Adolescent with HIV Disease

For reasons cited earlier, youth service workers, while heavily engaged in providing HIV prevention services, have little experience in dealing with the adolescent who is already infected with HIV. Adolescent-oriented HIV antibody testing services, HIV monitoring and treatment services, and psychosocial support services are either nonexistent or rudimentary at best. In all communities, appropriate and accessible medical, psychiatric, and social support resources should be identified for the population of youth who may be or are already infected. These resources should be affordable, confidential, and developmentally appropriate; service providers should also reflect the racial, ethnic, and lifestyle mix of the youth being served.

With the growing awareness that HIV disease is a chronic condition that may be manageable, there are increasing reasons to support early testing and identification of serostatus, early medical intervention, and periodic monitoring of health status. No less than adults, adolescents infected with HIV should have access to appropriate monitoring and to available treatment options. While educators or counselors may not be the purveyor of these specific services, they play a crucial role in conveying a medically accurate understanding of the chronic nature of HIV infection, in advocating for the development of appropriate testing and health care services, and in channeling potentially infected adolescents into appropriate care services. An emphasis on prevention must not occur at the expense of helping those already infected with the virus.

Do Scare Tactics Work?

Many of the HIV prevention campaigns developed for both adults and adolescents are grounded in the association between HIV and death. Grave markers and skulls and crossbones have been depicted on many posters and it is commonly believed, profoundly so by the "concrete-thinking" adolescent, that when one is infected with HIV, one dies. In light of emerging evidence that HIV disease can be a chronic, manageable condition, the use of these scare tactics needs to be re-evaluated. Most adolescents, and many adults as well, will not be able to reconcile two conflicting messages: 1) that HIV kills and 2) that one can learn to live with HIV. If the premise of relationship building is honest exchange, the call for employing scare tactics must become increasingly weak. At the same time, there is no consensus that fear campaigns are effective in promoting behavior change. All service providers are encouraged to tackle this difficult issue and to develop an approach which is an accurate and forthright reflection of emerging medical information.

Conclusion

Adolescents are not young adults. In the space of a few short years, adolescents experience profound developmental shifts in their bodies, in their reactions to changes in their bodies, and in their ability to reason, to name a few. In order to be a successful adult, the adolescent must accomplish several developmental tasks, including the achievement of a personal identity, the achievement of some degree of autonomy, and the development of new relationships with family and friends which reflect that increasing independence. Adults taking on the challenging task of educating and counseling adolescents must understand fully these developmental processes in order to deliver a message which has some hope of motivating behavior change. Messages, services, and arguments which appeal to an adult population will have little or no impact on youth; logic alone and the threat of negative future consequences will not be heard outside the context of a youth's everyday life.

In the case of HIV, adults, and most youth, are aware of the behavioral changes required to reduce transmission. The power to make those difficult behavioral changes rests with the youth themselves, and it is the basic task of adult providers to create an environment in which responsible decisions are generated by youth. The building of trusting relationships in which clear, honest, nonjudgmental, and knowledgeable information is delivered, will have the best chance of helping adolescents make decisions by which the risk of HIV transmission will be minimized. Attempts to change behavior by quick and easy approaches, by "one-shot" encounters, by behavioral sanctions, or by social control ignore the developmental needs of the adolescent and will frustrate providers by their ineffectiveness.

Working with adolescents is not easy, but it can be enormous fun; even the most patient adult, however, will have mixed results. Changes will occur slowly, and the expectations of both the providers and the community must reflect this reality. Adult providers cannot accomplish these changes alone. Community support and public policy are needed to support rational approaches to stemming the unchecked transmission of HIV among adolescents.

■

References

1. Zelnick M, Shah F: First intercourse among young Americans. Family Planning Perspectives 1983; 15(2):64-70

2. Zelnick M, Kantner JF: Sexual activity, contraceptive use, and pregnancy among metropolitan-area teenagers: 1971-1979. Family Planning Perspectives 1980 September/October; Vol 12:230-231 and 233-237

3. Hayes CD (ed): Risking the Future: Adolescent Sexuality, Pregnancy and Childbearing, Vol. 1. Washington, D.C., National Academy Press, 1987

4. Brindis C, Jeremy R: Adolescent Pregnancy and Parenting in California. San Francisco, CA, Center for Population and Reproductive Health Policy, Institute for Health Policy Studies, University of California San Francisco, 1988

5. House Select Committee on Children, Youth, and Families: Fact Sheet: AIDS and Teenagers. Washington, D.C., U.S. Government Printing Office, June 18, 1987

6. Bell TA, Holmes KK: Age-specific risks of syphilis, gonorrhea, and hospitalized pelvic inflammatory disease in sexually experienced U.S. women. Sex Transm Dis 1984; 11:291

7. Johnston LD, O'Malley PM, Bachman JG: Psychotherapeutic licit and illicit use of drugs among adolescents: an epidemiological perspective. J Adolesc Health Care 1987; 68:36-51

8. Brooks-Gunn J, Boyer CB, Hein K: Preventing HIV infection and AIDS in children and adolescents: behavioral research and intervention strategies. American Psychologist 1988; 43(11): 958-964

Editor's Notes

Page 249. Youth and adolescents continue to place themselves at risk for HIV infection in large numbers. Gay identified youth who do not scrupulously practice safer sex are at particularly high risk because of the extent to which infection is already present in gay male communities. Yet, as with other groups at risk, prevention efforts can be successful and are urgently needed (see DiClemente et al and Cates below).

Updated References

DiClemente RJ, Durbin M, Siegel D, et al: Determinants of condom use among junior high school students in a minority, inner-city school district. Pediatrics. 1992; 2:197-202

Cates W: The epidemiology and control of sexually transmitted diseases in adolescents. In: Schydlower M, Shafer MA, eds. AIDS and Other Sexually Transmitted Diseases. Philadelphia, PA: Hanley & Belfus, Inc, 1990: 409-427

■

Janet Shalwitz, MD, is the Director of Forensic Youth Medical/Psychiatric Services for the City and County of San Francisco, Department of Public Health, and Assistant Clinical Professor, Pediatrics, University of California San Francisco, California. **Ken Dunnigan, MD, MPH,** *is the Director of Health Center 1, a division of the San Francisco Department of Public Health.*

Double Jeopardy: Hemophilia and HIV Disease

Donna DiMarzo, MSW, MPH

"The AIDS virus is the greatest challenge which people with hemophilia, as a group, have ever faced. Although heat-treated blood products offer hope for the future, we must live with the knowledge that a very large number of people with hemophilia had already been infected with HIV before heat treatment was developed. We are somewhat encouraged that, for reasons medical science has not yet learned, persons with hemophilia seem to be developing AIDS and ARC at a slower rate than might be expected. Meanwhile, those of us who may have been exposed to the virus must learn to cope with our fears and anxieties. At the same time, we must do everything we can to stay as healthy as possible. We must learn to meet the challenge AIDS has presented to us and get on with our lives."

The Editors, AIDS News, Vol. I, No. 1, June 1987. Published by the Northern California Hemophilia Foundation.

Overview of Hemophilia

Hemophilia is a genetic, sex-linked coagulation disorder which results in delayed blood clotting. It is transmitted from the mother to her male offspring at the time of conception; it is a relatively rare condition which occurs once in approximately 10,000 live births.

Persons with hemophilia have deficiencies in clotting factor proteins. Most common is Hemophilia A, or Classical Hemophilia, caused by a deficiency in Factor VIII. Less common is Hemophilia B, or Christmas Disease, caused by a deficiency in Factor IX.

Depending upon the level of deficiency of these proteins and the clinical severity of the disease, hemophilia is also classified as mild, moderate, or severe. In mild hemophilia, excessive bleeding may occur after surgical or dental procedures, or following significant physical trauma. Those with mild hemophilia may only need to be treated minimally during their lifetime. In contrast, severe hemophilia is characterized by spontaneous bleeding into joints or muscles, often resulting in chronic impairment of mobility. Individuals with severe hemophilia usually require prophylactic treatment with factor products.

Epidemiology of HIV Disease in the Hemophilia Community

Concentrates of clotting factor are produced from large plasma donor pools obtained from as many as 10,000 - 15,000 individuals (1). Consequently, the risk of HIV infection to persons with hemophilia who required treatment with factor products in the United States was quite high. Many were exposed to HIV as early as 1978, and by the end of 1984, 70-85% of hemophiliacs had been infected with the virus (2). (See Editor's Notes, page 266.)

In October 1984, heat treatment of factor concentrates, coupled with widespread screening for antibodies to HIV in donated plasma and blood, had significantly reduced and largely eliminated the risk of exposure to HIV for persons with hemophilia.

Since 1981, the number of reported cases of AIDS to the Centers for Disease Control (CDC) has increased steadily (2). As of March 1, 1989, 845 cases of AIDS in adults and adolescents with hemophilia, and 84 cases of AIDS in children with hemophilia, have been reported to the CDC (3). Although the absolute number of persons with hemophilia who have acquired AIDS is small relative to other populations at risk, the proportion of AIDS is higher for people with hemophilia than for any other subpopulation (4).

Seroprevalence rates for antibody to HIV among the estimated 20,000 hemophilics in the U.S. have been reported to be 70% overall and as high as 90% for individuals with severe hemophilia (5). Although these rates are staggeringly high, the majority of individuals with hemophilia remain well and are asymptomatic.

Considerable speculation exists among researchers regarding what factors may account for the relatively low incidence of AIDS in this group. One theory suggests that those with hemophilia were exposed to inactivated virus in clotting factor concentrates and, therefore, are less likely to develop an active virus infection (5). Other researchers believe that the low incidence of AIDS in this group reflects the route of HIV transmission. They suggest that the intravenous infusion of commercially prepared factor concentrates results in a less even pattern of exposure to HIV than for sexual transmission or transmission through IV drug use (2). However, neither of these theories adequately explains the fact that despite the relatively low incidence of AIDS in individuals with hemophilia nationwide, there is mounting evidence of progressive HIV-induced immunologic deterioration (6).

Psychosocial Issues

Individuals with hemophilia who are seropositive, who have become symptomatic, or who have been diagnosed with AIDS experience a similar spectrum of feelings, concerns and fears that confront others affected by the AIDS epidemic. There are, however, issues which appear to be specific to the hemophilia community and which require special consideration.

The most obvious issue setting this group apart from all others is their pre-existing medical disorder. Hemophilia is a chronic, potentially life-threatening condition that requires a unique set of coping mechanisms for the individual with hemophilia and his family. For many, these coping mechanisms are functional and adaptive, enabling individuals and families to deal with the unpredictability of painful bleeding episodes, frequent and often lengthy hospitalizations, prolonged absence from school or employment, and chronic physical disability. For others, the stress of coping can bring about family disorganization and an increased tendency for parents to unwittingly encourage dependency, passivity, and helplessness in children with hemophilia.

In those hemophilics who exhibit dependent or passive-aggressive personalities, additional problems are common. These men are often without adequate support systems, and have not developed adaptive coping skills. They frequently experience considerable emotional distress and isolation, and the need for mental health care is particularly evident as these men begin to confront the threat of AIDS.

Denial is probably the primary defense mechanism used to cope with the threat of AIDS. Historically people with hemophilia have utilized and refined this defense to cope with stressors associated with a medical condition which remains largely misunderstood. From the child with hemophilia who denies his condition so that he may participate in the activities of his peers, to the adult whose denial of his HIV antibody status allows him to continue planning for the future, denial is an adaptive response that supports the development of self-esteem and hope.

Paradoxically, denial can also become dysfunctional when it interferes with medical treatment or when it prohibits the individual from acknowledging the risk of transmitting HIV to sexual partners. Although many HIV-positive men with hemophilia have acknowledged their risk and have made health-promoting lifestyle changes, many others continue to deny their risk, as evidenced by the increasing incidence of sexual partners who have seroconverted (7).

HIV infection in sexual partners of hemophilic men is of grave concern to health and mental health providers. Education, coupled with psychosocial counseling, has been minimally effective in promoting behavior change in this community (8). For those who have adopted safer sex behavior or abstinence from sexual contact and/or intimate relationships, it has been at the cost of high levels of emotional distress (8). Many adults and adolescents with hemophilia have expressed significant feelings of loss associated with changes in their sexual behavior and intimate relationships. Clinical work with some hemophilic men suggests that, despite a self-concept of being "different" or "disabled," sexuality has been one part of their lives where they have felt "normal."

In addition to the emotional stress placed on the infected individual, the AIDS epidemic has taken an enormous toll upon the parents of HIV-infected hemophilic children. Because hemophilia is a genetically inherited medical condition, it is not uncommon to have more than one male child in the family with the disease. Many families, therefore, face the potential loss of multiple children to AIDS.

Obstacles to Forming a Community Support Network

Although the hemophilia community consists of approximately 20,000 individuals nationwide, it is significant to note that unlike the gay community, there is little evidence of "community" or history of grassroots organizing. The absence of a cohesive, organized community has had an enormous impact on the development of a system of internal support, advocacy and community psychosocial services. Since the appearance of AIDS, Hemophilia Treatment Centers (HTCs), local hemophilia foundations, and other hemophilia-specific groups have attempted to mobilize hemophilics and marshal needed services. Unfortunately, geographic dispersion, isolation, and the fear of discrimination all have contributed to the further isolation of hemophilics. With the exception of a core group of seropositive hemophilics and their family members who have maintained high levels of visibility and activity despite concerns about discrimination, the majority of seropositive hemophilics only access HIV-specific mental health services within their hemophilia centers.

It is worth noting that both traditional and creative attempts at reaching hemophilics who may be isolated and in need of AIDS-related information and/or psychosocial support have had limited impact. To date, supportive and therapeutic groups, educational workshops and forums, peer outreach, and social support activities have attracted only a small percentage of those with hemophilia who are HIV infected. Although it appears that one-on-one intervention may be the most effective way of providing HIV-related mental health, psychosocial and educational services to hemophilics and their families, Hemophilia Treatment Centers have been unable to reach large numbers of hemophilics with these services. Constraints on the centers include inadequate staffing and an inability or unwillingness of staff to provide for home visits and/or flexible hours.

The relationship between HTCs and the hemophilia community has historically been ambivalent and complex. HTCs, which provide comprehensive medical and psychosocial services, are in a unique position to address the needs of the hemophilia community; in many states, hemophilics who seek supplementary, state-funded medical insurance "must" receive care from an HTC, limiting their choice of health care providers. Additionally, prior to the availability of home delivery of factor concentrates, hemophilics were reliant upon HTCs for their factor supply. Viewed by some in the hemophilia community as "forced dependency," this situation, coupled with the paternalism of the traditional medical model, has led some hemophilics to withdraw from HTC care.

The complexity of the relationship between HTC staff and the hemophilia community is also evident in the "bond" that often exists between medical providers, hemophilics and their family members. These relationships, characterized by mutual affection, trust and concern, have ironically, in some instances, created barriers to providing timely, ethical and effective psychosocial intervention. The denial seen in many patients regarding their seropositivity is at times even more pronounced in the providers caring for them.

Clearly, HIV infection in hemophilics and their sexual partners has had an enormous impact on the medical community. The emotional toll on providers has been significant; not only are many of their patients considered "friends," but some providers chose hemophilia as a specialty because they did not wish to work with terminal illness. As one provider poignantly stated, "The AIDS epidemic is more than I bargained for. I would have gone into oncology if I had desired to work with dying children." A combination of blurred provider-patient boundaries, anger in providers at having AIDS "imposed" upon them, and denial have left some health care staff ill prepared to deal with the complex and multiple psychosocial issues that accompany HIV disease.

For the mental health clinician working with an individual with hemophilia or a family member, it is important to consider homophobia as a barrier to accessing services. Homophobia appears to be fairly common in the hemophilia community and has an impact on the use of any services perceived as "gay oriented." This attitude is of particular concern in areas where there is a dearth of psychosocial or concrete services for those affected by HIV infection; it may be that the "only" resources available are those linked to the gay community.

Conclusion

The psychosocial issues confronting the hemophilia community and the barriers to providing responsive, effective intervention are many and complex. For mental health professionals working with this population, sensitivity and insight to these issues, coupled with a recognition of the need to challenge traditional methods of offering mental health services, are vital. Developing creative mental health programs and supporting mobilizing efforts in the hemophilia community can have far- reaching effects for this underserved population.

■

References

1. Williams J, Glader B: Statement Before the House Select Committee on Children, Youth and Families. February 21, 1987, Berkeley, CA
2. McGrady GA, Jason JM, Evatt BL: The course of the epidemic of acquired immunodeficiency syndrome in the United States hemophilia population. Am J Epidemiology 1987; 126:25-30
3. Centers for Infectious Diseases, Division of AIDS: HIV/AIDS Surveillance Report. Atlanta, GA, Centers for Disease Control, March 1989
4. Agle D, Gluck H, Pierce G: The risk of AIDS: psychologic impact on the hemophiliac population. Gen Hosp Psychiatry 1987; 9:11-17
5. Andrews CA, Sullivan JL, Brettler DB, et al: Isolation of human immuno-deficiency virus from hemophiliacs: correlation with clinical symptoms and immunologic abnormalities. Pediatrics, November 1987; 3(5):672-677
6. 1986 update of HIV seroprevalence, seroconversion, AIDS incidence and immunologic correlates of HIV infection in patients with hemophilia A and B. Blood 1987; 10(3):786-790
7. HIV infection and pregnancies in sexual partners of HIV-seropositive hemophilic men—United States. Morbidity Mortality Weekly Report, September 1987; 36(35):593-595
8. Parish KL, Mandel J, Thomas J, et al: Psychosocial and Sexual Adjustment to AIDS Risk Among Adults with Hemophilia. Poster Presentation at the Fourth International Conference on AIDS Stockholm, Sweden, June 1988

Editor's Notes

Page 261. HIV infection of blood products is now extremely rare. However, the number of diagnosed AIDS cases among adults with hemophilia has doubled in the past four years; among children, the number has tripled.

■

Donna DiMarzo, MSW, MPH, was the Northern California Coordinator of the AIDS Help and Prevention Plan and a Clinical Social Worker in the Comprehensive Hemophilia Treatment Center, University of California San Francisco Medical Center. She is presently the Social Work Coordinator for the HIV Center for Children and Their Families at St. Luke's/Roosevelt Hospital Center, New York, New York.

The AIDS Bereaved: Counseling Strategies

Amy Weiss, MS, MFCC

Losing a significant other to death is considered one of the most stressful events in a person's life, and even in the most uncomplicated of circumstances, the psychological tasks of grief work present the survivor with multiple challenges. The loss of someone to a death from AIDS can be especially difficult, and the subsequent bereavement process can become complicated. This article will review the process of normal grief, briefly describe complicated bereavement, and address some of the factors which differentiate the experiences of the AIDS bereaved from the experiences of others.

Normal Grief

Bereavement, or the state of grieving that accompanies a loss, is not an illness; it is a natural, healthy response. Bereavement is experienced in all cultures, observed in many species of animals, and can result in a broad range of physical and emotional symptoms. No one will necessarily experience all of them, nor must all be present for grief to be considered normal. However, understanding that many kinds of feelings are to be expected can make the experience of grief much more manageable.

When loss occurs, usual patterns of routine behaviors are disrupted. People stop doing the things they ordinarily do. Studies have shown that acute grief constitutes a definite syndrome, with both psychological and somatic symptomatology. The signs of grief may either appear immediately or be delayed; they may even appear to be absent. Symptoms may be distorted, exaggerated, or highly variable and will differ among individuals and according to different circumstances.

Grief affects a person socially, emotionally, spiritually, physically and behaviorally, and can produce both positive and negative states. The range of somatic symptoms that may occur in normal grief include tightness of the throat, choking, shortness of breath, the need for frequent sighing, an empty feeling in the abdomen, muscle weakness, chills, and tremors. These bodily sensations may be accompanied by intense mental distress: tension, loneliness, and anguish. The bereaved person's perceptions may also become disorganized to a degree that events seem unreal. Survivors may describe periods of hallucinations or even euphoria. They may describe a heightened perceptual and emotional sensitivity to persons and events in the immediate environment and may also become preoccupied with images of the deceased. Hostility, irritability and a feeling of general restlessness are common. Sometimes the bereaved talk incessantly about the deceased; sometimes they may talk about everything but their confrontation with loss and the details of the death.

Other commonly experienced feelings include guilt or anger in addition to sadness, longing, loneliness and sorrow. Grief produces feelings of anger and outrage at the injustice of the loss and frustration and a sense of impotence at the inability to control events.

The Process of Grieving

A number of models have been suggested to understand the various processes associated with grief. These models suggest a linear progression that people follow as they work through their grief. However, grieving is a highly individual experience, and while some individuals will follow the process outlined below, most often grieving is a circular process that sometimes omits various stages altogether.

A useful model for understanding the process of working through an experience of grief can be summarized in three phases. The first stage is a period of shock that usually lasts from the time the survivor learns of the death until the final disposition of the deceased body. This is traditionally the time when the community of family and friends supports the survivor through the funeral, memorial service or other ritual, and expressions of sympathy are frequent and freely given. The survivor often describes this period as one in which there is little time to appreciate the fact that the loss is real, and the absence of the loved one is often experienced as temporary or unreal.

The second stage is a period of working through intense grief. Although there is much variation in this stage, it usually lasts from several weeks to several months or longer. During this phase somatic symptoms are common and the bereaved person frequently withdraws from external events. Emotional suffering is acute and marked by crying spells, pangs of longing for the deceased, and frequently strong feelings of anger. These feelings are frequently accompanied by a sense of personal inadequacy and a feeling of being unable to take care of the details of living or to simply "go on" without the deceased. Survivors also begin to re-evaluate their social network as they are forced to greet the world as a single person. Paradoxically, this is a time when survivors are often left alone with their grief, since the formal rituals around death and dying have been completed.

The third stage is a period of re-establishing physical and mental balance. Survivors no longer experience the constant and acute physical or emotional turmoil of the second phase, and life begins to return to some semblance of normal. Sleep patterns and appetite return, and the survivor begins to once again participate in the outside world. Eventually, successful completion of the grieving process means the survivor is able to emotionally reinvest in activities, interests, and perhaps even a new partner.

Complicated Grief

The normal grieving process following a loss can become complicated by a variety of factors. Clinically, it is the degree of symptoms rather than the duration that is the most helpful when making this distinction—for example, when the normal sadness of grieving develops into clinical depression, or when anxiety over being alone develops into phobic avoidance of the home that was shared with the deceased. The delayed grief reaction is another type of complicated grief in which an individual develops a full grief reaction many years after an earlier loss that was not adequately grieved at the time. This reaction is usually initiated by a new loss or some other triggering event. Another situation in which complicated grief may occur is when the loss is sudden and totally unexpected, such as in an accident. These survivors may become debilitated by severe symptoms of grief and become unable to function.

The practitioner should be alert to the development of any of the following symptoms in survivors: the continued use of the present tense when talking about the deceased, or continually reporting that people seen at a distance or in crowds are commonly mistaken for the deceased. Making daily references to death, tombs or graveyards in a ritualistic manner, or the reporting of establishing daily rituals of relating to the deceased, are also signs that the grieving process may not be proceeding normally. Finally, the continued denial of the reality of the death should be a cause for concern, and while any of these symptoms may transiently occur as a normal part of the grieving process, the continued presence of such symptoms may suggest that an episode of normal grief may be developing into a more serious problem. Should these symptoms persist, a referral to a mental health professional is warranted.

AIDS Bereavement

The bereavement process for AIDS-related deaths is complicated by a number of special issues in addition to those commonly raised by the grieving of any loss. While AIDS bereavement can and often does follow all the stages of normal grief, these special features make the possibility of complicated bereavement more likely and the need for special interventions with these individuals more important. In addition to these special issues, each individual's response to losing someone to AIDS is highly personal and depends on the personality of the survivor, the relationship to the deceased, and the survivor's support system. Factors that differentiate AIDS bereavement from other kinds of grief are discussed below.

Stigma

Whether one has lost a spouse, lover, son, sibling or friend, grieving an AIDS death includes some degree of stigma. The disease draws attention to a number of cultural taboos—most specifically, sex and death. When grief is linked to such taboos, normal bereavement may be disrupted. For example, parents may not be aware of a son's homosexuality or an adult child's history of drug use. This information may be learned at the same time as being told that their son/daughter is dying of AIDS. There is often little time to process the meaning of this information. Consequently, parents may repress their feelings and reactions during the crisis period prior to death and have to address this significant emotional material during the time of bereavement.

Biological families often experience isolation when they return to their communities following a loss to AIDS. Some parents and siblings appear to identify with the stigma associated with homosexuality or drug use and an AIDS diagnosis, and choose to embark on a "coming out" process. They choose to clearly and honestly explain the family crisis, often encountering fear, hostile reactions, and moral judgments from others. Others feel it necessary to keep secret the fact of the death or at least the circumstances of the death, for fear of expected rejection and ostracism from their friends in the workplace or community. This fear of rejection often keeps family members from pursuing traditional channels of support during and after the loss, leaving the family isolated and frequently angry and resentful both at their community and often with their son or daughter, who not only died prematurely, but who died from this socially unacceptable disease. Parents frequently remark, "I wouldn't dare tell anyone for fear of hurting our son's memory or our own standing in the community. We know what our neighbors think."

Homophobia

Many gay and bisexual men become alienated from their families in the process of dealing with their sexual identity as "gay." Some are rejected outright by families, churches and synagogues and are told they are "sick and repulsive." Even in the closest of family relationships, sharing the news of one's homosexuality causes stress and strain. Many gay and bisexual people leave their families of origin to find a more hospitable and accepting environment for their life-style. Consequently, many gay men are far from kinships or biological families when they are diagnosed with HIV or AIDS or suffer a great loss. Furthermore, the same religious institutions that have been rejecting of gay men are exactly the traditional sources of support needed at times of bereavement, and thus, traditional rituals around grief and loss are often inappropriate to meet the needs of this community. New and creative rituals are being developed to meet the needs of the

AIDS bereaved. For example, the Names Project, a gigantic quilt made up of individual squares representing individuals who died of AIDS, is a beautiful and effective tool in assisting individuals grieving a loss to AIDS.

A related issue is the lack of legitimacy given to gay relationships and the multitude of problems with families of origin that can ensue after the death for the surviving gay partner. Partners of people with AIDS who have not received proper legal counsel are left vulnerable with no legal estate entitlement or protection. Biological families have the legal right to their dead kin's estate. Unfortunately, the courtroom can become the stage wherein the powerful feelings of anger, anguish and grief are acted out. Partners and family members misdirect the anger generated from their profound loss onto one another. This can be prevented by prompt social work and legal intervention when the person with AIDS is clear of mind and able to execute a will and determine his beneficiaries. However, the extra burden of these kinds of contentious feelings on the bereaved can considerably impact the bereavement of the survivor.

Worry about Health Status

Another issue that separates AIDS-related bereavement from other kinds of bereavement is that those who are AIDS bereaved are also very likely to be at risk for the development of the disease themselves. By the nature of the very intimate relationship that establishes the bereavement, the surviving loved one may also be HIV infected, or may already be symptomatic with HIV-related illnesses. These individuals, then, face not only the task of grieving the loss of their partner but also face anticipatory grieving of the loss of their own health. These individuals are at very high risk for complicated bereavement and require careful evaluation and ongoing support.

Stress of Caregiving

An additional and related issue that sometimes complicates AIDS-related bereavement is the survivors' fatigue resulting from caring for the deceased during the last months of life. The work required to keep the dying person fed, clean, and medicated appropriately along with the emotional strain and disruption of usual life activities can be overwhelming. Survivors who have provided these services are not only physically and emotionally tired, but they also frequently feel guilty that they didn't "do more" while the loved one was still alive and blame themselves for having any personal needs during that time that may have taken them away from the caretaking duties.

Multiple Loss

Individuals coping with the loss of a partner may also have lost many friends to AIDS. This applies specifically to gay and bisexual men and less so to biological families. These men are in the eye of the epidemic, and many experience bereavement overload not unlike the traumatic stress syndromes seen in soldiers who witnessed multiple deaths during wartime or in those who survived life in the concentration camps during World War II. It is not uncommon for some gay men in urban areas with high AIDS mortality to have lost their entire support system. This factor can contribute to delayed grief.

Suicidal Ideation

Suicidal ideation, attempts and completions appear to be more common among the population struggling with AIDS than in other groups facing terminal illnesses. An individual diagnosed with HIV infection who is grieving the loss of a partner might be at higher risk for suicide than other groups of bereaved. Having watched the partner die, anticipating the process for themselves, and fearing there will be no one left to care for them contribute to thoughts of suicide.

Alcohol and Substance Abuse

Significant problems with drug and alcohol use exist within the gay and bisexual male community. Those who have particular problems are at increased risk for relapse or increased use during the bereavement process in an attempt to anesthetize the pain of grief. The bereaved may also feel there is no longer any reason not to drink now that the loved one is gone, or he may unconsciously wish to punish himself for "failing" to care for the loved one well enough and may return to drinking or other drug use. These issues must be evaluated and addressed during this period, and attendance at Alcoholics Anonymous and other peer support programs should be actively encouraged.

Age and Stage Differences

The average age of people with AIDS is 36. The normal developmental tasks for 36-year-old adults are to create successfully intimate relationships and occupational satisfaction. Instead, gay and bisexual men are catapulted to the psychological tasks of old age and watching their friends die. Erik Erikson, in his landmark work on developmental psychology, has said that the identity of this period is a working through of all previous identifications in the light of the one inescapable reality—that the future is death. If the tasks are well integrated, the favorable outcome is wisdom; the pitfall, despair and isolation.

Conclusion

Healing is an individual as well as a community affair. Healing the pain of secrecy and isolation comes from reinvolvement in the community either as a helper, volunteer, professional, or recipient of services. Every hospice program has a bereavement program which serves the needs of people grieving the loss of someone to AIDS. There is great need for community education and much room for everyone's involvement.

The Chinese write the word for crisis with two characters; one means danger and the other, opportunity. The AIDS crisis in our communities across the United States and the globe certainly represents both physical and emotional danger—one laced with multiple loss, much suffering and agony. Yet there are opportunities as well—opportunities for increased understanding and intimacy in the family, in the gay community, and among nations and cultures. There is an opportunity for a "bridge of tears" to create compassion and understanding of our shared humanity.

In this chapter, the special aspects of grieving a loss to AIDS have been discussed. Bereavement is a personal crisis and represents a psychological turning point. Erikson has described such a "turning point" as a "crucial period of increased vulnerability and heightened potential." This seems to be especially true for those dealing with AIDS-related bereavement. Mental health professionals are in a position to help individuals confronting this crisis resolve their grief and help to make the process of bereavement more manageable.

■

Suggested Reading

De Spelder LA and Strickland AL: The Last Dance, Encountering Death and Dying. New York: Mayfield Publishing Co., 1983.

Worden, William: Grief Counseling and Grief Therapy: A handbook for the mental health practitioner. Palo Alto, Springer Publishing Co., 1982

Kübler-Ross E: On Death and Dying. New York, Macmillan Publishing Co., Inc.,1969

Erikson E: Childhood and Society (2nd Edition). New York, W.W. Norton and Co., 1963

■

Amy Weiss, MS, MFCC (Master of Science in Rehabilitation Counseling and Marriage, Family and Child Counseling), has a private practice in San Francisco. She is the former Bereavement Coordinator for the AIDS Hospice Program of the Visiting Nurses Association in San Francisco.

■

HIV, Stress and the Health Care Professional

Mary L. S. Vachon, RN, PhD and Jeanne Dennis, MSW

While considerable research into the cause, prevention, and treatment of HIV spectrum disorders has been conducted since the first description of the disease, very little work has been forthcoming on the stress experienced by professionals who care for people with AIDS (PWAs). The research that has been conducted on caregiver stress suggests that a considerable portion evolves from relationships with colleagues and problems within the work environment (1). Similar findings have been reported in a large study of stress in health care providers working with the critically ill and dying (2).

In a large study of AIDS-related stress in one hospital (3), staff felt they did not have sufficient knowledge to care for the physical needs of PWAs. They felt even less prepared, however, to deal with their emotional needs. The caregivers expressed concern about possible transmission of HIV through accidental needle sticks, through giving CPR, and through airborne transmission. Forty-two percent of those interviewed felt that hospital workers should not be required to care for PWAs although 94% felt that "AIDS patients have as much right to quality medical care as anyone else." About one quarter of those surveyed felt they had a relatively high risk of contracting HIV because of their job; almost half felt that working with AIDS was one of the most stressful parts of their duties; over one third were not comfortable with PWAs, and 41% said that no disease concerned them as much as AIDS. In addition, caregivers exaggerated the proportion of the time they spent in AIDS work and considered this to be among the more stressful aspects of their work. (See Editor's Notes, page 288.)

Furthermore, investigators found that AIDS phobia in health care workers was positively related with homophobia and AIDS stress. They hypothesized that AIDS phobia and ultimately AIDS stress were heightened by negative attitudes about homosexuality, but there was no evidence that homophobic staff avoided PWAs. The researchers suggested that staff would have the most difficulty during the transition period before they were accustomed to dealing with PWAs.

In another study, researchers surveyed a large group of California physicians and found significant information deficits (4). They found that one third of the physicians surveyed acknowledged feeling a moderate or good deal of discomfort in having homosexuals in their practice. On the basis of their findings, the researchers concluded that a significant proportion of California physicians, including those in the two metropolitan communities that have the second and third greatest number of AIDS cases in the United States, could not be expected to appropriately diagnose, counsel, or refer patients at high risk, or to provide adequate advice and reassurance to their patients.

Given the relative paucity of specific data available on the sources of stress among professional caregivers (including indigenous paraprofessionals), their manifestations of stress and the coping mechanisms they employ to decrease their stress, the authors used the opportunity at a seminar on stress and AIDS during an international symposium to generate data on caregiver stress and coping.

Sample

Data for this paper was gathered from a number of different sources. These included a convenience sample of approximately 125 health care professionals and volunteers who attended workshops at a North American Conference on Care of Terminally Ill Persons with AIDS held in 1987, and individual interviews with a convenience sample of caregivers in New York, Toronto, Hawaii, Africa, and Japan. Many, but by no means all, of the caregivers interviewed were involved with hospice or palliative care programs.

Design

The caregivers who attended the workshops were shown a model of occupational stress based on the Person-Environment Fit

Model derived from work done at the Institute for Social Research at the University of Michigan (5). In the Person-Environment Fit Model, both job satisfaction and occupational stress are viewed as the result of the interaction between the persons holding a particular job and the environment in which they are employed. The model is presumed to be dynamic. The fit between the person and the environment is not static but needs to be constantly reassessed.

Using the model, caregivers were asked to comment on the stressors they experienced within their work setting; how factors from their personal lives influenced their response to these stressors; how their stress was manifested, and what they did to cope with their stress. Similar information was gathered from discussion with and observation of colleagues in other settings.

Demographic Variables

Little is known about the implications of the fact that many, if not most, of the caregivers providing direct care to PWAs are themselves young and often, at least initially, inexperienced in the care of seriously ill persons.

The caregivers interviewed for the present study spoke of how their own age affected their response to PWAs. An older nurse said that she always tried to care for the PWAs herself because "I'm not too sure about the issue of contagion. The young nurses are thinking of getting pregnant and I don't want them to take the potential long-term risk." One's own sexual preference may also affect one's response to PWAs. Heterosexual caregivers were sometimes homophobic and wanted to avoid gay PWAs. Often, too, their sexual partners became threatened when they knew the health care worker had contact with PWAs. On the other hand, gay and lesbian caregivers spoke of finding that this work involved their total life and community. For some, dealing with PWAs led to coming out within their professional role in a way they had not previously considered (6).

Gay and lesbian caregivers also spoke of the difficulty they experienced because they were simultaneously dealing with both "patients" and friends with the disease. In addition, those at high risk wondered if they were foreseeing their own future—except that for them the future might eventually be gloomier, since there might be no one left to give them the care they now gave to others (7).

Of course, HIV does not only affect the homosexual community. As is becoming increasingly more obvious, the future PWAs are likely to be from Black and Latin communities. Given that the typical higher status health professional is white and middle class and minority groups in health care have often been relegated to lower status jobs, there may be some difficulty in caring for these groups. This becomes particularly true when such PWAs are disproportionately apt to be drug users and less than cooperative in the traditional health care system. Caregivers working in smaller areas where there have not been many PWAs spoke of the difficulty they had with confidentiality when a community member was being treated for AIDS.

Personality and Value Systems

Some caregivers found that contact with PWAs whose lifestyle was different from that of the caregiver was fairly threatening. For example, a hospice nurse related the experience of entering the room of a gay man with AIDS whose lover was in bed with him, holding and comforting him. The young man's parents were also in the room sitting together quietly. The young nurse felt she was sensing tension and awkwardness on the part of the parents and was keenly aware of her own discomfort at seeing the two men in bed together with the parents of one looking on. She accomplished the clinical task she needed to and then quickly left the room. Her training and experience as a senior hospice nurse had shaped her ability to facilitate communication and ease tension in most situations. However, her own emotional responses to this particular situation immobilized her.

Personal Support System

The personal support system of caregivers often serves as a stressor instead of providing support (2). In working with people with AIDS, this was certainly the case. Young physicians said that their parents, who had once been pleased to introduce them as "My daughter/son the doctor," were now ashamed to mention their work. This was particularly true if the physician was gay and the parents had not acknowledged this fact within their own social network.

Some caregivers felt particularly torn between the requirements of their professional role and their social network obligations.

Spouses sometimes forbade caregivers to work with PWAs. If the caregiver then did so, some, especially those in small towns, found that their colleagues would sometimes "report" them to their partner, leading to interpersonal conflicts. In addition, caregivers, especially those who had cared for very few PWAs, sometimes found their colleagues who were not caring for AIDS patients would not share drinks with them at mealtime. This was in marked contrast to their usual behavior and led to a feeling of social isolation.

Some caregivers worried about inadvertently bringing AIDS home to their family members, especially their children. They expressed concern that the long latency period of HIV might eventually turn up unexpected methods of transmission and these caregivers would have inadvertently been responsible for having passed it on. Some caregivers from smaller towns said that their children's friends were no longer allowed to play with them if the parents were known to be working with PWAs.

Caregivers in the gay community who had friends who then became patients found their network members sometimes did not appreciate the fact that certain aspects of the relationship were now confidential. These caregivers also found it difficult to deal with the strain inherent in the dual roles of friend and professional caregiver.

Work Environment Stressors

Previous research has shown that many of the stressors in work with critically ill and dying persons derive not so much from one's clinical work as from factors in the work environment (2). While the present research was not conducted in such a way as to allow for measurement of differences among various work environment stressors, it was certainly clear that a number of the stressors mentioned did evolve from the work environment. Caregivers spoke of team communication problems that often involved conflicts between those of different sexual preference or those with different value systems around issues such as the prolongation of life. They also had difficulty with inadequate staffing, deficient equipment, and even inadequate education to handle the problems with which they were confronted.

Illness-Related Variables

Much of the difficulty with AIDS evolved from the dual facts that the disease attacks young people and has devastating manifestations and symptoms. Caregivers spoke of what seemed to be the particular cruelty of a disease that would place large purple spots all over the face of an actor or model or would take away the ability to speak from someone who always prided himself on being articulate. They also had difficulty with the neurologic manifestations of the disease, particularly irrational and angry behavior. It was often not clear what behavior their patients could actually control.

Culpability and Fear

There were also different responses to PWAs based on caregivers' feelings about the culpability of the persons involved. In situations in which a patient's behavior, directly or indirectly, led to the disease, there was sometimes a tendency to "blame the victim."

In situations where the disease was iatrogenic, caregivers often felt quite guilty. Particular problems were experienced by staff in clinics for hemophilics. These clinicians often felt responsible for indirectly causing the disease through transfusions. Their feelings of responsibility sometimes led to their finding it quite difficult to give needed sexual counseling to patients. They did not want to have to say, "Not only might you die because of the blood products we gave you to keep you from bleeding to death, but in addition you will have to alter your sexual practices and should probably not have children." Some caregivers did not give the needed advice, and the disease spread through families. Staff in a Catholic hospital were told they were not to advise the use of condoms to seropositive hemophilics.

Patient-Family Variables

Numerous concerns arose for caregivers as they worked within patient-family-friendship systems that challenged caregivers' firmly held beliefs. Often ethical issues arose, such as the health care provider who was at high risk. If such a person were in a position in which there was the risk of blood-to-blood contact or in which he or she had to make quick life and death decisions in isolation, should there be an ethical obligation to be tested and, if positive, to alter one's clinical practice? What were the obligations of a colleague who suspected that someone might be neurologically impaired as the result of an HIV infection? What were the obligations of the health care professional to the partner of someone who is HIV positive when the positive person refuses to tell his/her partner?

Caregivers were also concerned with the spouses of young seroconverted individuals who refused to take sexual precautions. This was especially clear with the spouses of hemophilics, who sometimes said that if their spouse were to die then they would want to die as well, and so they were prepared to take the risk.

Conflicts that arose between the family of origin of the PWA and his or her partner often caused considerable discomfort for staff. These problems became particularly acute when questions of legal next of kin and power of attorney had not been resolved before the patient became seriously ill and/or neurologically impaired. Caregivers needed to become aware of the bonds of love and dependency that arose within the traditional and nontraditional friendship and kinship systems of those with AIDS.

Facilitating communication is the core of most psychosocial interventions in hospice care, and the "conspiracy of silence" in families is a concept with which most caregivers are familiar. The secrecy and silence that surrounds the diagnosis of AIDS presented numerous clinical and ethical challenges. Situations were often complicated, and it was not always clear what approach caregivers should take. Particularly difficult situations arose when the diagnosis of the disease, or the terminal phase of the disease, was the occasion of the family of origin's having to confront the fact that their child had been living an alternative life-style.

There were a number of other patient issues that also caused caregiver stress. These included: feelings of guilt and responsibility, depression and suicidal ideation, anger and acting out behavior, and dealing with death.

One of the beliefs, perhaps myths, that hospice has espoused suggests that someone who is pain free wants to live or that individuals whose quality of life is good do not want to end their lives. Many PWAs, however, have seen friends and lovers die of the illness and know that the final stage is difficult and may involve wasting, skin lesions, and dementia. They do not want to subject others to having to care for them in that condition, or they may feel there will be no one left to care for them. For such PWAs, suicide may become a real option for consideration and an area for psychosocial intervention requiring advanced counseling skills. This was also an area in which teams found that they differed considerably. Some caregivers felt that suicide was an option, and others felt that it was a moral wrong.

The goal, albeit an ideal one, of hospice caregivers is to help patients put things in order, get closure on relationships, feel centered within themselves, and have a peaceful death. All of this tended to take more effort and work for both patient and caregiver when the dying person was young. This work required skillful intervention on the part of caregivers, who often struggled to help their patients maintain hope when this was appropriate and to help them prepare for death when this was inevitable. Unfortunately, the nature of the disease meant that death sometimes came much sooner than expected.

Occupational Role

Hospice staff experienced role conflict as they cared for PWAs who were still involved with active treatment. They felt that in originally choosing to work in hospice care, they would no longer be involved with the prolongation of life through technology. However, even though they recognized that a goal of hospice was to enable people to live and die the way they chose, such staff still had difficulty dealing with those who chose to die.

Younger residents felt that their general medical education was suffering from the biased exposure they were receiving to young, critically ill and dying PWAs (8). It was often even more difficult to deal with the symptoms involved in the care of these patients and the use of aggressive intervention, with which caregivers had little experience. Caregivers in one hospice were totally unprepared to deal with the pain experienced by some PWAs; many had been told that pain was not a problem with AIDS.

Work Environment

A lack of basic equipment, such as rubber gloves, and a lack of trained staff to care for PWAs also created difficult work environments. For those working in hospices or other settings in which care was provided to people with problems other than AIDS, there was sometimes difficulty in deciding what percentage of resources should go toward caring for PWAs and what percentage should go to other patients. Caregivers found it difficult to work in settings in which they felt that colleagues were giving inferior care to PWAs, feeling that they were to blame for their disease.

While team communication problems were not the major difficulty in those surveyed, such problems certainly existed. For example, caregivers spoke of colleagues who were not willing to share the load of caring for PWAs, and at times there were problems between direct caregivers and administrators regarding realistic expectations of what could be accomplished and how many hours caregivers could be expected to work. Particularly when caregivers were members of the gay community, there was sometimes the feeling that no sacrifice was too great, and caregivers often worked long hours for no extra recompense. This became a serious problem as some of these same caregivers began to succumb to AIDS themselves. When they were no longer available to work long hours, others were not necessarily prepared to provide the same kind of time.

At other times, administration refused to let gay caregivers work with PWAs, feeling that they would somehow be unable to be objective in the care they offered.

Interventions for Caregivers

Study subjects reported various personal means of coping with lifestyle management. A healthy diet, regular exercise, a moderate amount of sleep, time for oneself, and a good support network provided a basic foundation for handling the stresses of AIDS work. In addition, it was very helpful to have hobbies or activities outside of the work situation.

Having a belief system that gives meaning to one's work was reported to help many. For some this was a religious commitment, for others it was a belief that what they were doing was at least making some difference in this very difficult situation. Many caregivers said they took personal responsibility for making sure they had the knowledge and professional competence necessary to cope with the disease. Most acknowledged that being able to set some limits on their clinical work was important if they were to be able to continue to work in the field. This involved their feeling that they knew what they were doing, had some control over their work situation, and derived some pleasure from their work. Sometimes involved caregivers left for a brief vacation or leave of absence, but at other times caregivers had to decide that they had been in the field for as long as they were prepared to be at this point in time.

Coping mechanisms within the work situation were also crucial. A sense of knowing what one's team was trying to do, giving support to one another, and learning together was an invaluable coping mechanism that often took much work to accomplish. Staff selection involved having team members with different capabilities and capacities and whose motivation for working in the area was not too neurotic. Successful teams often had members of different age groups and with different previous professional experience. In addition, teams had to decide if sexual preference would be of concern in staff selection.

It was important in many settings to have staff members with whom PWAs could identify. Often this required bringing in those who had lived a similar lifestyle. In work with drug users, it was often helpful to have former users available as staff. In situations involving difficulties between the PWA and partner, or friends and the family of origin, it was often helpful to have different staff members deal with the PWA and his/her friendship network while another caregiver dealt with the family. Caregivers could then work together to try to bridge the gap between the two groups. Offering bereavement services was an important coping mechanism for many teams. It had to be recognized, however, that not all caregivers who could work effectively with PWAs could also do bereavement work. Different settings worked out different approaches to bereavement care. For some, it was helpful to have separate women's groups, as well as separate groups for families and lovers. Other programs found that they could mix the groups.

Administrative staff needed a firm commitment to making sure that caregivers were properly trained and regularly updated in the rapidly expanding knowledge available regarding the care of PWAs. Appropriate policies had to be developed regarding decision making in the areas of treatment cessation and Do Not Resuscitate Orders. In addition, there had to be careful thought given to issues involving the use of scarce resources. Policy development in the area of confidentiality was also essential. Caregivers cannot be expected to work in environments in which the proper equipment to care for PWAs is not available. Organizations had to develop policies regarding whether or not they were prepared to go into their local communities to educate local citizens about AIDS and the care they were giving to PWAs. Whenever community education programs were held, there had to be a strong commitment to totally preserve the confidential nature of the relationship with PWAs. Being able to become involved in community outreach programs provided a break for some care-givers, while for others it was just an additional burden.

Conclusion

While there are numerous anecdotal accounts of the stress that caregivers working with PWAs experience, there is little research available on the subject. This chapter has attempted to begin to look at some of the stressors that caregivers experience in a systematic way. Hopefully, it will provide a basis for future quantitative research.

The qualitative data obtained in this study indicate that the stress experienced by caregivers working with PWAs is both similar to and different from the stress experienced by those working with patients with other diseases. Both groups experienced significant difficulty with various issues in the work environment and with issues related to their occupational roles. Those working with AIDS do, however, have somewhat more difficulty with the manifestations of the disease: with fear of contagion, with feeling that their professional education might be compromised, and in dealing with complicated family situations. In addition, those working with HIV spectrum disorders are more likely to be at risk of developing the same health-related problems themselves. This fact tends to lend an additional pressure to the field and to mean that certain caregivers may well experience significant distress as they work with people with whom they can so strongly identify. This situation can lead to the development of "survivor guilt" as staff members begin to wonder why the PWA and not the caregiver is the person affected.

The major stressors identified in this chapter involve those that derive from the caregivers' own personal background, value system and personal support network and the stressors that evolved from the work environment. Work-related stressors involve dealing with the spectrum of manifestations of HIV-related disorders as well as dealing with issues related to the manner in which the disease was contracted. Relationships with PWAs and their personal support networks are often complicated and can lead to caregivers' feeling impotent and uncertain about how best to deal with the stressors involved. One's occupational role often involves role strain and uncertainty about decision making and helping PWAs to live with their own choices. Significant stressors within the work environment also involve such issues as team communication problems and unrealistic expectations of what caregivers could accomplish.

Given that the stressors derive from both the person and the work environment, coping strategies must also be developed at both the personal and environmental levels. Personal coping mechanisms involve life-style management, developing a personal philosophy that gives meaning to one's professional role, as well as being able to get away from the work situation. Organizational coping strategies involve effective team work and staff selection, expanding roles such as bereavement counseling and community education, as well as good working relationships with administrative staff.

Work involving those with HIV-related disorders is challenging and potentially stressful. The recognition of the sources of stress and some suggested coping strategies outlined here will hopefully enable caregivers to continue to care and to give.

■

References

1. Bennett JA: Nurses talk about the challenge of AIDS. Am J Nursing 1987; 87:1150-1155

2. Vachon MS: Occupational Stress in the Care of the Critically Ill, the Dying and the Bereaved. Washington, D.C., Hemisphere, 1987

3. O'Donnell L, O'Donnell CR, Pleck JH: Psychosocial responses of hospital workers to acquired immune deficiency syndrome (AIDS). J App Soc Psychology 1987; 17:269-285

4. Lewis CE, Freeman HE, Corey CR: AIDS-related competence of California's primary care physicians. Am J Public Health 1987; 77:795-799

5. French JRP, Rodgers W, Cobb S: Adjustment as person-environment fit, in Coping and Adaptation. Edited by Coelho G, Hamburg D, Adams J. New York, Basic Books, 1974

6. Lewis A: Development of AIDS awareness: a personal history. Death Studies 1988; 12:371-379

7. Pearlin LI, Semple S, Turner H: Stress of AIDS caregiving: a preliminary overview of the issues. Death Studies 1988; 12:501-518

8. Zuger A: Professional responsibilities in the AIDS generation. Hastings Center Report 1987; 17:16-20

Editor's Notes

Page 276. Risk to the health care worker of providing care to people with HIV has recently taken on an additional dimension with the emergence of airborne pulmonary tuberculosis, particularly when it becomes multi-drug resistant (see Dooley et al below). To date, there have been no reported TB-related deaths of health care workers but several providers have become infected and received treatment (see Nichols below).

Updated References

Dooley SW, Castro KG, Hutton MD, et al: Guidelines for preventing the transmission of tuberculosis in health-care settings, with special focus on HIV-related issues. Morbidity and Mortality Weekly Report 1990; 39(RR-17):1-29.

Nichols S: Mt. Sinai School of Medicine, Personal communication, October 1992.

■

Mary L. S. Vachon, RN, PhD, is Senior Mental Health Consultant, Department of Social and Community Psychiatry, Clarke Institute of Psychiatry, and Associate Professor, Department of Psychiatry and Behavioral Science, University of Toronto, Toronto, Ontario, Canada. Jeanne Dennis, MSW, is Administrator, Visiting Nurse Service Hospice, New York, New York.

■

Too Many Casualties: HIV Disease in Gay Men

Michael Helquist

The AIDS epidemic has burned itself into the consciousness of gay men for nearly a decade. To make a difference in the lives of these men, and to help them make sense of that experience, counselors and health care workers must consider how to provide a caring, therapeutic response in working with this population.

It is certainly easy to see why health care providers might choose not to get involved with AIDS. Yet health care providers who want to get involved or cannot avoid working with AIDS will have to address inevitably many issues that they would rather avoid. There is no escape.

This paper will not attempt to give an exhaustive or all-inclusive description of how AIDS affects gay men; it will highlight some of the major stress points that may bring clients to the services of mental health practitioners. It will not describe specific interventions so much as it will illustrate the experiences that gay men face today.

The Gay Community Response to AIDS

Observers from outside the gay community may be surprised to learn of the ongoing, sometimes raging debate within the gay community about whether gay people should retain or release their "ownership" of AIDS as an issue. While the historical and epidemiologic link between AIDS and high-risk sex between men is obvious, outsiders may not realize how much gay men and lesbians have shaped and defined how AIDS is perceived and dealt with in the world. Gay people have defined how we talk about AIDS, how we argue over the issues, and how we develop medical and social services in reaction to AIDS. Perhaps the best way to explain the response is by contrast: the gay community has invested as much energy and commitment to AIDS prevention and care as the various governments, as least in the early years, have avoided the issue.

AIDS has reshaped and redefined what it means to be gay in the Western world, to such a degree that the gay community struggles to understand where to draw the line. Does it boost or undermine efforts to secure civil rights and to obtain protection from violence and discrimination? Is it important that public health officials emphasize the threat of HIV to heterosexuals while they downplay the continuing high incidence of HIV disease among gay men? Fundamentally, gay people question whether the authorities will pay even grudging attention to their needs if the community, in a sense, "lets go" of the issue.

Counselors and health care providers may encounter gay men whose lives have been touched by HIV disease in any number of ways. The earliest mistake would be to anticipate that gay people have responded to AIDS in some uniform way. The themes are common, the responses and the impact highly individualized.

Thousands of gay men in North America, Western Europe, and Australia were among the first to recognize and respond to the threat of AIDS. They formed organizations to respond to that threat: first with educational programs and then with social services, legal aid, emotional support, and more recently, by organizing underground drug trials and staging demonstrations against intractable government regulations. Their efforts infused these men with a sophisticated knowledge of AIDS, the health care system, clinical care, and biomedical politics. In the midst of all this activity, these men saw their lovers, colleagues, and friends struggle with and die from the disease. Many physicians find that their patients know as much, if not more, about the latest scientific reports and clinical procedures than they themselves do.

New practitioners in the field of AIDS care could reasonably feel intimidated as they approach gay clients who may be bringing this history to the counseling session. Yet these men come looking for assistance, not primarily for a colleague who has lived through "the AIDS wars."

Other gay clients will not have been so intimately involved with AIDS organizational efforts; they will likely respond to the threat or reality of HIV disease from more of an individual rather than community perspective. They will be scared to death, worn down with worry and grief, or stymied in their efforts to get on with their lives under the cloud of AIDS.

Finally, counselors should remember that AIDS has had its most profound impact to date on a certain generation of gay men. Much as the Vietnam war has taken its greatest toll on those who were on the front lines of service or dissent, AIDS has to date hit primarily gay men in their 30s and 40s. Younger gay men, gay adolescents, and older men may enter this time of AIDS without the direct knowledge of the urban gay culture of the '70s or the heavy tolls on their social networks and families.

The reality of AIDS for gay men is the same as what being gay means today: a variety of outlooks, values, lifestyles, political affiliations, and sexual histories. Counselors will become increasingly effective if they make the effort to understand the range of experiences gay men bring to counseling sessions.

Textures of Gay Life

With all of their diversity, gay people can still lay claim to a community with a shared understanding of what is held in common. The notion and reality of community provides a context within which people can understand their daily lives, their hopes and disappointments—even the discrimination they encounter. AIDS has not and likely will not destroy the gay and lesbian community although the future toll of the disease threatens to claim tens of thousands of gay lives. The history of the AIDS epidemic already holds untold numbers of examples of how gay people have strengthened their own extended family, making their political and cultural institutions vibrant and determined, and their personal bonds deep and resolute.

Writer Edmund White observes that the gay community has followed "a terribly speeded up itinerary":

> To have been oppressed in the '50s, freed in the '60s, exalted in the '70s, and wiped out in the '80s is to have experienced a frightfully rapid evolution.

Those gay people who need counseling will represent all, several, or perhaps only the latest of the decades described above, each with its own telling marks. Counselors should recognize and, perhaps, take some comfort in knowing that there exists a vibrant and open community to which gay clients can be referred for the support and services they need.

Even while fortified by their "strength in numbers," individual gay man who are moving through time in step with AIDS may find their days have no rhyme, no reason of their own. Just as gay couples have had few role models to help them define their relationships, gay men find that the meaning of their daily lives is wide open to the unknown. For them each day holds more than the normal share; each phone call can bring news of an acquaintance just diagnosed, each morning newspaper can announce the early death of a well-known hero, each visit with a friend can reveal that another has just become blind. For many men the tragedies and deaths have piled up; after five or ten or twenty deaths faced in your 30s and 40s, another can stun but without much resonance.

With so much uncertainty and fear overshadowing their days, gay men must find their own ways to cope, to not sink into a constant demoralized state that robs them of a present as well as a future. One gay man who has experienced all that AIDS can offer summed up both the lack of direction and the determination to go on. He said simply, "There are no rules, there are no guidelines; you must move toward the light."

At nearly every turn, men who are trying to live a responsible life with respect for human values confront hatred, anger, discrimination, violence or threats of it, and an insidious denial of their existence and contribution to society. They hear the Catholic pope describe their lives as "an intrinsic moral evil" and fundamentalist leaders declare that AIDS is God's retribution. At international AIDS conferences, public health officials acknowledge them as people with HIV disease, not as gay men, who have created state-of-the-art AIDS prevention programs. Government funding agencies, which have never provided much money for specific AIDS education programs for gay men, decide that efforts must now "shift" to other populations. In 1987 the U.S. Justice Department reported that gay people are probably the most frequent victims of violence. Finally, gay people are encouraged implicitly to hide their identity and their relationships, an undertaking that places severe strain on one's well-being and mental health.

What this widespread response to gay people represents is an institutional prejudice that robs them of their humanity, making them targets of violence and discrimination while it chips away at their self-respect.

Counselors will find a full range of adaptations among their gay clients to this societal prejudice. Some men have never explored how they have internalized this external homophobia, yet they struggle with poor self-esteem. During the early years of the AIDS epidemic, gay men were hesitant to acknowledge how many of their friends and lovers were being lost to government and bureaucratic neglect, fearing perhaps that they would not "know what to do with the anger." Many gay men have only reluctantly relinquished their striving to be the "best little boys in the world."

More recently, gay and activist organizations have formed to channel this anger and energy, forcing the government to stream-line their drug review programs and to allot funds to some of their educational projects. With this anger out in the open, observers question whether these "outbursts" and demonstrations are ap-propriate and productive.

Counselors may find that this anger, whether kept under wraps or expressed, is a creative force that their clients can channel to help them make needed personal changes and cope with the demands of living with the realities of AIDS. Again, an appro-priate therapeutic response includes both understanding and respect for what it means to be a gay man today.

In contrast to the pain and anger many gay men feel, there is often a profound appreciation and joy for the good things that life continues to offer. The comfortable afternoons with friends, the surprise at a new relationship blossoming, the unexpected help from colleagues and strangers in time of illness, as well as the pleasures of travel, nature, and the arts—all these provide a bright companion to the darker influences that inhabit the lives of gay men. Counselors may find their own attempts to acknowledge and express their deepest feelings challenged by the powerful example of their gay clients.

Familiar Life Passages

Even in a time of AIDS, gay individuals must pass through familiar passages in life. Gay males of all ages may face the decision about whether to come out of the closet and how far; they must deal with relationships—entering, enduring, improving, and leaving; they must lose parents and other loved ones not due to AIDS; and they must find what it means to age.

Coming out as a gay person always has profound implications on the life to follow; the impact is often different depending on one's age at the time. But the pressure and tension and fear preceding coming out are usually the same for all. Teenagers who know that they are gay face two options: they can be honest and risk being scorned at school, on the streets, and at home, or they can lie and undermine their feelings of personal worth while they endure a crushing loneliness. The toll on teens can be especially heavy: the Youth Suicide National Center estimates that the suicide rate among U.S. gay teens is 30% to 40%. Many teens leave home, or are forced out by their parents, and live on the streets as runaways, becoming vulnerable to prostitution, drugs, and violence.

A great many gay men chose not to come out earlier in life, and now they feel the threat of being forced out of the closet by their fear of AIDS or possible diagnoses. These men often struggle with the feeling that their lives are missing something, that they are not validated fully in the community. Yet to come out today to parents, relatives, and others means having to address all the likely questions about AIDS as well. The prospect has not become easier with age, and support from friends and a counselor can play an important role in the process.

Relationships take on special meanings, sometimes difficult ones, in this time of what many gay men refer to as "the plague." Negotiating safe sex and dealing with the always troublesome issue of intimacy pose formidable challenges to gay men. Some have internalized society's accusations that they are to blame for AIDS.

Yet with so many challenges to relationships today, gay men find the whole notion charmed, enchanting, and deeply powerful when they are so "lucky" to find happiness in a new or enduring relationship. Counselors can expect to encounter a full range of relationship issues and lessons with many of their gay clients. Perhaps in this area more than in others, counselors can find their practice yielding more opportunities than expected in professional and personal growth.

Gay men have changed profoundly with AIDS in their midst, and that fact usually overshadows the other reality for gay men moving through the '70s, '80s, and '90s: the exuberantly sexual population of the early years is aging. Observers comment that since the advent of AIDS, gay men have become more responsible (a comment in itself that negates the responsible lives led by gay men of all ages before AIDS appeared). The issue is not so much responsibility as it is changes and a maturity that comes with age.

Aging brings all the usual questions about the meaning of the life that remains, what is important, what can be changed, and, sometimes for the less optimistic, what is the use? AIDS, of course, has forced all these questions much earlier in life, and men in their 30s now struggle with questions that should not have confronted them for a decade or so more. Counselors will find a profound challenge to help these men evaluate their lives and determine what is important for their futures.

Conclusion

Counselors should know that their skills are sufficient to the needs of their gay clients. This society raises people to be homophobic; the real issue is whether counselors are willing to learn and to move along a continuum of greater understanding and respect. Counselors need not be intimidated by dealing with gay men in this time of AIDS, but they should remember to work with their clients as people threatened by illness, not defined by it. Gay men face an uneasy survival, knowing that the worst may be yet to come. Many live with a certain stoicism, finding that sadness colors their every day. Yet AIDS has given many a life a jolt that pushes them to find even greater meaning in their lives and provides ever more powerful lessons to those others willing to learn.

■

Michael Helquist is Director of AIDSCOM, an international prevention project managed by the Academy for Educational Development, Washington, D.C. He has been a consultant to the World Health Organization, the Centers for Disease Control, and various AIDS organizations.

VIII
Case Vignettes

■ **Adam: A Man with AIDS**
Judy Macks, MSW, LCSW

■ **Jim: A Man in Denial**
Judy Macks, MSW, LCSW

■ **Greg: A Seropositive Gay Man**
David Silven, PhD and Thomas J. Caldarola, MA, MFCC

■ **Gary: A Married Man**
David Silven, PhD and Thomas J. Caldarola, MA, MFCC

■ **David: A Potential Research Subject**
Joyce M. Johnson, MA, DO

■ **Teresa: A Pregnant Adolescent**
Michael Shernoff, MSW, ACSW

■ **Sam: A Teenage IV Drug User**
Michael K. Baxter, MSW

■ **Jack: A Psychiatric Inpatient**
Jay W. Baer, MD

■ **Carla: A Recent Widow**
Marsha Blachman, LCSW

- **John: A Man with Hemophilia**
  Donna DiMarzo, MSW, MPH

- **Mario: A Recent Immigrant**
  Yvette G. Flores-Ortiz, PhD and Hugh A. Villalta, MA

- **Nicholas: A Heterosexual Alcoholic**
  Terry Tafoya, PhD

- **Randy: Shame and Loss of Face**
  Kiki Wu Yen Ching, MSW, LCSW and Richard Daquioag

- **Reed: A Physician's Assistant**
  Scott K. Morris, PA-C, BHSc

- **Shannon: A Blood Donor**
  Margo Nason, RN

- **Beverly: A Transfusion Recipient**
  Margo Nason, RN

■

Adam: A Man with AIDS

Judy Macks, MSW, LCSW

Part One

Adam is a 39-year-old black architect referred by his physician to individual counseling. Adam had complained to his physician of stress-related problems. He reported having difficulty concentrating, remembering appointments, and said, "I just don't seem to be thinking very clearly." Adam asked his physician for Valium to help him sleep at night. His physician honored his request and agreed that Adam's problems were stress related. He referred Adam to individual therapy to learn how to manage stress in his life.

Adam has been married for ten years. He has two children—sons, aged seven and four. Adam began noticing about two months ago that he was becoming very irritable at home and at work for no apparent reason. This change coincided with his difficulty concentrating and with his memory problems. Adam also noticed this past month that his work was suffering. He said his drawings were not always accurate, and he could not account for this new development.

Over the course of several sessions of attempting to identify the sources of Adam's stress, he began to discuss family-related concerns. He has had a very happy marriage and loves his family tremendously. Recently, however, his wife confronted him about her fear that he was involved with another woman. Adam emphatically denied this accusation. Adam seems particularly uncomfortable discussing this issue. Only toward the end of the session does he begin to reveal the secrets he has been carrying.

Although Adam had not lied to his wife about being involved with a woman, he reveals that he has been having sexual contact with men during most of his married life. His wife doesn't know this. He feels tremendous guilt, and he does not want her to find out. The therapist becomes concerned about Adam's risk of contracting AIDS and begins to discuss risk factors with him. Adam says that he never considered himself at risk for AIDS because he is not gay. Adam becomes extremely agitated and anxious upon hearing that he could, in fact, be at risk for AIDS.

Key Concerns

1. The client first presents with vague complaints of stress-related problems, the origins of which are unknown.

2. The client's difficulties have begun to intrude upon his family life, his relationship with his wife, and his job. His stress level is likely to increase given these additional problems.

3. The client is at risk for HIV infection, and he may have already been infected. He is unprepared for this information and will likely be quite anxious about his risk.

4. Communication problems already exist between the client and his wife; the client faces even greater challenges with informing his wife of his sexual activities with men.

5. Memory problems, difficulty with concentrating, and changes in the client's drawing ability may be suggestive of neurologic impairment—if the individual is infected with HIV.

Counseling Plan

1. Develop a treatment alliance which will enable the client to explore all aspects of his life, including an inquiry into the full range of sexual activities.

2. Once the presence of risk behavior has been ascertained, obtain a detailed sexual history to determine degree of risk for contracting AIDS. The client may want to consider taking the AIDS antibody test.

3. Assess the client's level of knowledge about AIDS, HIV infection, transmission, risk reduction, and his willingness to follow safer sex guidelines. Assist in his developing a plan of action to reduce or eliminate his risk of contracting or transmitting the virus.

4. Provide the client information about the AIDS antibody test. Discuss the pros and cons of taking the test, particularly the considerations regarding how it might affect his sexual activ-

ity, his personal safety, and the safety of his wife and his sexual partners. Include a discussion of protection of his confidentiality. Discuss his ability to tolerate the emotional impact of being antibody positive.

5. Refer client for medical screening and for neuropsychological testing to assess whether presenting symptoms may be organically based and related to HIV infection.

Part Two

Adam decided to delay taking the antibody test; he said he still could not believe that he might have been exposed to something like AIDS. The therapist got Adam to agree to undergo a medical exam and neuropsychological testing. Adam said he was reluctant to see his current physician for this checkup. The therapist suggested other physicians (or a gay medical referral service) who were AIDS knowledgeable, culturally sensitive, and gay sensitive.

After thorough evaluation, Adam decided to take the antibody test. He returned for his follow-up appointment and informed the therapist that his antibody test was positive and that the results of his neuropsychological testing were consistent with early HIV-related dementia complex. Additionally, his physician called and told him that he had an opportunistic infection associated with AIDS. Adam kept repeating, "I don't understand; I don't know how this could be happening to me." He told the therapist that she was the first person he had told about his diagnosis.

Counseling Plan

1. Respond empathetically to the client's extreme agitation and shock regarding his AIDS diagnosis. Allow him plenty of time to discuss his feelings and the implications that his diagnosis will have on his life.

2. Review basic information about AIDS; add further information about the neurological complications with AIDS. Inquire whether the client understands his opportunistic infection and determine whether he is getting enough information from the physician.

3. Discuss AIDS prevention and specific risk reduction: how to avoid transmission of HIV during sexual activities. Emphasize the necessity of using condoms during sex with male and

female partners. Balance this discussion by emphasizing that sexual relationships are still possible for him.

4. Acknowledge the difficulty for the client of making these behavior changes.

5. Discuss possible risk to his wife and to his one-year-old daughter (mention that his daughter may not be at risk if he were infected after his child's conception). Discuss how and when the client can disclose this new information to his wife.

6. Work with the client's profound guilt about having contracted AIDS, having had sex with men, and having possibly infected his wife and child.

7. Recommend marital counseling for the client and his wife.

8. Assess the need for social services, financial benefits, medical insurance, legal advice, etc.

Discussion Questions

1. During the first session, the information given by the client did not necessarily reveal that he was at risk for exposure to HIV. What questions would you ask to determine the actual risk?

2. Under what conditions would you recommend that the client take the AIDS antibody test? If you choose to do this, at what point in the counseling process?

3. After the client reported to you his AIDS diagnosis, would you recommend that his wife and child take the AIDS antibody test? Why or why not?

4. What would you do if Adam had not been willing to discuss the diagnosis with his wife? What would you think and feel about this and how would you handle these reactions?

■

Judy Macks, MSW, LCSW, works as an independent consultant specializing in AIDS and organization development. Formerly the Director of Training for the UCSF AIDS Health Project, she has published extensively on the psychosocial aspects of AIDS and the impact of AIDS on providers.

Jim: A Man in Denial

Judy Macks, MSW, LCSW

Part One

Jim is a 34-year-old white gay man previously employed as a bartender and part-time delivery man. He was referred for evaluation of his depressed mood and vague suicidal ideation.

Jim's initial diagnosis of Kaposi's sarcoma (KS) was made four months earlier. His reaction was one of deep shock and significant denial. He reported that he was convinced that some error had been made, and he decided to ignore the whole matter. He did not return to the clinic in one month as requested, and he resisted his housemate's urging to seek professional guidance.

Over the next several months, Jim continued to talk and act as if nothing were bothering him. Recently he had noticed two dark spots on his leg that would not go away. It was at this point that he presented himself at the clinic for a second opinion. At the clinic he appeared physically fit and described himself as feeling fine. When pressed, however, he acknowledged a one-year history of night sweats, recurrent fevers, diarrhea, and swollen lymph glands. He was again diagnosed with KS, resulting in profound despondency. The clinic staff referred Jim for crisis intervention and counseling.

Past History

Originally from the East Coast, Jim has been living in California for the past ten years. He is single, something of a loner, has never had a primary relationship last more than six months, and has an eight-year history of speed use. He also drinks wine occasionally, primarily with dinner. He has been alienated from his family of origin since he was a teenager; he feels he can count on no support from them.

Six months prior to his diagnosis, he lost his job in a local bar, the third position that he has lost in the last year. He became depressed and, for a while, stayed with friends. In time, he went on General Assistance (GA) and moved into an inexpensive hotel. Jim stayed at the hotel for nearly six months. At the time of his diagnosis, he was living in the home of a woman who had befriended him.

During the first counseling session, Jim admitted to contemplating killing himself if his lesions became visible, especially if they were to appear on his face. During subsequent sessions, Jim vacillated between thoughts of suicide and denial of the consequences of his diagnosis.

Key Concerns

1. The client's suicidal ideation must be assessed and dealt with by the counselor and the clinic staff.
2. In the midst of his denial and depression, the client may seek solace in continued drug and alcohol use.
3. The client has very limited financial resources and few friends to provide him with emotional support.
4. The client feels immediately threatened by how the KS lesions could drastically affect his life; he senses that his whole self-image is at stake.

Counseling Plan

1. Acknowledge the client's shock, sadness, and concern over these recent events. Encourage him to express himself freely, supporting his comments as natural reactions to his situation. Encourage the client to consider these sessions as a safe place to be with his fears and concerns.
2. Discuss with the client his current living environment to determine how well he is taking care of himself. Does he need additional assistance with household matters—cooking, preparing meals, etc.? During this conversation, determine whether the client continues to use drugs and alcohol. How does the client feel about the likely impact of substance abuse on his current impaired health? Is the client willing to undertake a treatment plan to end his substance abuse?
3. Gently explore the depth of the client's denial, recognizing his right to think that he will improve and that he might begin a

new life. Assess whether the denial is having a negative impact on his personal health care.

4. Explore the importance of possible facial lesions to the client. Is there a way to lessen the client's reaction to such a possibility? Does the client have coping skills that will help him deal with such an event if it occurs?

5. Consider referring the client for psychiatric evaluation and the possibility of antidepressants.

Part Two

Jim began chemotherapy as his lesions began to increase. He felt nauseated and fatigued; during this time, he lost his appetite. Nevertheless, he began to talk of plans to return to the East. When the first lesions appeared on his face, he said he felt resigned and defeated. He did not speak of suicide but seemed extremely depressed. The clinic staff discussed radiation therapy with him, and he seemed to grasp at that option to be free of the facial lesions. The therapy led to his losing his facial hair and much of the hair on his head. The inside of his mouth became badly blistered. He complained of a "foul taste" in his mouth and was unable to chew food or eat anything solid. He lost nearly 30 pounds during the course of his treatments. Nine months after his diagnosis, Jim was emaciated and greying, chronically fatigued, and covered with lesions. He was also plagued by devastating and recurrent diarrhea.

Key Concerns

1. Many patients with AIDS come to a decision to forego treatment when the side effects of drugs and discomfort of the needed procedures are too much to bear. This is often a difficult decision for individuals to reach, depending on their sense of "not giving up" or "not letting others down." The counselor should be alert to these issues and should initiate discussions with the client about what is important to him and his feelings about the treatment of his condition.

2. The counselor may be the only person in this client's life to suggest that final plans be made. The client may need encouragement and information to complete a will and to outline his wishes for health care in the event that he becomes severely incapacitated or incompetent. (Some states offer a legal means

for doing this known as a "durable power of attorney for health care"). The counselor might also contact the family, if the client wishes, to help them determine what role they might take at this time.

3. The client has limited emotional and social support. Referrals to community and support agencies and emotional support groups should be made. The counselor may need to increase the frequency of visits.

4. After obtaining consent from the client to speak to the referring physician, the counselor should contact the physician for further information. The counselor should also help the client explore issues related to medical treatment. The client should be encouraged to speak to his physician about treatment options and prognosis. The counselor might act as intermediary and speak to the physician on the client's behalf if the client prefers.

Discussion Questions

1. In the latter stages of the client's illness, right before his radiation therapy and once the side effects cleared somewhat, if the client continued with his drug use, how would you deal with this? If the client said he was simply seeking some comfort from the drugs, how would you respond?

2. What criteria should be used to determine whether to be attentive (that is, making home or hospital visits) during the client's final stages? How can the counselor obtain support during these difficult situations?

■

Judy Macks, MSW, LCSW, works as an independent consultant specializing in AIDS and organization development. Formerly the Director of Training for the UCSF AIDS Health Project, she has published extensively on the psychosocial aspects of AIDS and the impact of AIDS on providers.

Greg: A Seropositive Gay Man

David Silven, PhD and Thomas J. Caldarola, MA, MFCC

Greg is a 30-year-old gay black man who has come in desperation to a community mental health agency for "some help and advice." At first he seems reticent to open up with the white counselor and is relieved to hear that the session is being kept in confidence. He then begins to tell his story, with stops and starts as he lets what he is saying sink in. It is obvious that he has not discussed much of this before.

Greg discloses that he has been HIV positive for the last year and that he has told very few people. "In fact, I only trust one friend with this and I'm afraid even he can't handle it.... Most of my other friends claim they're negative, and I'm afraid to tell them." Lately he has been losing sleep and obsessing about his HIV status at work, feeling paranoid that if people at work found out, he would lose his job. He expresses fear about the future stability of his insurance status as well.

The hardest part for Greg is his family. He just returned from an out-of-town weekend visit to see them and he found it "a bitch not to be able to share my dirty secret with them." When the counselor explores this situation further, he learns that Greg's family has "no idea that I'm gay, either—at least it's never directly spoken about." Greg then launches into an emotional story of his struggles with being a gay black man, feeling alienated within the black community and at times within the gay community as well. He laments that he has been single most of the time since he came out—relationships lasting only two to three months at best. "And now I feel like a leper....No one will come near me if I tell them I'm positive, so I don't tell them and then I feel guilty after sex."

At this point Greg grows silent and his eyes seem far away. The counselor questions him how he is handling his health, and Greg responds adamantly that he hasn't done much, but "I've been healthy all my life and still am." After a silence he admits his fear of developing symptoms. When asked about drug and alcohol use, he admits that he has been handling stress by smoking a small amount of pot daily and having three to four beers after work most days of the week. He denies having any addiction problems with alcohol or drugs, stating "I've always been able to handle a joint and a drink or two every day....Now I need it more than ever."

The counselor encourages Greg to return for at least a few more sessions while he is in this crisis period. Greg reluctantly agrees, hoping that he can "figure some way out to deal with my family and not have them get more messed up about this than I am."

Key Concerns

1. Greg's self-esteem and self-image issues appear to predate his HIV positive status. His feelings of alienation within the black and gay communities, as well as his feelings of contamination, continue to affect his relations with family, friends, and potential lovers, as well as his work environment. These issues need to be addressed if he is to open up and seek the help he needs.

2. Greg's isolation and fear of rejection have made any disclosure of his antibody status practically impossible. This situation is extremely stressful and may eventually affect his health. His work with the counselor is the beginning of a support system, and referral to an HIV-positive group support seems crucial at some point.

3. Greg's concern about his family's reactions to his being gay and HIV positive are overwhelming for him—a double coming-out process. He fears losing their support as well as upsetting them. Yet the isolation he experiences by withholding information from family feels equally distressing. He craves and needs their acceptance and support.

4. Greg's alcohol and drug use is a concern, especially in view of his HIV status. Though he denies it is a problem, he is using substances to distract him from other issues. This "gray area" level of substance use—in which the individual denies a problem but seems to be abusing—is a difficult one to confront. This client may reject the counselor who pushes too hard on this issue at first. A careful approach is necessary without avoiding the issue altogether.

5. Given the client's uncertainty about his job, his fear of the future, sense of isolation, and feeling of desperation, the possibility of suicidal thinking may be present and should be addressed directly.

Counseling Plan

1. Help the client build self-esteem by validating his concerns, normalizing them, and building on his strengths and survival skills. The question arises whether referral to a black gay therapist (if one is available) or to a gay support group is indicated and should be discussed with the client. The counselor's bond with the client is the important factor, and any referral needs to be made taking into account the client's needs and what is available in the community.

2. Encourage careful disclosure of his antibody status either in HIV positive support groups or by helping the client explore which friends might be best able to handle the information. Role playing can often be helpful to prepare for difficult disclosures.

3. Explore the family situation and help the client decide when, if, and how best to approach them—for example, starting with his closest relationship to establish initial support for himself, and developing a timeline for dealing with coming out about his sexual orientation and his HIV status. The client's substance use needs to be gently confronted and assessed. Use of adjunctive referral to other agencies might be helpful, as well as exploring the dangers of his substance use to his present health status and its influence on his isolation and self-esteem. This topic will most likely elicit some resistance and should be approached directly but with an understanding of his temporary need to use substances as a defense.

4. Help the client develop more sense of control over his situation by encouraging him to be more actively conscious of developing a health regimen, including working with a physician he trusts.

5. Long-range goals include working on self-esteem and self-image issues.

Discussion Questions

1. How might this client's race complicate this case for a non-black counselor? What steps might be taken to increase trust and understanding for the client, and how can these issues be best addressed?

2. How do you deal with "gray area" substance use when the client denies that he has a problem?

3. How would you handle this client's isolation and concerns about disclosure if working in a community where there are no relevant support resources available?

4. How do you handle long-term issues like self-esteem and self-image in time-limited counseling?

■

David Silven, PhD, is a clinical psychologist and Coordinator of the Prevention/Education Program of the UCSF AIDS Health Project in San Francisco. Thomas J. Caldarola, MA, MFCC, is a counselor for the AIDS Prevention Project and AIDS Family Project at Operation Concern and a member of the UCSF Prevention Team, UCSF AIDS Health Project, in San Francisco.

■

Gary: A Married Man

David Silven, PhD and Thomas J. Caldarola, MA, MFCC

Gary is a 40-year-old married man who lives with his wife and two children. He has a history of sporadic homosexual encounters over the past ten years, which he has not disclosed to any of his friends or family, including his wife. He seeks counseling one week after learning from his physician that he is seropositive.

Gary initially presents in the interview as guarded and reserved. After long silences following vague statements about being under stress, he recounts tearfully the painful news of a week ago, along with the dread he feels when contemplating the effects on his family life. He describes sleepless nights during the past week, dominated by ruminations about his future. He spontaneously acknowledges thoughts of suicide as "maybe the only way out at this point." He fears ostracism by friends and family, as well as discrimination at work and possibly the loss of his job. The question, "Is there anything left for me now?" repeatedly comes up. Gary describes being consumed with the fear that he has infected his wife and children. He has spoken to no one about the situation since his physician informed him a week ago. He mentions, almost in passing, that he has had unsafe sex with several men during the past week and that this only adds to his sense of shame and failure.

Gary continues to describe his utter shock at the news. He states he knows little about AIDS, having more or less assumed that he and his social network were essentially immune to the epidemic. He reports that he has no friends who are gay or who he feels confident would be accepting of his homosexual behavior. He expresses the fear that he will become sick and die any day. The counselor notes that Gary repeatedly refers to himself as having "AIDS."

At the end of the interview, Gary is reluctant to schedule a second appointment. He expresses embarrassment and shame about having talked about his situation, particularly his history of homosexual behavior, to the counselor. He states that he has never talked to anyone about his homosexual behavior, and that he realizes he has been avoiding facing the issue for many years.

Key Concerns

1. Gary appears to be experiencing an acute anxiety reaction characterized by rumination, sleeplessness, and dread. The risk of suicidal behavior should be considered substantial, especially in view of his extreme isolation at present.

2. Gary's usual social support system is suddenly seen as unavailable. This occurs at a time when he is highly distressed and particularly in need of support. It is unlikely that he is informed about other potential sources of social support in the community for HIV-positive individuals.

4. The client's wife is at moderate to high risk for HIV infection through sexual intercourse with the client, unless they have been following safe sex guidelines since the time that Gary himself became infected.

5. Gary is continuing to have unsafe sex, which puts others at risk of infection and places his own health status at further risk. This behavior may reflect his ignorance about HIV transmission or, more likely, the level of his denial. It may also be a function of his hopelessness and his suicidal wishes.

6. Gary has long-standing unresolved issues related to his sexual orientation. It is possible that he might have avoided examining these issues in any depth if his current crisis had not occurred. However, given the present circumstances, he must now face these issues, and in a context in which his defenses are already strained by many other stresses.

Counseling Plan

1. Crisis intervention is indicated to help the client stabilize and to prevent further self-destructive behavior. This client will benefit considerably from having the opportunity to simply air his feelings and concerns in the presence of an accepting and

empathic counselor. The counselor can also assist Gary in identifying potentially supportive friends, acquaintances, or extended family members who can help him through this difficult crisis period. Referral to available HIV positive support groups or organizations in the community which are set up to deal with HIV-positive individuals' concerns may be advisable. Providing information to correct faulty assumptions is likely to help in reducing some of the client's terror about such possibilities as impending death and possible infection of his children.

2. Suicidal risk should be carefully assessed on an ongoing basis. Referral to a psychiatrist for evaluation of the appropriateness of psychotropic medication should be considered. Assuring the client that his suicidal feelings are a common result of the hopelessness which seropositive clients experience may help to reduce the client's urge to act on suicidal impulses.

3. Couple or family counseling sessions should be considered to help the family integrate the news once Gary has disclosed his HIV status. His wife is likely to feel a great deal of fear, hurt, sadness, and anger, and it will be important to provide avenues for her to deal with these feelings. She is also likely to benefit from information and guidance in deciding whether to take the antibody test herself.

4. Gary probably needs to be educated about the potential added risk to his health if he continues engaging in unsafe sexual activity, as well as the risk of infecting others through this behavior. Furthermore, it should not be assumed that he has stopped engaging in unsafe sexual activity with his wife.

5. Once the immediate crisis period has subsided, the counselor will need to evaluate the client's motivation to work on long-standing issues related to sexual orientation.

Discussion Questions

1. If the counselor decides to refer this client to a support group for HIV-positive individuals, would it be preferable to refer to a gay-identified group? What if the only groups available are gay identified or primarily gay in membership?

2. How should the counselor balance the desire to stabilize this client, who is already in crisis, with the need to address the issue of disclosure to the wife and to others?

3. What kind of intervention would be appropriate if the client reveals that he is continuing to have unsafe sex with his wife without disclosing his antibody status?

4. How should the long-standing issues of the client's sexual orientation be addressed in the early stages of counseling?

5. On what basis does the counselor decide whether to offer individual consultation to the client's wife while continuing to work with the client?

■

David Silven, PhD, is a clinical psychologist and Coordinator of the Prevention/Education Program of the UCSF AIDS Health Project in San Francisco. Thomas J. Caldarola, MA, MFCC, is a counselor for the AIDS Prevention Project and AIDS Family Project at Operation Concern and a member of the UCSF Prevention Team, UCSF AIDS Health Project, in San Francisco.

David: A Potential Research Subject

Joyce M. Johnson, MA, DO

David, a 36-year-old gay white male, was diagnosed with HIV disease. His only symptom was lymphadenopathy and clinically he felt quite well. David had been in individual therapy with a social worker for about 18 months. As an adjunct to this therapy, the social worker referred him to a psychiatrist to focus on AIDS-related issues. Shortly after the referral was made, David, still feeling well, was diagnosed with Kaposi's sarcoma. Several friends suggested he enter a medication clinical trial. His decision about whether to pursue a pharmacologic treatment protocol became a therapeutic issue with the psychiatrist.

During treatment with the psychiatrist many issues surfaced. David had decided from the start that he was hesitant to enroll in a double-blind placebo-controlled trial, since he did not want to go through the evaluation procedures of a protocol (lumbar puncture, repeated blood tests, etc.) and not know whether he was receiving medication. Most of the trials for which David was potentially eligible required one or two weeks of hospitalization. Becoming a hospital patient had many meanings to David. Most of his friends with AIDS who entered a hospital died there. David felt he would be "captured" by the hospital and would lose the freedom to pursue his usual daily activities. David would also be isolated from his friends and support system. He tried to assess the likelihood that the protocol treatments and medications would be medically helpful.

David spent much time talking about "quality" versus "quantity" of life. He knew that he felt well. However, due to the medication toxicities and side effects, he knew he would probably feel "sick" if he entered a protocol. He was also realistic about the pain involved with intravenous lines, lumbar punctures, and other procedures. He decided these immediate discomforts would be tolerable if there were a high probability that he would later regain his current subjective state of health and have a better long-term prognosis. David realized that his apparent health was tenuous.

Feelings about death and dying surfaced. David expressed satisfaction with his present life: relationships with friends, closeness to his lover, progress in his job-training program. This satisfaction seemed to magnify David's difficulties in making a decision about entering a treatment protocol.

David decided not to enter a clinical trial. He felt resolved about his immediate AIDS-related concerns and terminated treatment with the psychiatrist. He continued individual therapy with the social worker. He went on a one-week vacation and then began receiving AZT. Fortunately, David remains well and continues with his remarkable spirit.

Key Concerns

1. Patients have many feelings about entering a treatment protocol, and these concerns are often not addressed by those managing the study.

2. A patient's attitude about and acceptance of HIV disease is often reflected in his attitude about entering a treatment protocol.

3. The potential benefits (medical, psychological, etc.) of a clinical trial should be weighed against its risks. These vary for each patient.

Treatment Plan

1. Continue medical management of Kaposi's sarcoma and monitor AZT treatment.

2. Continue individual therapy with the social worker. The social worker may want to participate in AIDS education programs to learn more about HIV disease.

3. The psychiatrist remains available for consultation with either the patient or the social worker.

Discussion Questions

1. What are some of the reasons patients enter clinical trials?

2. What is the role of informed consent in a clinical trial?

3. What is the role of "hope" when one faces death and dying?
4. How can various mental health professionals work together to provide HIV disease patients with the most comprehensive care?

■

Joyce M. Johnson, MA, DO, is an Assistant Clinical Professor, Department of Psychiatry, Georgetown University, Washington, D.C., a member of the American Psychiatric Association AIDS Commission, and a psychiatrist in private practice in Chevy Chase, Maryland.

Teresa: A Possibly Pregnant Adolescent

Michael Shernoff, MSW, ACSW

Teresa is seventeen years old and is referred for therapy by her guidance counselor at the high school she attends. She had always been an average student until this semester, when she began to fail most of her subjects and was caught cutting classes. Prior to the current semester, she was involved in various extra-curricular school activities.

She is the only child of parents in the midst of finalizing a separation after several years of trying to hold together a very chaotic household. Teresa admits to regular use of alcohol and marijuana and presents as a moderately depressed individual with mild suicidal ideation. During sessions, she often becomes tearful and discusses feeling sad, listless and lonely.

After several sessions, Teresa admits that for the past eight months she has been having intercourse with Tim, one of the boys at school. Her period is late and she worries that she might be pregnant. She has been too afraid to raise these concerns with Tim. Since fearing she might be pregnant, she has become depressed and has been avoiding him. In addition, she has not been in the mood to have sex since the onset of her concerns about being pregnant.

Though intelligent and somewhat informed about birth control, Teresa has not been to a physician or family planning clinic to confirm whether or not she is pregnant. She feels unable to confide in either of her parents since they are preoccupied with the separation. She is terrified of her parents' reaction if they ever found out. She feels strongly that neither of them would be supportive, understanding or comforting to her during this crisis.

In a recent discussion with Tim, he confided to her that he has been shooting up cocaine with his friends for the past year. She is confused by this information and is now afraid that perhaps she is incubating AIDS. She is not in love with Tim and does not wish to get married at this time. She does not want to have a baby, but having been raised Catholic, she is deeply conflicted about whether or not to have an abortion.

Key Concerns

1. Teresa may actually act on her suicidal ideation.
2. She is currently in a crisis due to the fact that she may be pregnant and/or exposed to HIV.
3. If she is not pregnant, she needs to be better educated about contraception.
4. Whether or not she has already been exposed to HIV, she needs to learn how to protect herself from contracting or transmitting sexually transmitted diseases that include AIDS.
5. Teresa may have become sexually active out of loneliness and as a reaction to unconscious feelings she has about her parents' separation.
6. She appears to lack the interpersonal skills and assertiveness necessary to control whether or not she engages in sexual intercourse.

Counseling Plan

1. Assess the seriousness of the suicidal feelings, and develop an intervention strategy if the client appears highly at risk of making a gesture or an attempt.
2. Refer client to a family planning clinic where she can receive gentle and sensitive pregnancy testing to determine whether or not she is pregnant.
3. Explore all of her feelings about the various options open to her if she is pregnant.
4. If the client is not pregnant, urge her to obtain education and counseling about birth control in case she decides to continue remaining sexually active.
5. It is important for the primary therapist not to take any stand on what type, if any, birth control the client should employ. The specifics of this are best left to the family planning clinic. But it is essential for the therapist to explore her feelings about "artificial" methods of contraception since she has been raised Catholic.

6. Once it has been determined whether or not the client is pregnant, begin to explore issues around taking the HIV antibody test. Be certain to stress that if she decides to take the test, it could be done anonymously.

7. Offer to have sessions with the client and Tim if she feels this would be helpful. Use these sessions as an opportunity to find out what Tim knows about safer sex and safer needle usage, and to begin to educate him about how to protect himself and his sexual partners from HIV.

8. If the client is not pregnant and has not been exposed to HIV, then the following issues can be raised:

    a) Begin to educate the client about the many different ways of being sexually active that do not have to include penetration or intercourse in order to achieve orgasm.

    b) Explore with the client her feelings about power and control in sexual situations, and work with her to devise ways of increasing her assertiveness in sexual situations. This can include role playing various situations where she sets firm limits about not engaging in intercourse.

    c) Provide the client with concrete methods of maintaining control in sexual situations that will result in her not going further than she feels ready, comfortable or able to. This can include suggesting frottage or mutual genital stimulation. If she decides against employing any method of birth control herself, practicing putting a condom on her boyfriend and masturbating him while he is wearing one can be one sexual technique they can safely employ.

Discussion Questions

1. If the client turns out to be pregnant or has been exposed to HIV, how do you help prepare her to disclose this information to parents she knows will be disapproving?

2. If the client has been exposed to HIV and is pregnant, what are the ethical issues that need to be raised in order to help her make an informed decision about how to proceed?

3. The therapist is a practicing Catholic, and has strong beliefs about artificial methods of birth control. Recognizing that if correctly used, condoms are generally effective in preventing

the transmission of HIV, and that not everyone will abstain from having intercourse until marriage, how can the therapist reconcile these two seemingly opposing realities?

■

Michael Shernoff, MSW, ACSW, is Co-Director of Chelsea Psychotherapy Associates in Manhattan and co-chairs The AIDS Task Force of The Society for the Scientific Study of Sex and the Task Force on AIDS and The Family of the American Orthopsychiatric Association. He is a member of the National Committee on Lesbian and Gay Concerns of the National Association of Social Workers.

Sam: A Teenage IV Drug User

Michael K. Baxter, MSW

Sam is a 17-year-old white male who has had repeated contact with the Juvenile Justice system since the age of 12. He is currently detained on charges of assault, his eighth charge to date.

On admission interview with the clinic nurse, Sam was noted to be "agitated, crying at times, explosive at others, and probably under the influence of speed, although denied." Medically, Sam presented with oral thrush, enlarged nodes in three sites, and a 10 percent weight loss since his last admission three months ago. He was generally in poor physical health.

During the past four years, Sam has been living primarily on the streets, moving from east coast to west coast with relative ease. He has had several short, unsuccessful stints living with one or the other of his parents during this time, which always resulted in his running away.

Sam was diagnosed with symptomatic HIV infection by his family physician prior to his last admission and was counseled at that time to take the AIDS antibody test for confirmation. The result of that test was positive. He was then referred to a local AIDS clinic and was seen once for medical assessment. After initial assessment, he again ran away from home and failed to return for follow-up appointments. He made contact with his counselor on two occasions when he was "tweeking" on speed and felt he was losing control. He made it clear that he was not interested in any medical treatment at those times, stating that he was fine.

Currently, his probation officer is looking for possible alternatives for placement, ranging from inpatient drug treatment to long-term detention in a juvenile facility. Neither of Sam's parents feel able to take him into their homes again at the present time, nor is it likely that the court would approve of such a plan.

Sam has stated to his counselor that he can't handle being locked up and is likely to "do something" if he doesn't get out soon.

He says he is willing to do anything to get out and would gladly go to a drug rehabilitation program if that were possible.

Key Concerns

1. Sam presents with serious medical concerns. Continued contact with medical providers will be essential.

2. Sam's medical condition is further compromised by his extensive drug use, around which he is largely in denial. Sam presents with a long history of using speed, cocaine, alcohol, and marijuana.

3. Sam has had no consistent living situation in several years. While several different placements have been tried with Sam in the past, none have worked out satisfactorily, nor is there any easy response to the present situation.

4. Finding services, medical care, and social support that are appropriate to this client may be difficult if not impossible. Utilizing the services of the local AIDS clinic proved to be rather uncomfortable for Sam, who is neither an adult nor identified as gay. Finding more comfortable services will be important to a successful intervention in this case.

5. Sam presents with serious psychological concerns, both generally and specifically related to being incarcerated. It has become clear that Sam is generally distrustful of authority, be it institution or person. He presents as someone unlikely to form any real bonds with those working with him. Of immediate concern are his suicidal threats; longer term concerns are his long-standing depression and personality problems that make it difficult for him to trust and to use resources available to him in a more positive way.

6. What are the placement consequences of Sam's involvement with the judicial system? It will be important to future placement to consider HIV status and what specialized services will be necessary. This will likely necessitate discussion with the judge and the probation officer.

Counseling Plan

1. If necessary, facilitate medical assessment. Explain to Sam prior to exam what exactly will be happening when he sees the

323 ∎

medical provider and what tests, if any, he may be asked to take.

2. Establish a good working relationship with the medical provider, and let Sam know that this is happening. The key is to always work *with* Sam, not do things *to* him; otherwise he will feel as if he really has no control over his life.

3. Begin to help Sam express his feelings about being HIV positive, how he sees this affecting his life, and what this means for his future (if indeed he can see that at all). Supportive counseling will be required daily while he is incarcerated. The primary concern initially will be to establish a relationship with him. Help Sam to seek alternatives to suicidal feelings, likely connected to his feelings of powerlessness at being incarcerated. It is essential to empower him to the extent possible. Help Sam explore the positive possibilities in his life; support the positive decisions he makes.

4. With Sam's consent, meet with available family members to assess their needs and to make referrals as appropriate.

5. Confer with the probation officer regarding possible placements, making suggestions as indicated. It is important to find out what Sam has told his probation officer and what he does or doesn't want you to discuss. The same holds true if it is necessary to talk to the judge hearing the case. These consultations should proceed slowly, and only after careful discussion with Sam.

■

Michael K. Baxter, MSW, is AIDS Program Coordinator, Forensic Youth Services, San Francisco Department of Public Health.

Jack: A Psychiatric Inpatient

Jay W. Baer, MD

Jack is a 38-year-old gay white man with no psychiatric history except episodic binge drinking and a two-month history of *Pneumocystis carinii* pneumonia. He was admitted to the hospital after he became disruptive in an alcohol treatment program. Clinically, he appeared to be suffering a manic episode and exhibited insomnia, hyperactivity, pressured speech, flight of ideas, mood swings, grandiose and religious delusions, auditory and visual hallucinations, markedly impaired judgment, and complete denial of his AIDS diagnosis. It was unclear if his symptoms were caused directly by HIV infection of the brain or were part of a reactive or "functional" disorder. A negative CT scan and lumbar puncture suggested the latter was the case. Jack improved moderately after treatment with antipsychotic medication; lithium was not used, as Jack had recent renal complications of AIDS. He was released ten days after admission, following a successful challenge in Superior Court of his mental health hold.

Jack was readmitted ten days later after increasing fatigue and severely impaired judgment rendered him unable to provide food, clothing, and shelter for himself. Treatment with antipsychotic medication was reinstituted. At first he continued to exhibit manic symptoms. On one occasion, he became threatening and required seclusion. He repeatedly abused the telephone, calling 911 so the police would rescue him, badgering friends, and trying to order everything from plane tickets to brass bands.

After a few weeks, Jack's clinical status began to change. Many of his "manic" symptoms diminished or disappeared; for the most part, he maintained his grandiose denial of his prognosis, although this was punctuated by periodic lucidity and acknowledgement of his illness. He began to show signs of dementia: decreased attention to grooming and common etiquette, disorientation, failing short-term memory, wandering, and deficits in visual spatial recognition. He had a number of medication complications, although he was able to tolerate a neuroleptic (Navane, thiothixene) and gradually required a lower dose. His dementia progressed rapidly, he grew weaker, and nursing assistance with basic activities was necessary.

Jack was placed on permanent conservatorship. Though he no longer required acute psychiatric hospitalization, he remained on the unit for nearly six months until he could be placed in a residential program with 24-hour care. He died ten days after discharge.

Key Concerns

1. When a patient with HIV disease develops new major psychiatric symptoms, the specific cause or multiple causes of these symptoms may be unclear.
2. HIV dementia can render a patient unlike the other patients on an inpatient psychiatric unit, leading to patient stigma and greater staff stress.
3. Violent behavior of HIV-infected individuals raises staff and other patients' anxiety even more than such behavior of individuals whose HIV status is unknown.
4. Response to psychoactive medications can be affected by advancing HIV brain disease.
5. Demented patients pose disposition problems due to inadequate subacute placement facilities.
6. People with AIDS can meet legal criteria for involuntary psychiatric treatment. Court rulings on these matters can be affected by judges' and attorneys' feelings about AIDS as well as whether the behavioral problems are deemed "medical" or "psychiatric."

Treatment and Counseling Plan

1. A full diagnostic workup is appropriate for an HIV patient with a radical change in mental status to rule out reversible causes of illness (for example, cryptococcal meningitis).
2. Psychoactive medications are employed for ameliorating target symptoms. Patients with dementia generally require low dosages and careful monitoring of side effects. The medication

treatment plan is revised as the patient's medical and psychiatric status evolves.

3. Consultation with HIV-knowledgeable medical staff is required for ongoing management of the patient's medical condition.

4. Individual patient confidentiality needs to be respected.

5. Mental health holds should be utilized according to clinical standards (inability to care for self) and not determined by diagnosis (HIV dementia).

6. The inpatient staff must receive ongoing education and support so they can manage competently the numerous issues that arise. These include containment of patients' fears of HIV transmission, diminution of the real risk of HIV transmission (for example, via needlesticks during seclusion episodes) and dealing with their own feelings regarding working with dying patients.

7. AIDS education for patients should become a regular component of the inpatient treatment milieu.

8. A relationship with a subacute facility should be cultivated for aftercare referrals; if no such facility exists, appropriate government officials should be lobbied to help with development of this service.

Discussion Questions

1. Is involuntary psychiatric treatment ethically justified in a patient known to have a terminal illness?

2. Is it appropriate to mainstream HIV patients into general psychiatric wards, or should they be cared for in speciality "HIV only" areas?

3. How can mental health professionals better define the etiology of mental illness in patients infected with HIV?

4. How can staff best be prepared and supported in this difficult work?

■

Jay W. Baer, MD, is an Assistant Professor of Psychiatry, Tufts University, School of Medicine, Boston, Massachusetts.

Carla: A Recent Widow

Marsha Blachman, LCSW

Carla is a 37-year-old black woman. She lives with her two sons, Ray (age 15) and Mark (age 13), in a two-bedroom apartment in a large U.S. city. Most of her extended family—parents, siblings, and in-laws—reside in a different part of the state. As with many families, they have a history of both closeness and distance.

Carla married Ricky, her high school sweetheart, when she was 19 years old. She had not dated much prior to their relationship. Ricky worked in construction and earned a moderate income. Carla loved him especially for his kind and quiet manner. Three years ago Ricky suddenly became ill and was hospitalized. The doctor told Carla that Ricky had advanced cancer, and he was dead within 25 days.

The family found it difficult initially to adjust to Ricky's death. Since there were no relatives nearby, Carla and the children turned to each other for emotional comfort. The boys missed their father and, fortunately, found a school coach that got them involved in team sports. This helped ease their sadness. Carla got a new secretarial job which was not very interesting, but she needed more pay and secure benefits and the change boosted her spirits.

Carla and several co-workers attended a noontime talk on "AIDS and the Workplace." Now that the boys were older, Carla wanted to start dating, yet she was hesitant because of all the wild rumors about "catching" AIDS. After the talk, a co-worker suggested they go together to an anonymous test clinic to take the HIV antibody test so that they could make sure there was nothing to worry about. Carla was certain she didn't have any risk but agreed to go along with her friend. She thought she might feel more confident about pursuing an attractive co-worker in her office if she took the test first.

Two weeks later Carla returned to the test site for the results. She was stunned and confused when the counselor told her she had tested positive for HIV infection. They reviewed the risk factors again, and Carla was certain a mistake had been made. She could not believe this was happening to her and insisted on having the test repeated.

The following days passed for Carla as if she were in a waking nightmare. She lied to her co-worker, saying she had decided not to go back to get the test results; she didn't dare tell anyone what was happening. She became sullen, teary, and slept poorly. She noticed she stopped hugging the boys and spent less time with them at night. Finally, it occurred to her to call the doctor who had cared for her late husband Ricky. She asked him to review Ricky's medical records for any indication that he might have had AIDS. The doctor agreed and shortly called back to say that this closer look was very revealing. He was now of the opinion that Ricky had actually died of AIDS and not cancer. Carla returned to the anonymous test site for results of the second test; she still tested positive for HIV.

During this interview with the counselor at the test site, Carla asked several questions: What does being HIV positive mean? Will she die quickly like Ricky? Is she any danger to her sons? What if she is unable to work? What medical care is available? The counselor attempted to answer these questions in a general way and provided a list of referrals for more concrete information.

Carla was unable to pursue these referrals for the next eight months. She continued to go to work and keep up with family obligations until, quite run-down, she became sick with the flu. The suddeness of the illness reminded her of Ricky's death and AIDS. In a panic, she searched unsuccessfully for the list of resources from the post-test counselor. Not knowing what else to do, she phoned the local suicide prevention hotline. The worker gently calmed her down and recommended a social worker trained to deal with AIDS issues. Carla agreed to seek help and immediately called for an appointment.

Key Concerns

1. Carla displays an emotional numbing brought on by shock and disbelief. Her initial response reveals an avoidance of thoughts and feelings about being infected. This reaction could be potentially life threatening.

2. Withdrawal, especially from family members during a time of crisis, often reflects fears of infecting others or, conversely, fears of being rejected or discriminated against.

3. Carla has experienced extensive losses and must now consider planning for her own needs and the needs of her sons.

4. Carla exhibits depressive symptomatology with the potential for suicide that requires thorough evaluation and treatment planning.

Counseling Plans

1. Develop a therapeutic alliance that will enable communication and exploration.

2. Evaluate for suicidal risk and follow through with appropriate interventions. Ask about past and current drug and alcohol use.

3. Explore negative and positive aspects of antibody status disclosure, especially as this relates to building a support system and decreasing isolation. Explore her feelings about talking with her sons and other family members. Refer the client to an HIV positive support group for women and/or families, if available. If none exists, try to introduce client to another seropositive woman, perhaps through the local AIDS service organization.

4. Discuss the delay in seeking services. Assess whether denial might lead to problems with personal health care and treatment options.

5. Examine client's feelings about her husband's "mysterious" death and attitudes toward her own mortality. Allow for feelings of grief, anger, and guilt to surface in a safe, contained relationship.

6. Explore self-esteem and identity issues (for example, being a black single parent, an HIV-positive female, and sexuality). Encourage emotional expression.

7. Encourage the client to identify successfully with previous coping skills. Enhance her options by suggesting and teaching problem-solving and stress-reducing methods.

8. Assess the client's current level of knowledge about HIV infection and AIDS, prevention and risk reduction. Create

with her a manageable plan to decrease and eliminate potential harm to others. Acknowledge the difficulties in making behavioral changes. Provide useful literature as indicated.

9. Determine financial, medical, spiritual, and social needs. Refer her to available resources.

10. Provide hope and optimism for ongoing health and adjustment to the many challenges brought on by the threat of AIDS.

Discussion Questions

1. What are the specific cultural issues to be considered in working with an HIV-positive black (or any other ethnic minority) female?

2. Would you involve Carla's children in treatment planning? If so, how would you work with the family?

3. How might you address Carla's shock over being diagnosed HIV positive? How strenuously would you challenge denial as a defense mechanism?

4. What should the therapist's role be regarding disclosure concerns? How might you structure the sessions to address the concrete implications as well as the symbolic meaning that "coming out" has to Carla?

5. What kinds of community resources are available to women and minorities with AIDS-related concerns?

6. What is known about heterosexual transmission and, specifically, female to male? How and when might this information be useful to Carla?

■

Marsha Blachman, LCSW, is Women's Services Coordinator, UCSF AIDS Health Project, San Francisco, California.

John: A Man with Hemophilia

Donna DiMarzo, MSW, MPH

John is a 40-year old Pacific Islander with severe hemophilia, referred for evaluation following a new diagnosis of *Pneumocystis carinii* pneumonia. He is seen in his hospital room, tearful and moaning, "I can't believe this is happening to me. . . . It can't be true."

John has been a patient at the Hemophilia Treatment Center since his arrival in the U.S. ten years ago and is well known to the psychosocial staff. He has had multiple, serious bleeding episodes requiring hospitalization. Despite his hemophilia, he has been able to maintain fairly steady employment as a clerk. His wife, Anne, also works full time. Although both John and Anne appear to be "Americanized," they have maintained many of their culture's traditional values, beliefs and practices.

John was initially referred to the social work service for assessment of chronically depressed mood, feelings of hopelessness, and low self-esteem. Clinical assessment revealed classic symptoms of dysthymia—chronically depressed mood, irritability, low energy level, low self-esteem, limited social interaction, and feelings of hopelessness and despair.

John related a history of chronic depression beginning in childhood. His presentation was further complicated by a dependent personality disorder, seen frequently in children and adults with chronic illness. As a child, John was dependent on his mother, who now resides with him, and later, on his wife Anne. He describes Anne as his "right hand" and states he would not be able to live without her. John has few social contacts and has been obsessive about hiding his hemophilia from friends and employees.

Clinically, John has been difficult to engage—he avoids eye contact, responds minimally, if at all, to questions posed, and evokes sympathy rather than empathy. John is known to be HIV positive.

Key Concerns

1. John's dual psychiatric diagnosis of dysthymia and dependent personality disorder have reduced his ability to cope effectively with his hemophilia, suggesting that he may not have the emotional resources to cope with a new diagnosis of AIDS.

2. John historically has been resistant to psychosocial intervention and support and has been a difficult client to engage in a relationship.

3. John's cultural beliefs and practices have not allowed him to adopt safer sex practices—specifically, to use condoms. John's wife, Anne, may have been exposed to HIV infection.

4. John's fear of discrimination and ostracism relating to his hemophilia has prompted his secrecy about his disease, thereby limiting social contacts and the availability of a support system. It is likely that his secrecy will extend to his diagnosis of AIDS.

5. John is excluding his children from knowledge of his diagnosis. This exclusion may engender feelings of anger and remorse in his children when they eventually learn of his illness. Additionally, this will preclude them from providing support to their father or seeking support for themselves.

Counseling Plan

1. Become more knowledgeable about patient's cultural and religious values, beliefs and practices, particularly as they relate to death and dying issues, marital relationships, sexuality and child-rearing practices.

2. Develop a trusting relationship with John by providing active listening, emotional support, and assistance with concrete services.

3. Offer psychosocial services to patient's wife and family.

4. Coordinate psychosocial intervention and maintain communication with medical providers in the hemophilia and AIDS clinics.

5. Discuss risk reduction/safer sex practices, and encourage John to involve his wife in counseling.

6. Explore John's reluctance to share his diagnosis with his children and the potential outcomes of both withholding and sharing this information with them.

Discussion Questions

1. How might the patient's cultural and religious beliefs, values and practices influence his emotional responses to an AIDS diagnosis, and to his perceived risk of transmitting HIV to his wife?

2. Given the patient's dual psychiatric diagnosis and, now, a dual medical diagnosis, what specific concerns might you have regarding the patient's ability to process and cope with a life-threatening medical illness?

3. How will you address John's fears and concerns about sharing his illness with family members and friends in an effort to marshall his support system, given the realities of discrimination?

4. Should John continue to dismiss the need for behavior change in his sexual relationship with his wife, how will you address this with him? Would you approach his wife without his consent? If so, how might this affect your relationship with John?

■

Donna DiMarzo, MSW, MPH, was formerly the Northern California Coordinator of the AIDS Help and Prevention Plan (AHPP—a regional AIDS education and risk reduction project) and a Clinical Social Worker in the Comprehensive Hemophilia Treatment Center, University of California San Francisco Medical Center. She is presently the Social Work Coordinator for the HIV Program for Children and Their Families at St. Luke's/Roosevelt Hospital Center, New York, New York.

Mario: A Recent Immigrant

Yvette G. Flores-Ortiz, PhD and Hugh A. Villalta, MA

Mario is a 30-year-old immigrant Mexican male admitted to the AIDS ward with a diagnosis of *Pneumocystis carinii* pneumonia (PCP). Mario is married with two adolescent sons. He denies use of IV drugs; and although he admits to homosexual relations, he denies being gay. His wife, Veronica, is aware of Mario's sexual relationships with men, which she "guessed" because of the "types" of men her husband befriended. Veronica admits that she and her husband discussed his relationships with men on several occasions, but she was not comfortable talking about it, so she stopped bringing up the subject. Mario became ill two weeks ago; Veronica treated him at home with herbs and medicines obtained in Mexico. Mario was assumed to have the flu.

Mario and Veronica are both told of his diagnosis. She does not want the children to know their father has AIDS, and she herself refuses to believe it. The medical staff perceives her as being in denial. They are monolingual Spanish speaking, so a bilingual worker is assigned. The worker explains to Veronica how Mario was infected, her own risk, and the course of the illness. The worker also provides her with social service information. Veronica appears to have difficulty understanding the information and focuses on whether certain herbs might cure him. She decides to take the HIV antibody test herself; the results are negative. The children visit their father on the ward and, since they are bilingual, they clearly understand that this is an AIDS ward. Veronica, however, insists the children should not be told their father's diagnosis.

Mario has been the primary provider for the family; Veronica has been a homemaker. Since Mario's illness, the family has not had enough money for rent or food. Veronica wants her husband cured as soon as possible so the family can get back to normal.

Special Considerations

1. **Generational level.** Are individuals first- or second-generation American immigrants or are they foreign-born? This can be ascertained by inquiring about country of origin, length of residence in the United States, and migration patterns (that is, whether the person came first to a border state or migrated to the border state from another state).

2. **Immigration status.** Undocumented individuals may avoid health providers for fear of deportation.

3. **Region of origin.** Individuals from rural areas may have had little access to health care prior to migration and thus rely primarily on home remedies. Those from large cities may be dissimilar, in terms of health practices, to urban U.S. residents. An important area to assess is the distance from the country or culture of origin. Often gay Latinos feel they need to make a choice between their sexual preference and their ethnic group, thus distancing themselves from family, friends, and other potential sources of support.

4. **Language preference and fluency.** The extent of knowledge of English, the level of comfort in speaking in English or Spanish about health, illness, and sexual practices will directly affect interactions with health care providers.

5. **Family and social supports.** Do individuals have other relatives in the area, including extended families, friends, and neighbors who can be a resource? Do they live in an ethnic neighborhood? Do they belong to a church? Does the patient wish to contact family members in the country or city of origin? Traditional Latino cultures consider the family institution important; thus, family members most often attempt to find solutions that guarantee the survival of the family.

6. **View of health.** How are illnesses and health explained? What role do traditional beliefs that illnesses are caused by imbalances in diet or interpersonal relations, spirit possession and punishment from God for specific transgressions, play in the individual's life?

7. **Cultural beliefs and attitudes about homosexuality.** Attitudes toward homosexuality vary; however, there is a predominant view of homosexual relationships as deviant or

sinful. Often gay people will not label themselves or "come out" publicly. While some men may engage in homosexual relations, they may not consider themselves gay or bisexual. Attitudes regarding permissible sexual behavior often differ for men and women, with men having more freedom to experiment than women.

8. **Health practices.** Use of herbs, folk remedies, over-the-counter prescriptions, and use of needles for injection of vitamins and other medicines is common in Latin America. Drugs, drug use and addicts tend to be viewed negatively. Often drug use among the middle class and more affluent is denied. For patients infected with HIV through needle sharing, disclosure of the illness implies acknowledgement of drug use, which in and of itself may be stigmatizing.

9. **Religion and religious beliefs.** The person's own understanding of God and theology may be a source of strength or conflict. For example, some individuals view homosexuality as sinful, despite their own sexual orientation, and AIDS may be viewed as a punishment from God, and death as the ultimate act of contrition.

10. **General level of acculturation.** This may range from monocultural Latino to quite acculturated to Anglo attitudes, behaviors and values. The level of acculturation may influence whether Western explanations of illness are accepted or understood as well as one's comfort level in discussing sexual practices or topics considered taboo.

11. **Family organization.** How are roles defined within the family? Who makes the decisions (including who is told about the illness)? Who is primary provider? What is the role of the eldest child? What is the role of the extended family, including "compadres" (co-parents, typically godparents of children) and friends?

12. **Socioeconomic status.** The level of education, income, and class in country of origin for immigrants influence socioeconomic status. These factors help determine the level of economic stress and possible sources of support for the family.

Case Discussion

Mario, Veronica and the children are an immigrant family. The family has migrated only recently to the United States. The process of migration typically prompts a crisis with several losses: of family, status, familiar places, and material possessions. The period of adaptation after a migration can tax severely the coping mechanisms of a family. This family is facing a new crisis: the husband is critically ill with a disease the wife has trouble under-standing and accepting. AIDS is still a stigmatizing illness among Latinos, and the wife is likely to feel shame, anger and guilt. She is unwilling to tell the children, who could be a source of support for her and her husband.

The couple appears to have a traditional marriage in which the husband is the primary provider and the wife's main role is that of mother. The family has a traditional value orientation, particu-larly with regard to taboo subjects (the wife is very uncomfortable with discussion of sexual issues, even with her husband), sexual roles (the man has extramarital relationships which are tolerated by his wife), and health beliefs (the wife has relied primarily on herbal medicines).

Furthermore, Mario's acute medical crisis shifts the role of pri-mary parent and major decision maker to Veronica, yet she may have little experience making independent decisions. In addition, the couple appears ill equipped to handle the financial impact of the illness. Veronica may have to become financially responsible for the family, yet she may not have the necessary education or skills to do so. In working with this family in the early stages of hospitalization, the focus of the interventions will be on the wife, as the husband is critically ill.

Key Concerns

1. Difficulty of the wife in accepting the diagnosis.
2. Socioeconomic situation of the family.
3. Management of the husband's illness by the family.
4. The mother's refusal to tell the children.
5. As recent immigrants, they may lack a social support system of family and friends.
6. How has the family coped with other crises in the past?

Counseling Plan

1. Provide the family with appropriate social, financial, cultural, and informational resources.

2. Frame all recommendations, interventions, and advice in terms of their benefit to the family as a whole.

3. Provide Veronica with an opportunity to discuss her changing role in the family. Do not challenge her denial initially, work with it gently by reiterating the facts of Mario's illness simply and precisely.

4. Offer Veronica an opportunity to express any feelings of shame, anger, fear, and sadness. Explain the possibility of a referral to a support group of women in similar situations.

5. Discuss the intrafamilial resources, including the children, on whom she may rely. Help her explore the benefits of telling the children. They may be able to help her carry the emotional and financial burden. They may already know about their father, and talking about their own fears and related feelings may help them.

6. When he is able, discuss these same issues with the husband. Determine whether Mario and Veronica wish to talk with one another about the future (his prognosis, his health needs, how to provide for the family as he convalesces). Assist them in determining when and how to tell the children or other family members.

7. Act as an advocate for the family, serving as a cultural broker who can explain hospital policy and other information to them.

8. Treat this patient and family with utmost respect, including use of formal language and sensitivity in discussing taboo issues. Provide them with education and information that may help them integrate the news of the illness and identify ways to cope.

■

Yvette G. Flores-Ortiz, PhD, is a professor at the California School of Professional Psychology in Berkeley/Alameda, California, and has a private practice in Berkeley, California. Hugh A. Villalta, MA, is a counselor at the Shanti Project and has a private practice in San Francisco, California.

Nicholas: A Heterosexual Alcoholic

Terry Tafoya, PhD

Nicholas is a 30-year-old Native American male, divorced father of one. He is an unemployed carpet layer with a serious drinking history who was recently found to be HIV seropositive after consulting his physician for a variety of complaints, including unusual skin rashes, weight loss, general weakness, and easy bruising. Nicholas denies ever having sexual contact with other men and has a history of multiple female sexual partners. He seeks help from a variety of AIDS service agencies upon learning he is seropositive and is found to be depressed, anxious, rejected by his ex-wife, drinking heavily, and complaining of increasing fatigue.

Nicholas was originally from a small village in rural Alaska. There were several siblings in his family of origin. Following the death of his parents before he was ten years old, the children were all placed in foster care. Nicholas was the only one placed with non-Indian foster parents. Throughout his adult life, he has moved extensively across the United States and often joined Native American organizations in an attempt to establish his "Indianness." This included working with the American Indian Movement (AIM) and spending time with traditional spiritual leaders. The result of these attempts backfired and only emphasized his sense of not actually "belonging." He was even told by a traditional Native elder that he should leave the spiritual encampment and return to the city. This rejection was apparently influenced by Nicholas' short temper and long history of using alcohol and marijuana nearly every day.

Throughout his experience at the Native American clinic, Nicholas was hostile, angry, and depressed. He largely refused to admit his substance use was a problem and while agreeing to participate in a support group, he complained loudly to anyone who would listen that all AIDS support groups available were either "homosexual or Christian" and he could not identify with either.

It was not unusual for him to call the AIDS coordinator of the Indian clinic at 3:00 a.m. to complain about the lack of services, or for him to contact the executive director or board members of the clinic to insist that enough was not being done.

In the beginning the reaction of the clinic was to attempt to involve him in helping set AIDS policy goals, but his inexperience with understanding how systems operate, and his inconsistency in establishing recommendations (for example, adamantly supporting extensive HIV antibody testing, and then reversing himself on this), led many of those involved to question his mental health and the relevance of his service to the clinic. Nicholas has also served on a number of panels as an HIV-positive patient to discuss minority needs and concerns involving AIDS. It was also recently disclosed that he was contacting women he met as a result of his public presentations, utilizing them in much the same way as he has used the AIDS coordinator, calling them early in the morning to state dissatisfaction, particularly after drinking episodes.

Case Discussion

Seeking help from established AIDS agencies is not considered typical for recently diagnosed Native Americans. Help is usually sought first from the family or the Native American community. However, Nicholas did point out that little was being done to provide culturally sensitive service to Native Americans. He went to the local urban Indian clinic and, in a very confrontational style, accused the clinic of "not doing anything about AIDS for Indians." Nicholas was the first HIV-positive Native to come into contact with the clinic. Although an AIDS coordinator had been appointed, and the clinic was working with a coalition of minority AIDS groups, preparing culturally relevant posters and brochures, at that point there was indeed, as Nicholas pointed out, "Nothing about AIDS" displayed in the clinic. At that time, HIV antibody testing was not provided through the clinic. Since then, new priorities have been established by the Indian Health Service and local health officials, resulting in HIV antibody testing services, blind testing for seroprevalence, and free condom distribution at the clinic.

Although Nicholas is not the most typical Native American with HIV Spectrum Disease (a more representative individual would be a gay or bisexual male), he exhibits some interesting qualities and experiences relevant to treatment issues. Since he is literally the first Native American in the Pacific Northwest to "come forward" about his condition, he was viewed by some clinic staff as a valuable resource for providing AIDS education to the Native community.

This situation has been difficult for the clinic, as well as putting Nicholas in the awkward position of having a lifetime of rejection from the Native community for being "too white" in his behavior and upbringing, and then having immediate recognition as the "Indian expert" on the Native AIDS experience.

His rejection of therapeutic assistance seems to be tied to denial related to substance abuse. He has repeatedly turned to supportive Native women, who have no professional training or experience, and who have difficulty setting limits on the nature and extent of their help. This is very indicative of a community trying to organize itself in a crisis mode, to meet the stated needs of a Native man in need, even when those stated needs do not always represent the best interests of the patient.

In addition, Nicholas' experience emphasized the need for strongly coordinated service delivery efforts and utilization of available resources. It is also clear that this case indicates the need to have AIDS policy issues and coordination in place in agencies before the first patient shows up needing services. Finally, Nicholas also illustrates two problems that are common in the Native American community: alcoholism and the issue of non-acceptance when an individual feels that he or she does not "belong" either in mainstream society or in one's racial community. The subsequent problem of isolation can be severe.

Key Concerns

1. Nicholas' continued denial of his substance abuse and treatment for depression.
2. The need to arrange ongoing social services and medical follow-up.
3. The lack of support from any family members or other identifiable peer group.
4. Nicholas' continued acting out and intrusive behavior with clinic staff.

5. Nicholas' verbal skills and ability to mislead case managers about treatment.

6. Lack of supportive services for heterosexuals with HIV infection.

Counseling Plan

1. Develop staff consensus on treatment plan to avoid misunderstanding and pitting one staff member against another. Decide whether and under what circumstances Nicholas should be asked to participate in AIDS forums sponsored by the clinic.

2. Identify a primary therapist. Attempt to formulate an agreement on treatment goals: Nicholas' substance abuse must be confronted directly.

3. Consider contracting with Nicholas regarding his participation in substance abuse treatment. Establish consequences for failure to follow through.

4. Clinic staff need to agree on limits to be placed on Nicholas' interaction with staff. For example, all calls should be referred to the primary therapist.

5. Attempt to identify other Native American substance abuse treatment groups.

6. Once sobriety is attained, reassess for depression. If still significant, consider referral for medication.

■

Terry Tafoya, PhD, is Director of Training, National Native American AIDS Prevention Center; Professor of Psychology, Evergreen State College; and Clinical Faculty, Harborview Community Mental Health Center, University of Washington Medical School.

Randy: Shame and Loss of Face

Kiki Wu Yen Ching, MSW, LCSW, and Richard Daquioag

Randy is a 31-year-old gay male of Chinese/Filipino descent. He is a first-generation American, born and raised in Honolulu. Five years ago, he moved to San Francisco to pursue a Master's Degree in Computer Science. He is one of six children and has two older sisters and one younger brother living in the Bay Area. For the past year, Randy has been living with Harold, his lover of two years. Harold, a forty-year-old Caucasian male, is a real estate agent. Randy's family members avoid the subject of his sexuality and relationship with Harold.

Upon Harold's insistence, Randy began psychotherapy shortly after he developed complaints of sleep disturbance and diminished appetite, which began six months ago, after he learned he was antibody positive. Harold, who took the antibody test at the same time, received a negative result. Randy reports frequent periods of tension in his relationship with Harold. When Harold attempts to discuss Randy's health status and treatment and other HIV-related matters, Randy becomes defensive and withdraws into silences that can last for several days at a time. In their last conflict, the two disagreed about the disclosure of Randy's HIV status: Harold wanted to discuss it with friends and Randy felt his privacy was being violated.

During the course of therapy, Randy expresses fears of failing the family expectations of carrying on the family line as the eldest son, of becoming dependent on his family rather than taking care of them, and of bringing shame to the family if his HIV infection were to progress to AIDS. Additionally, Randy experiences personal shame. He feels that fate has singled him out, as he knows of no other Asian men who are HIV positive, which increases his sense of isolation from the Asian community. Randy is also ashamed of feeling needy. He is concerned about future financial problems, medical expenses and becoming a burden to his lover and family. He has difficulty communicating these concerns and feels angry at people for not knowing what he needs. "They should know what I need, without my having to ask. I wouldn't think of putting people in that embarrassing position. If people were really sensitive, they'd know it's hard to ask for help." If he were to become ill, Randy expresses a fantasy of disappearing to a location where his partner and family wouldn't find him.

Randy maintains a fatalistic attitude toward life and is resigned to the idea that he will die in four or five years. He is dissatisfied with his medical treatment but feels unable to communicate his frustration with his physician. He is confused by medical terminology and feels his physician does not take time to explain his medical condition. Consequently, he fails to keep his appointments. Randy is accustomed to various culturally sanctioned treatment modalities, such as herbal therapy and acupuncture. He is uncertain if they can be integrated with Western medicine and is also concerned that the pursuit of alternative therapies will involve disclosing his HIV status to members of his community.

In therapy, Randy attempts to squash irrational thoughts and unacceptable feelings, such as thinking that he is being punished for not meeting family obligations and feeling resentful that his lover is seronegative. His usual manner is polite and congenial, frequently denying the existence of problems and responding in a confused fashion to the therapist's efforts to explore emotional issues. He spends a great deal of time talking about concrete details. He is reluctant to show his emotions, as he equates this with weakness, and challenges the value of focusing on feelings in therapy. He is uncomfortable talking about sex, and topics of illness and death are avoided because he was taught that verbalizing them would bring about their occurrence.

Key Concerns

1. Randy's fear of bringing shame to his family exacerbates his isolation and lack of support.
2. He is not engaged in his medical treatment and does not see it as beneficial.

3. His discomfort with affective expression can result in somatization, confounding a clear distinction between HIV-related symptoms and psychosomatic symptoms.

4. Because Randy and Harold have different communication styles, conflicts within the relationship are not resolved.

5. Cultural attitudes related to direct expression of needs create obstacles to the client's needs being addressed.

Counseling Plan

1. Acknowledge and respect the client's experience of bringing shame upon himself and family, while reaffirming that he is not to blame for his situation. Appreciate that Asian-Americans are conflicted by two cultural value systems, the Asian system requiring one's personal needs to be put aside in deference to the larger good of the family, and the American system emphasizing individual autonomy. The client should be given support for the choices he has made and will continue to make within this continuum. Reassure him that other Asian-Americans experience similar conflicts, and attempt to connect him with other gay Asians. Encourage him to test his family's ability to respond positively to his situation. Is there a family member he can imagine approaching? Identify, develop, and utilize potential sources of support, with emphasis on the concept of kinship systems. Expand the client's extended family network to include church, social organizations, etc., which Asians traditionally rely on in times of crisis.

2. Asians are taught to respect, without question, institutional authority, such as the medical profession. Encourage the client to take a more active role in asking medical questions and participating in his own treatment planning. Role playing may be helpful. Help the client identify the benefits of both Western and alternative therapies, calling upon the healing traditions of his culture. Assist him in becoming familiar with the social service system.

3. Given conflicting cultural norms and communication styles, normalize the client's difficulty in expressing emotions. Give the client control by reinforcing his power to regulate the pace of his affective expression, while facilitating the process. Asians

typically experience public display of feelings as a "loss of face" in contrast to the value placed on the ventilation of feelings in Western psychotherapy. Work with the client to learn ways to express his feelings. Asians often experience emotional and psychological stress in the form of physical ailments.

4. Focus on "here and now" material, and use the therapeutic relationship to assist the client in developing his ability to communicate his HIV experience. Gently push him to begin talking to his partner about his HIV concerns. Work to determine what kind of support he might need while rehearsing how he might go about asking for support. Help him identify alternative ways of coping. The couple may need to be referred to couples counseling to strengthen their problem-solving ability. Their communication patterns and role distributions may have functioned adequately until the couple system became overloaded by HIV stressors. Help client retain control and autonomy without excluding his partner and potential others from involvement.

■

Kiki Wu Yen Ching, MSW, LCSW, Department of Public Health, is a social worker for the San Francisco Community Mental Health Service and a board member of the Gay Asian Pacific Alliance Community HIV Project (GCHP). Richard Daquioag is a social worker with the UCSF AIDS Health Project and a board member of GCHP.

■

Reed: A Physician's Assistant

Scott K. Morris, PA-C, BHSc

Reed is a 38-year-old physician's assistant with over ten years' experience. For the past eighteen months, he has been working in an HIV Clinic. He had inserted and removed hundreds of needles without incident and always followed CDC guidelines for preventing exposure by wearing gloves and using proper technique. On this occasion, he was removing a 22-gauge butterfly needle from the arm of an asymptomatic HIV-positive person. After he had successfully removed the butterfly from the patient's arm, his attention was distracted as he went to place it on his work table. The needle flipped up, penetrating his glove and into the palm of his hand. As soon as he had bandaged the site on the patient's arm, he immediately removed his gloves and washed the area with Hibiclens soap solution. Reed was up to date on his tetanus immunization and had completed a series of Hepatitis B vaccine. He reported to Employee Health, where an HIV antibody test was run and subsequently reported as negative. Despite the fact that Reed knew that the risk of seroconverting after a single exposure was approximately half of one percent, he nonetheless elected to enter into a post-exposure zidovudine protocol.

Key Concerns

1. The employee's status has suddenly changed. Now he is a statistic, one of several thousand health care workers who have been exposed to HIV on the job. Despite knowing the odds of seroconverting, he worries that he could be in that half of one percent that become positive.

2. He has already decided to confront his current antibody status by being tested and is relieved to know that he is negative. He knows that, however remote, the chance does exist that he could seroconvert.

3. Now he must decide who, if anyone, he should tell about his exposure. Should he tell his new wife of six months, and if he does, how will she react? Should he tell his co-workers, and what will their reaction be?

4. He needs to talk to someone about these worries and decisions that he has to make.

Counseling Plan

1. Determine how he has coped with working in an HIV Clinic full time. Has he had any reservations about working with this population group or fears about occupational exposure?

2. It is apparent that his level of knowledge of HIV transmission is high and that he is also aware of the low probability of seroconversion after a single exposure. These statistics should be reinforced by the counselor.

3. Support within his unit will undoubtedly be high. A counselor should attempt to elicit what support will be forthcoming within the home setting. How knowledgeable is Reed's wife about HIV and its transmission?

4. Suggest that he and his wife meet with the counselor together to discuss any fears she may have or that they may have together.

5. Consider whether more intense therapy is needed over time for either Reed or his wife. Are they interested in ongoing sessions to help manage their anxiety?

Discussion Questions

1. How far would you take the discussion regarding seroconversion?

2. Would you ask him what he would do if he did seroconvert or just emphasize the low probability?

3. Would you recommend his wife come in for antibody testing?

■

Scott K. Morris, PA-C, BHSc, is Clinical Coordinator, AIDS Clinical Trials Unit, Duke University Medical Center, Durham, North Carolina.

Shannon: A Blood Donor

Margo Nason, RN

Although all potential blood donors are carefully screened for possible HIV-related risk factors, they do not receive the same counseling process as those tested at an alternative test site (ATS). The ATS client is encouraged to do a "benefit-risk" analysis in deciding whether or not to take the HIV antibody test. At blood banks, the purpose of the screening process is to ensure the safety of the blood supply. In most states, positive test results must be given within a designated period of time from the donation date, and the main thrust of counseling and referrals takes place at this later time.

The counselor at the blood bank sent a certified letter informing Shannon of her positive HIV antibody status. When Shannon did not call to make an appointment to discuss these results, the counselor personally contacted her by telephone. Shannon sounded very casual but agreed to an appointment time the following day. When this appointment time had come and gone, the counselor called again, this time waking her at noon. Shannon explained that she had overslept, and scheduled another appointment for the following day. Shannon asked if she could bring her boyfriend, and the counselor agreed.

Shannon was a lovely 18-year-old blue-eyed blond. She was dressed fashionably and casually, much like other teenage girls her age in San Francisco. Well mannered, soft-spoken, and somewhat shy, Shannon showed no overt signs of concern about the information contained in her letter. Nine months previously, when she was 17, Shannon had been recruited to donate blood at her high school. The first donation tested negative for antibodies to HIV and was transfused. It was shortly after this initial donation that Shannon and her mother, a single parent with a new romance taking much of her time, began fighting. Soon, for Shannon, home was an unpleasant place to be. Shannon had a part-time job after school, where she was attracting the attention of the male employees her age. The most sympathetic to her plight was Kevin, a young man of 19 who soon persuaded Shannon to live with him. She and Kevin moved in together and began a sexual relationship. Although Shannon had received sex education, including AIDS prevention information, at her high school, the couple's method of birth control was "the withdrawal method." Four months later, Shannon donated blood a second time, only this time the blood tested HIV positive and was discarded. By California state law, Shannon was notified 60 days later.

When interviewed for risk factors, Shannon denied any IV drug use; in fact, the only significant change in Shannon's life since her initial donation was her sexual relationship with her new boyfriend. Kevin denied any bisexual relationships; however, he indicated he had previously used IV drugs, but he denied ever sharing needles. He had had casual sex with several female partners and was not sure of their risk factors. At this time, Kevin requested that he be tested, and Shannon asked that she be given another HIV antibody test to rule out any possibility of lab error.

By now, Shannon and Kevin seemed anxious to leave and get on with their day. In case they were going to have sexual contact before their appointment scheduled the following week (or in case the couple failed to keep their next appointment), the counselor felt it necessary to provide safer sex information before they left. Shannon especially seemed unaware of the potential risks to a child should she become pregnant. Both Shannon and Kevin appeared to be very uncomfortable talking about sexual matters, so they were also given literature to read when they were able to be more receptive to this information.

Although they were late, Shannon and Kevin kept their second appointment. Shannon was informed there had been no error on her test, and Kevin was informed that his test was also positive. They were unable to look at one another, and then Kevin announced that they needed to leave to get to work on time. When the counselor asked Shannon how she was feeling, Shannon looked down at her left wrist and replied, "I think I need to buy a new watch."

Key Concerns

1. The client is unable to take in or comprehend this new information; this denial could be life threatening.

2. The client has a questionable understanding of basic AIDS information, safer sex guidelines, and birth control issues.

3. This young client needs to begin to develop problem-solving skills and coping strategies to handle this life-threatening news. This is a task at odds with her stage of development.

4. The client has a limited support system and is currently estranged from her only family member, her mother.

Counseling Plan

1. Assess the client's level of comprehension regarding HIV infection.

2. Obtain a complete risk factor history.

3. Determine other important factors in the client's life, including social and emotional support structure. Identify appropriate support service options for the client and the couple.

4. Determine if the client has medical coverage. Discuss the advantage of receiving periodic health exams with a knowledgeable physician. Discuss confidentiality issues.

5. Provide both verbal and written information on safer sex guidelines and other HIV-related topics. Be sure the client knows how to use condoms and that she has access to them.

Discussion Questions

1. How would you help this young client express the emotional impact of her positive antibody status?

2. What are the specific considerations in counseling an HIV-positive woman who has just turned 18 years old and wants "to think about other things" appropriate to being a teenager?

3. What would be the best approach for providing persuasive birth control information to a client this age?

4. What are the unique needs of a client who has not had pre-test counseling and is virtually unprepared for the impact of positive HIV test results?

■

Margo Nason, RN, is a Counselor and Researcher at Irwin Memorial Blood Bank in San Francisco.

Beverly: A Transfusion Recipient

Margo Nason, RN

Although all potential blood donors are carefully screened for possible HIV-related risk factors, they do not receive the same counseling process as those tested at an alternative test site (ATS). The ATS client is encouraged to do a "benefit-risk" analysis in deciding whether or not to take the HIV antibody test. At blood banks, the purpose of the screening process is to ensure the safety of the blood supply. In most states, positive test results must be given within a designated period of time from the donation date, and the main thrust of counseling and referrals takes place at this later time.

Beverly is a 36-year-old woman, married and the mother of a four-year-old daughter, Jenna-Rain. At the time of her blood donation, Beverly considered herself to be "a full-time Mom." She and her husband, Russell, recently became owners of their first home. It was at this time that the 60-day rule of notification was applied and Beverly was informed of her positive HIV test results.

Russell had been a long-term donor at the blood bank. A friend's child who had leukemia needed O+ blood; and since both Beverly and Russell had O+ blood, Russell encouraged Beverly to be a "designated donor" for this child in need. Beverly decided to help but was also a "little nervous." She had had a transfusion in 1982 during the last trimester of her pregnancy, and she was vaguely concerned about her risk of HIV infection. Except for this low, but nevertheless potential risk, there were no other factors in her history to exclude Beverly from donating. Her donation was screened and confirmed to be HIV positive, and her unit of blood was discarded. Sixty days later, Beverly learned that she had been the recipient of HIV-positive blood—before AIDS was well known to the public and before the HIV antibody test had been made available to blood banks.

Beverly came to her first counseling session with her husband at her side. First came the tears and then Beverly's utmost concern:

"What about Jenna?" Beverly felt that she could ultimately cope with her own infection, but she could not bear to know that she had infected either Jenna or Russell. Jenna had, of course, been exposed to the same HIV-positive transfusion; in addition, she had enjoyed breast-feeding for almost an entire year. But Jenna was a radiant, robust, outgoing four-year-old with no history of health problems. Still, Beverly and Russell now had to consider whether or not to have their daughter tested. Other issues began to emerge. It was presumed that Russell was HIV negative all along or otherwise the blood bank would have notified him previously. (To protect the blood supply, Russell was informed that he was no longer eligible to donate.) Still, he wanted to be tested again to have baseline results before he and Beverly began practicing safer sex. And what changes would "safer sex" bring to their marital life, and what about having another child? Later, Beverly would say that her menstrual blood had always been a positive symbol of her womanhood and fertility and how painful it was to view this blood instead as being potentially lethal.

Beverly began to consider where, besides Russell, she would find emotional support. She had always been the strong one in her family—now, how would her parents and siblings react? If her friends found out, would they still allow their young children to play with Jenna? Would Beverly still be allowed to participate in her daughter's co-operative nursery school? Beverly was eager for referrals and acknowledged her need to talk with other women and share her feelings. So began Beverly's personal journey until ultimately she asked, "What can I give to this epidemic?" which led her eventually to do such things as speak publicly at local conferences on issues related to women and AIDS.

When Beverly and Russell bought their home, part of the plan had been that she would return to work and share this new financial burden. Would she be able to do her share, and how could she safeguard her health? Beverly began to talk a lot about her priorities and organize her life around the things that really mattered to her. "It's funny," she says, "but now I really do stop to smell the roses."

Key Concerns

1. What will be the long-range impact of this information on Beverly's marriage?

2. Beverly is uncertain about telling her family and friends and worries about their reaction.

3. The client must incorporate this new information into her self-image as a healthy person. She worries about her ability to maintain her responsibilities as a wife and mother.

4. The client is uncertain about how to or whether to make long-term plans.

Counseling Plan

1. Obtain history of the client's risk factors and assess level of HIV awareness, transmission, and prevention.

2. Acknowledge the client's feelings of shock and anger and her fears and concerns for her immediate family. Guilt may also be a factor if her husband or child are also infected.

3. Since there was no formal pre-test counseling, discuss such issues as confidentiality and legal concerns. Explore "if, when, and how" to tell others of her antibody status.

4. Advise a medical checkup to determine overall health and any possible symptoms of HIV.

5. Offer follow-up counseling, telephone contact, and other referrals for support services for women and for transfusion recipients.

Discussion Questions

1. What are the special considerations involved when a client has not had formal pre-test counseling?

2. What information should the client have to help make a decision about HIV testing for her daughter?

3. What unique issues might occur for a client who is infected through a prior blood transfusion?

■

Margo Nason, RN, is a Counselor and Researcher at Irwin Memorial Blood Bank in San Francisco.

Appendices

■

Appendix A
Natural History of HIV Disease

William Lang, MD

Since the description of AIDS in 1981, when epidemic Kaposi's sarcoma and *Pneumocystis carinii* pneumonia were first reported in otherwise healthy gay men, HIV has been isolated and established as the cause of AIDS. Since that time, the natural history of HIV infection has become increasingly better defined. The purpose of this discussion is to describe the stages of HIV infection, and the expected course and outcome of each of these stages. The relationship of each stage to the basic science of the disease will also be described.

Stage 1: Acute Infection

The natural history of HIV disease can be readily divided into three stages, the first of which is infection. In order for infection to occur, an individual must first be exposed to HIV-infected material through high-risk sex, needle use, contaminated transfusion, or from infected mother to fetus. Exposure to the virus does not always result in infection, but infection can never occur without exposure. Certain kinds of exposure carry significantly higher risk of infection than others. For example, transfusion recipients of HIV-infected blood almost always become infected. Babies born to HIV-infected mothers, on the other hand, become infected during pregnancy only about 30%-50% of the time. Similarly, certain types of sexual activity have been shown to carry a higher risk of infection than others. Receptive anal intercourse, for example, whether homosexual or heterosexual, has been shown in a number of studies to be the most efficient method of sexual transmission of HIV. Additionally, infection from heterosexual intercourse appears to occur more readily from men to women than from women to men, but is quite unpredictable.

The number of exposures required to result in infection also varies. Sometimes infection occurs with relatively few or perhaps even a single exposure, while in other situations, infection does not occur despite a high number of exposures. In very rare situations, infection of a caretaker has occurred from caring for an HIV-infected person. So far these have only been observed when caregivers have exposed their open cuts to significant amounts of HIV-infected body secretions (such as blood or stool or become infected through occupational exposures, most often due to needlestick injuries or when caregivers have exposed their open cuts to significant amounts of HIV-infected body secretions (such as blood or stool or wound drainage). No documented case of HIV infection has been reported from living day to day with people who are infected with HIV even though thousands of people with AIDS or HIV infection share their homes with family and friends.

Infection, then, occurs only when HIV successfully enters the body and incorporates itself into host cell DNA. In most individuals who become infected the virus multiplies rapidly and spreads widely throughout the body. Sometimes, though not always, this stage of initial infection is accompanied by an acute flu-like illness with fever, muscle aches, rash, swollen lymph nodes, sore throat and headache within a few weeks of exposure. Usually, however, infection occurs without the individual having any awareness of illness, and it is most often detected either by a positive HIV antibody test, or quite a bit later in the course of HIV infection (in the last stage) when severe immune depletion results in serious illness.

The end of this first stage of HIV infection is usually marked by a significant reduction in the number of T helper-cells in the blood of infected persons. While individuals' experiences may vary, generally, T helper-cells, an important component of the immune system, fall by approximately one third of their usual value, from an average of about 1000 cells per microliter to about 650 cells per microliter, during the first year of infection. The number of T-helper cells then usually falls more slowly, suggesting that the body's immune defenses are having some success in fighting the virus. One frequent physical manifestation of this immune response is swollen lymph nodes around the neck, in the armpits, groin and elsewhere. This finding is seen in more than half of infected individuals and usually persists for long periods. Altogether the first stage of infection probably occurs over 6-12 months.

Stage 2: Latent Infection

The second stage of infection is best characterized as silent infection. Most individuals during this stage feel well and have little if any indication of infection. When signs of infection are present, they are usually confined to swollen lymph nodes or perhaps complaints of fatigue, which are difficult to distinguish from the fatigue of chronic anxiety. Quite often infected people are indistinguishable from uninfected people at this stage except for changes in laboratory values.

During this second stage, and throughout all stages of infection, the HIV antibody tests remain positive. Probably the most important laboratory test during this phase is the T-helper cell count, which usually continues to fall slowly but progressively.

This stage of disease is monitored by following the patient's symptoms and physical exam as well as a number of laboratory tests. These blood tests include T helper-cell counts; beta$_2$ (B$_2$m) microglobulin levels, a measure of lymphocyte fragments thought to be indicative of lymphocyte destruction; and the p24 antigen. When p24 antigen is detectable, or when B$_2$m levels are rising, there is a substantially higher chance that a severe illness will develop in the following year or two.

A falling level of T-helper cells, rising beta$_2$ microglobulin or the presence of p24 antigen can mark the end of this second or latent stage of HIV infection. This stage usually lasts an average of three to five years, although many have remained in this latent stage for nine or ten years and some even longer. The antiviral drugs zidovudine (AZT), didanosine (ddI), and zalcitabine (ddC) can lengthen the time individuals remain in this stage. By using the monitoring tests outlined above, physicians now have a rational basis by which to make decisions about when to begin treatment with AZT; for example, when T helper-cell counts fall to the level of approximately 500 cells per microliter, most physicians would evaluate the overall status of the patient and consider starting treatment with AZT.

Stage 3: Clinical Disease

The end of the latent second stage and the beginning of the clinical third stage of HIV infection is often blurred. However, when T helper-cell counts fall below 200, the immune system is no longer functioning well enough to ward off certain illnesses. These illnesses are caused by organisms that generally do not cause disease in healthy individuals, but take advantage of poor host defenses and cause one or more of the "opportunistic infections," such as *Pneumocystis carinii* pneumonia (PCP), that have come to be associated with a diagnosis of AIDS. Some of the

Table 1. Stages of HIV Infection

I. Acute Infection
    a. Requires exposure to the virus
    b. Viral infection and spread
    c. Early immune response and development of antibodies
    d. "Flu-like" syndrome possible
II. Latent Infection
    a. Lack of physical symptoms except lymphadenopathy/fatigue
    b. Low level of viral activity
    c. Progressive loss of T helper-cells, rise in beta$_2$ microglobulin
    d. Fall in p24 antibody, appearance of p24 antigen
III. Clinical Disease
    a. Development of opportunistic infections and tumors

manifestations of the third stage—increased fatigue, oily skin rashes, and hairy leukoplakia (a viral infection that causes a milky white coating on the tongue)—are very subtle, and it is often difficult to pinpoint their onset. Other phenomena such as shingles (a painful viral infection of the nerve tracts) or Idiopathic Thrombocytopenia Purpura (ITP or low platelet counts) may occur and then resolve while the individual becomes asymptomatic again. Nonetheless, as this stage progresses, T helper-cell levels continue to fall and clinical manifestations of immune suppression become more obvious. For example, the occurrence of thrush, or oral candidiasis (a fungal infection in the mouth), or a marked worsening of herpes infections is usually a clear signal of the immune system's progressive debility. From this point, a major opportunistic infection such as PCP or a tumor such as Kaposi's sarcoma usually occurs within months to a year or two.

Progression to this third stage of clinical disease occurs in approximately 80% of people who have been infected for ten years. In the one study which has observed infected people for this long, 50% have developed AIDS and another 38% have developed symptomatic HIV infection. Most researchers fear that even more people will go on to develop overt disease as the duration of infection stretches out past this ten-year mark. Overall, this last stage of infection lasts from a few months to as long as several years, but on average, death occurs within 18-36 months.

In 1993, the Centers for Disease Control amended the definition of AIDS to include those with less than 200 T helper-cells. In addition, the definition added HIV infected people with any form of tuberculosis (an increasingly common serious illness among people infected with HIV), those with recurrent bacterial pneumonia, or infected women who develop cancer of the cervix. This amended definition is beneficial in giving a better picture of the scope of the HIV epidemic in the United States, but it does not change the course of the three basic stages of infection as described above.

Table 2 . Laboratory Evaluation of HIV Infection

Detection of Infection

HIV Antibody - establishes presence or absence of viral infection

Measures of Severity of Disease

T Helper-Cell Number - important immune cells directly affected by HIV infection

Beta$_2$ Microglobulin Level - pieces of lymphocytes found circulating in the bloodstream

p24 Antigen - Viral particle present in bloodstream with increased levels of HIV activity

Treatment

Fortunately, there have been some developments that have had a clear-cut beneficial impact on the short-term outcome of this third stage of HIV infection. AZT has come into widespread use since it was shown in 1986 to lengthen the lives of people with AIDS (PWA's) and symptomatic infection. Many PWA's taking the drug feel better and survive approximately 12-18 months longer than those not taking AZT. Nonetheless, the duration of benefit of AZT is limited, and most people with AIDS progress to more severe disease and death in spite of treatment. In addition, because AZT has significant potential toxic side effects, not everyone can take it for prolonged periods.

ddI and ddC, like their chemical cousin AZT, have recently been approved for use in late stage HIV infection. Although there has been no proof as yet that they will prolong life, especially after prolonged AZT use, they have shown the ability to increase T helper-cell counts and diminish p24 antigen levels. They also have the benefit of not causing the same kinds of toxicity as AZT and, therefore, are particularly useful for people who can't tolerate AZT.

Recent studies have combined AZT with ddI or with ddC resulting in a rise in T helper-cells (ddI and ddC have not been used together because

Table 3.   Management of HIV Infection

Monitoring

Allows assessment of immune status and estimates risk of opportunistic infection.

Prophylaxis

Oral antibiotics, especially trimethoprim/sulfa and Dapsone or aerosolized pentamidine lengthen the time to occurrence of PCP in moderately and severely immunocompromised people.

Treatment

Zidovudine (AZT) is effective in prolonging life and improving well-being for a period of months to years in most moderately to severely immunocompromised people. Toxicity is a potential limiting factor.

Didanosine (ddI) and zalcitabine (ddC) are now available for use when AZT no longer prevents a decline in T helper-cells, or is not well tolerated.

Other treatments remain unproven.

Treatment for specific infections and tumors is often effective at least for a limited period of time. Treatment is usually more effective if infections are detected and treated early.

they cause similar toxicities). This approach is logical and combination therapy has promise with AZT, ddI and ddC as well as with newer experimental drugs.

Another area of progress in the treatment of late stage HIV infection has been the development of drugs for opportunistic infections and cancers. These new drugs have provided alternatives for patients allergic to standard treatments as well as improvements in effectiveness and safety. They also are being used effectively as preventative measures to decrease the chances of recurrent or new opportunistic infections.

Earlier treatment, before the development of signs of late stage disease, is another relatively recent trend. Most doctors now recommend starting treatment with AZT when T helper-cells fall below 500. Aside from the benefit of decreasing serious complications of HIV disease, AZT also has a much lower likelihood of serious side effects in this healthier group of people. Other forms of treatment—to inhibit viral growth and improve immune function—are being actively pursued in research settings, and by individual physicians and people with HIV.

In the meantime, physicians have become much more adept at monitoring the effects of HIV infection and treating some of its manifestations. Knowledgeable doctors see their infected patients at regular intervals depending on the patients' particular circumstances. By monitoring T helper-cells, beta$_2$ microglobulin, and p24 antigen as well as by a careful history and physical examination, physicians can determine the stage of infection and provide a rough estimate of how much time there may be before the infection progresses to a more serious illness. For those with signs of more advanced immunodeficiency, prophylactic treatments aimed at forestalling the development of opportunistic infections have become standard care. Antibiotics such as Septra or Dapsone or aerosolized pentamadine provide a significant degree of protection against PCP. More frequent monitoring also allows earlier recognition and treatment of many HIV-related illnesses.

In summary, this description of the natural history of HIV infection is an overview of a process with many individual variations. While in the majority of individuals each of these stages is retrospectively discernible, there are exceptions to the rule. There are cases in which infection has resulted in a prompt and rapid decline in helper cells progressing to AIDS within a year. There are also cases in which HIV infection has been present for many years without progressive decline of immune function. Nevertheless, for the majority of those infected with HIV, the natural history of this disease is relatively well understood and stands as a challenge for all to find a means of more effectively altering its course.

■

Bibliography

AmFAR Directory of Experimental Treatments for AIDS and ARC. New York, Mary Ann Liebert, Inc. Publishers, 1987-1993

Centers for Disease Control: 1993 Revised Classification System for HIV Infection and Expanded Surveillance Case Definintion for AIDS Among Adolescents and Adults. MMWR 1992; 41;(RR-17): 1-18

Centers for Disease Control: Public health service statement on management of occupational exposures to HIV, including considerations regarding zidovudine post-exposure use. MMWR 1990; 39;(Supp. RR1)

Chamberland ME, Bell DM: HIV transmission from health care worker to patient: What is the risk? Ann Intern Med 1992; 116:871-872

Fox R, Eldred L, Fuchs E et al: Clinical manifestations of acute infection with human immunodeficiency virus in a cohort of gay men. AIDS 1987; 1:35-38

Graham NMH, Zeger SL, Park LP, et al: The effects on survival of early treatment of human immunodieficiency virus infection. New Eng J Med 1992; 326(16): 1037-1042

Gwinn M, Pappaioanou M, George JR, et al: Prevalence of HIV infection in childbearing women in the United States: surveillance using newborn blood samples. JAMA 1991; 265:1704-8

Lang W, Perkins H, Anderson RE, et al: Patterns of T-lymphocyte changes with human immunodeficiency virus infection: from seroconversion to the development of AIDS. J Acq Imm Def Syn 1989; 2(1):63-69

Levy J: Mysteries of HIV: challenges for therapy and prevention. Nature 1988; 333:519-523

Moss A, Bacchetti P, Osmond D, et al: Seropositivity for HIV and the development of AIDS and AIDS related conditions: three year follow up to the San Francisco Hospital cohort. Br Med J 1988; 296:745-750

Padian N: Heterosexual transmission of acquired immunodeficiency syndrome: international perspectives and national projections. Rev Infect Dis 1987 (Sep-Oct); 9:947-960

Richman D, Fischl M, Greico M, et al: The efficacy of azidothymidine in the treatment of patients with AIDS and AIDS-related complex: a double-blind, placebo-controlled trial. New Eng J Med 1987; 317:192-197

Winkelstein W, Lyman D, Padian N, et al: Sexual practices and risk of infection by the human immunodeficiency virus: the San Francisco Men's Health Study. J Am Med Assoc 1987; 257:326-330

■

William Lang, MD, is Clinical Director of the San Francisco Men's Health Study and Vice President of Clinical Research for ViRx, Inc., in San Francisco.

Appendix B
Information About Your Test

(Note: This information is provided as a sample of the kind of material that should be made available to those receiving a positive antibody test. This brochure is used at the Anonymous Test Sites in San Francisco.)

You have tested positive for HIV infection. You may be feeling scared, confused, or angry. Along with these emotions, you may have many questions about your health condition and its impact on your life. We hope these pages will help answer some of your questions and identify resources that will help you cope.

Meaning of Positive Test Results

1. *Does being antibody positive mean I have AIDS or ARC?* No. The test does not diagnose AIDS. But it does mean that the virus that causes AIDS is in your body and that you can spread the disease to others.

2. *What does testing HIV positive mean?* A positive test result means that you have been infected with the virus that causes AIDS (Acquired Immune Deficiency Syndrome) and ARC (AIDS-Related Complex) conditions and that your body has produced antibodies against the virus. The test does not directly detect the presence of the virus, called the HIV virus (Human Immunodeficiency Virus). Instead, it detects the presence of antibodies, which indicate the presence of the virus. Some of the terms used to refer to this positive condition are HIV positive, antibody positive, or seropositive.

3. *If I have antibodies, doesn't that mean I have antibodies that are fighting the HIV virus?* Yes, but unfortunately the kinds of antibodies that your body produces are only effective for a limited time in fighting the virus.

4. *Will I get AIDS or ARC?* Based on what is known right now about the progression of HIV infection, your chance of developing AIDS or AIDS-related symptoms in the future is probably quite high. Recent studies indicate that most people infected with the HIV virus will develop AIDS or AIDS-related symptoms within seven to twelve years of infection. The critical issue is when—and that is where you can help yourself. (See the "Staying Healthy" Section.)

5. *Could my test results have been wrong?* **Probably Not.** If your test was done at a San Francisco County Alternative Test Site (ATS), your blood has tested positive in four (4) separate tests. ATS blood samples are first tested using a test called the ELISA, which is a highly accurate test. If the sample tests positive, it is retested two more times with the ELISA. If it still tests positive, another test called the IFA (immuno-fluorescent assay) is performed. If the test result is positive on all four of these tests, it is concluded that the sample is positive.

6. *Can I be retested?* **Yes.** You can repeat the test as often as you like, but based on what we know about HIV infection, once your blood test is positive it will continue to be positive.

What Now?

1. *Why me?* We don't know why some people who are exposed to the virus become infected, while others who are equally exposed to the virus do not. The fact that you have antibodies to HIV in your blood simply tells us that you were exposed to the virus at some time in the past and became infected.

2. *Am I contagious to others?* **Yes.** The virus can be transmitted through sexual contact involving body fluids (semen and vaginal secretions), by activities that can lead to the exchange of blood (such as sharing needles when using drugs), and from a mother to her unborn or nursing baby. There is no evidence that HIV can be transmitted by casual contact. It is safe to continue working, to share eating utensils, to hug your friends, and to live in close quarters with others. (See the "Stopping the Spread of the Disease" Section for more information.)

3. *My partner is not positive; is (s)he immune?* **There is no known immunity to HIV infection.** We know that some people who have engaged in high-risk behaviors test negative. However, we don't know if they will continue to test negative. We urge all people to avoid exposing themselves and others to the virus.

4. *What do symptomatic and asymptomatic mean?* A person is described as symptomatic when(s)he is HIV positive **and** has symptoms related to HIV infection. Some of these symptoms are swollen lymph glands, a yeast infection in the mouth (candidiasis), or chronic fevers or diarrhea. **A person can be symptomatic and not have AIDS.** To be diagnosed with AIDS, a person must have specific symptoms that meet the requirements of the AIDS diagnosis. A person is described as asymptomatic when(s)he is HIV positive but does not show any symptoms.

Whom Should I Tell?

1. *Should I tell others that I'm HIV positive?* It is important for most people to have others they can talk to for support. However, you should be careful that your results are shared only with persons you can trust to keep the information confidential. Discrimination has occurred in employment, housing, and obtaining insurance coverage. You should give careful thought to what could happen if your test results become common knowledge. Since there is no risk to others through casual contact, it is not necessary to inform your boss, co-workers, or casual acquaintances that you are positive.

2. *Should I tell sexual and/or needle-sharing partners?* Consider informing partners who might not otherwise know that they may have been exposed to the virus. If past or present partners are not aware of their risk for infection, they cannot make an informed decision about taking the test, taking care of their health, or preventing the spread of the disease. Some individuals feel that telling partners risks the confidentiality of their HIV status, and these persons simply make a commitment to safe behavior.

3. *What should I tell my partner(s)?* We encourage you to discuss safe sex practices and to agree on what kinds of sexual activities you will practice and which ones you will not. If you are an IV drug user, talk about the importance of using clean needles. (See the "Staying Healthy" Section for more information.)

4. *Should I tell my doctor and dentist?* Before telling your doctor and dentist, ask them how they will record the information. Decide if their method is acceptable to you. Also before telling your current doctor, you may want to find out if (s)he has experience treating HIV infection. If not, you may want to change physicians, which will eliminate the need to share this information. (See the "Medical Follow-Up" Section for more information.) **Cautions.** Recent changes in state law give doctors the power to inform your partners of your HIV status. In addition, if your HIV status is in your medical record, it may affect your insurance coverage. **Why You May Want to Tell.** Your doctor and dentist can both watch for signs or symptoms of HIV-related illnesses. Also, advances in medical treatments are being made, and it is important for your doctor to actively assist you in dealing with the HIV infection.

5. *Will information in my medical chart about my HIV status be confidential?* A Word of Caution. Insurance companies have access to medical records and have been known to cut off coverage to persons with HIV infection. All information contained in medical records is available to insurance companies when you apply for health, life, or disability insurance. An insurance company's

knowledge of your positive test may result in the denial of future requests for coverage or benefits. Dentists and physicians can keep your HIV status in a special section of your chart (or in a separate chart) that is not released to insurance companies. Explore with your physician his or her willingness to keep HIV antibody test results (and the results of other tests that indicate antibody status) out of your records. You might ask: "If I tested positive, would you find it necessary to document that in my record?"

Medical Follow-up

1. *Should I see a doctor?* **Yes.** It is important that you see a physician who is knowledgeable about HIV infection as soon as possible. There are treatments available that may help to delay the onset of symptoms. Don't wait to go to the doctor unitl you feel sick. If you are not feeling well, you should see a doctor immediately.

2. *What will the doctor do?* The doctor will probably want to give you a complete physical exam to determine your current health status and to establish baselines against which changes in your health can be measured.

3. *What should I do if I don't have a doctor?* If you have health insurance, you can call the Bay Area Physicians for Human Rights (415-673-3189) for a referral to a doctor who is HIV sensitive. Unfortunately, if you do not have health insurance and cannot afford to pay for medical care, your options are more limited. (See Appendix C: National AIDS Support Organizations.)

4. *What kinds of additional tests should I take?* Some of the special HIV-related tests that your doctor might recommend include the following:

   - A skin test for tuberculosis (TB), called a PPD.
   - A blood test for syphilis, called a VDRL.
   - A test for intestinal parasites (particularly for persons who have anal sex).
   - Tests that are used to measure your immune status and monitor the progression of the HIV infection. Such tests include the T4, which counts the number of T4 cells in your blood; the p24, which looks for the presence of p24 (a part of the AIDS virus) in your blood; and the $Beta_2$ Microglobulin, which is a test of the destruction of cells in your blood. Please note that there is some controversy about the use and meaning of some of these tests, so you will want to work closely with your doctor on these matters.

5. *Won't my insurance be cut off if I take additional tests?* **A Word of Caution.** If you can afford it, you may want to pay cash for AIDS-

related tests and not have these tests appear on your insurance form. Even if the results of these tests are normal, insurance companies have been known to deny coverage to people who take these tests.

6. *Should I start drug treatments?* There is a growing consensus that early intervention with antiviral treatments may slow the progression to AIDS. For this reason, some HIV-positive people (especially those with AIDS-related symptoms) choose to take the FDA-approved medication AZT or other experimental drugs and treatments. Project Inform (415-558-9051) provides extensive information regarding new drug treatments that are currently being studied and used by leaders in the HIV treatment field. In all cases, talk with your doctor before starting any treatments or experimental drug protocols.

7. *What about alternative healing?* Many HIV-positive people choose to use a variety of alternative healing resources, either alone or in conjunction with traditional Western medicine. Acupuncture, chiropractic medicine, nutritional supplements/special diets, massage/bodywork, visualization, hypnosis, meditation, and spiritual exploration are among the treatments used.

8. *How will I know if I start to get sick from AIDS?* AIDS is actually a term that includes several different kinds of illnesses. Although the progression of HIV disease from the asymptomatic condition to full-blown AIDS usually follows a pattern of progressive illness, the pattern varies in each individual. Some common early symptoms are fever, night sweats, or a persistent cough. These conditions may worsen, or you may develop other symptoms. **If you start to feel sick, see a doctor immediately. If you do not have insurance, contact the Centers for Disease Control (CDC) National AIDS Hotline (800-342-2437). They will direct you to the nearest county facility.**

Staying Healthy

1. *What should I do to stay healthy?* There is still much to be learned about why some people who are HIV positive develop AIDS and others do not. Follow a "common sense" approach to taking an active role in maintaining your health:

   - *Sleep.* Get enough sleep.
   - *Diet.* Eat a balanced diet.
   - *Exercise.* Exercise regularly.
   - *Stress.* Reduce the stress in your life. Seek out a stable support system and, above all, work at maintaining a healthy outlook and a positive attitude. The AIDS Health Project (415-476-6430) offers a variety of groups for stress reduction, health promotion, and emotional support.

- *Drugs, etc.* Limit the use of tobacco, alcohol and other drugs. These drugs can suppress your immune system and weaken your body. If you use IV drugs and must share needles or syringes, flush the works twice with bleach followed by twice with water.

- *Sex.* Always insist on safe sex.

2. *What about exposure to other diseases or to vaccines to prevent diseases?* Protect yourself from exposure to diseases or to live vaccines, such as polio or measles vaccines. Live vaccines cause a mild case of the disease being vaccinated against. This mild disease could be harmful to someone who has HIV infection and a weak immune system. If you have a child who is due for a vaccination, consult your physician about risks associated with your exposure.

3. *Since I am already HIV positive, can I have unsafe sex with another person who is also positive without hurting myself?* No. As an HIV positive person, you need to do everything possible to stay healthy. Your good health is your best protection against the development of AIDS and AIDS-related symptoms. There are many strains of the HIV virus. Unsafe sex exposes you to these other strains and to other sexually transmitted diseases. If you are having sex with someone who is also HIV positive, you should **always** be practicing safe sex. It is protecting both of you. Remember, your health is dependent on maintaining a strong immune system. When you are exposed to viruses, your immune system is further weakened.

Stopping the Spread of the Disease

1. *What should I do to prevent infecting others?* Do not do anything that allows your blood or sexual body fluids to be transferred to another person.

- Do not have unsafe sex.

- Do not share IV drug needles.

- Do not donate blood or plasma for transfusion, sperm for artificial insemination, or body organs for transplantation. If you are listed as an organ donor, remove that designation from your driver's license.

- Do not share toothbrushes, razors, acupuncture or tattoo needles or other items which may be contaminated with blood.

- Do not leave accident surfaces uncleaned. If you have an accident that results in bleeding, wash surfaces with soap and warm water. For surfaces that require special care, wash with one part bleach to ten parts water.

2. *Can I still have sex?* **Yes.** But you need to practice safe sex in order to protect yourself and to keep from spreading the disease to others.

3. *What sexual activities are considered safe?* Any activities which don't involve sharing body fluids—semen, blood, vaginal secretions and breast milk—are safe. Kissing, hugging and mutual masturbation are safe.

4. *What sexual activities are "probably safe"?* Anal and vaginal sex using a condom and nonoxynol-9 are probably safe. Use latex condoms and water-based lubricants. As an added protection, it is recommended that the receptive partner use a spermicidal foam with nonoxynol-9. Sexual activity in which the exchange of bodily fluids is stopped by a condom or barrier is probably safe. Oral sex on a man is also probably safe if it is done with a condom, or without putting the head of the penis in the mouth. Oral sex on a woman is probably safe if it is done with a barrier that keeps vaginal secretions from coming in contact with the partner.

5. *What sexual activities are "unsafe"?* Unprotected (no condom) anal, vaginal, and oral sex is **unsafe.** Always use a condom when having anal and vaginal sex. Always use a condom or barrier when performing oral sex and bodily fluids are involved. Unprotected oral sex, whether performed on a man or woman, is considered unsafe when bodily fluids come into contact with a partner. When performed on a man, it is unsafe when pre-ejaculate or semen (cum) enter the mouth. When performed on a woman, it is unsafe when vaginal secretions enter the mouth.

6. *What do I do if I like to drink and do casual drugs?* The best choice is to stop drinking and using drugs. People who are intoxicated or "high" are more likely to do things that place them at risk of contracting or transmitting HIV. For example, if you are "high," you may be more inclined to have sex without condoms.

7. *What do I do if I am an IV drug user?* Get help to stop using. Sharing needles and syringes is the surest way to pass the AIDS virus from the blood stream of one person to another. If you haven't stopped shooting drugs, don't share your needles. If you must share your needles, clean them first.

Here's how to clean a needle:
- Flush the needle two times with bleach.
- Then flush the needle two times with water.
- **DO NOT** shoot or drink the bleach.

8. *What if I can't stop using IV drugs?* Get help. Most people need help to beat an addiction.

Special Considerations

Pregnancy

1. *I want to get pregnant. Should I? A Word of Caution.* It is estimated that there is a 30%-50% chance of a woman passing the AIDS virus on to her baby. The virus can be transmitted while you are pregnant, when you give birth, or through breast-feeding. Most physicians recommend that women with a positive test result not become pregnant until more is known about AIDS and pregnancy. Talk with your partner, doctor, a health worker, or an AIDS information agency.

2. *What do I do if I am already pregnant?* It is possible to transfer this infection to your unborn child during pregnancy even if you remain healthy. At some point, you will probably want to notify your doctor, since your HIV-positive status could influence your health care treatment needs. Before sharing your results with your doctor, first explore their willingness to keep your positive test results out of your (and your baby's) permanent medical records.

3. *I am positive and just had a baby. Could my child also be HIV positive?* Yes. There is a 30%-50% chance that the AIDS virus will be transferred from you to your baby (see above). Talk with your doctor about whether your child should have the antibody test. Also, since HIV has been found in breast milk, your doctor will probably recommend that you bottle-feed rather than breast-feed your baby.

A Final Word

The news that you have been infected with HIV is not easy to receive. It is important that you establish a close relationship with someone you can trust so that you can speak openly about your feelings, problems and any fears you might have.

If you want a referral to an AIDS-sensitive mental health professional or peer support group, call the AIDS Health Project at 415-476-6430. Ask about our "Positives Being Positive" peer support program.

The U.S. Public Health Service has made AIDS and AIDS virus-related illnesses its number one priority. Scientists all over the world are working to find ways to eliminate this disease. A great deal of progress has been made in a short period of time. There is every reason to expect that these advances will continue.

■

Information About Your Health *is published in pamphlet form by the AIDS Health Project (AHP) for distribution to persons who test positive at the Anonymous Test Sites in San Francisco. AHP, Box 0884, San Francisco, CA 94143-0884, (415) 476-6430.*

Written by Neil Seymour, MFCC. Edited by Peter V. Campos and Eileen Eya. Portions derived from materials provided by the Contra Costa AIDS Program.

Appendix C
National AIDS Support Organizations

AIDS Action Council
1875 Connecticut Avenue,
NW, Suite 700
Washington, DC 20009
(202) 986-1300

American Associations of
 Physicians for Human Rights
Medical Expertise
 Retention Program
273 Church Street
San Francisco, CA 94114
(415) 255-4547

American Foundation for AIDS
 Research (AmFAR)
733 Third Avenue, 12th Floor
New York, NY 10017-3204
(212) 682-7440

American Hospital Association
Advisory Committee on
 Infections within Hospitals
840 North Lakeshore Drive
Chicago, IL 60611
(312) 280-6000

Centers for Disease Control
National AIDS Hotline:
(800) 342-2437
Spanish line: (800) 344-7432
Hearing Impaired line:
(800) 243-7889

Lambda Legal Defense
 and Education Fund
666 Broadway
New York, NY 10012
(212) 995-8585

National Gay and Lesbian
 Task Force
1734 14th Street, NW
Washington, DC 20009
(202) 332-6483

National Center for
 Lesbian Rights
1663 Mission Street, 5th Floor
San Francisco, CA 94103
(415) 621-0674

National Hemophilia Foundation
Soho Building
110 Greene Street, Suite 303
New York, NY 10012
(212) 219-8180
FAX: (212) 966-9247
H.A.N.D.I.: (212) 431-0906

National Institute of Allergy
 and Infectious Diseases
Office of Research Reporting and
 Public Response
(301) 496-5717
Clinical Trials: (800) 874-2572

National Lesbian and
 Gay Health Foundation
P.O. Box 65472
Washington, DC 20035
(202) 797-3708

National STD Hotline:
(800) 227-8922

National Task Force on
  AIDS Prevention
631 O'Farrell Street
San Francisco, CA 94109
(212) 749-6700

National Association of Black
  and White Men Together
2261 Market Street
Box 506
San Francisco, CA 94114

Project Inform
1965 Market Street, Suite 220
San Francisco, CA 94103
National: (800) 822-7422
Hotline: (415) 558-9051
Office: (415) 558-8669

Public Health Service
AIDS Clinical Trials
Information Service
(1) (800) TRIALS-A

World Health Organization
525 23rd Street, NW
Washington, DC 20037
(202) 861-3200

Canada

AIDS Committee Toronto (ACT)
P.O. Box 55, Station F
Toronto, Ontario M4Y 2L4
CANADA
(416) 926-1626

Australia

AIDS Action Committee
GPO Box 5074
Sydney 2001
Australia
(02) 211-1177

New Zealand

New Zealand AIDS Foundation
P.O. Box 6663
Wellesley Street
Auckland, New Zealand
(09) 33-124

Appendix D
Updates: New Issues

Since *Face to Face* was first published in 1989, two new psychosocial issues have arisen affecting, in particular, communities that have weathered the epidemic since its genesis. Multiple loss and relapse to unsafe sex occur after years of watching people die and abstaining from once cherished but now dangerous sexual activities. We include here two articles, published in 1992 and 1993 in our eight-page, monthly review *FOCUS: A Guide to AIDS Research and Counseling*, that address these concerns.

Coping with Multiple Loss

Tom Grothe, RN, MA and Leon McKusick, PhD

Many people engulfed by the AIDS epidemic can no longer tally the number who have died. Mothers who have seen HIV spread through their families, friends close to a gay community besieged by the epidemic, health care workers who have watched dozens of their patients die: all have struggled with this continuing pain. In Africa, where whole families and lineages have been wiped out, grief affects entire countries.

Urban gay men, in particular, are subject to multiple loss, and mourn not only those who have died, but also all the ways their lives have been diminished by the deaths of so many. They have lost leaders and role models; their fondness for their past—the time before the epidemic; and their hopes for the future. And, of course, many gay men mourn the loss of health even before they become ill.

Research on gay men in San Francisco reveals increasing levels of depression with each year of the epidemic, and also a greater likelihood of depression among men experiencing a higher number of deaths and among men who are HIV-infected and symptomatic.[1] Another study indicates that social support is crucial in mitigating symptoms of depression in men with AIDS:[2] ironically, the deaths that cause the depression also deplete the social support networks necessary to deal with multiple loss. In response to such data, health professionals are developing ways to help those overwhelmed by multiple loss.

Bereavement Theory

Bereavement theory offers insights when searching for tools to alleviate the turmoil of multiple loss. For example, William Worden identifies four progressive tasks of bereavement:[3] to accept the reality of the loss; to experience the pain of grief; to adjust to an environment in which the deceased is missing; and to withdraw emotional energy and reinvest it in another relationship. While these tasks are essential, they are based, like most bereavement theories, on the experience of one death causing pain and followed by healing. With AIDS, however, the dying continues, and if the bereaved were to feel the ongoing pain of multiple losses, they would never get beyond acute grief.

In some cases, this psychological flooding of emotion incapacitates rather than heals, and to defend against this flooding, some people become emotionally numb. These alternatives to coping with massive loss have been identified before as the two phases of post-traumatic stress syndrome: intrusive-repetitive and denial-numbing.[4] While in most cases multiple loss does not cause post-traumatic stress syndrome, the similarities of these phases can offer ways to work with the multiply bereaved.

Mardi Horowitz suggests that mental health practitioners encourage individuals in the denial-numbing phase to reexperience their feelings by retelling the traumatic events.[4] To respond to the intrusive-repetitive phase, during which clients may feel overwhelmed with emotion, therapists should provide leadership and external structure. They should encourage clients to reduce stresses and even suppress painful emotions.

While suppressing emotion may seem to limit psychological work, Verena Kast suggests a way therapists can continue ongoing, in-depth work without focusing on a client's pain.[5] She believes people can learn as much about themselves by examining their joys as they do by examining their sorrows, and she encourages therapists to help clients create autobiographies of joy. By searching for and exploring past moments of joy and connection, clients are able to recreate these emotions. Kast also notes that even during hard and painful times, there are quiet joys to be cherished.

Viktor Frankl, a concentration camp survivor who lost his family in the Nazi holocaust, developed a school of existential psychotherapy to respond to questions like, "What is the purpose of my suffering?" His theories may be particularly meaningful to those who are multiply bereaved. Frankl believes meaning in life is derived in three ways: creating a work or doing a deed; experiencing something or encountering someone; and, when we can no longer act, being aware of the attitude we take toward unavoidable suffering, the courage and grace we are able to summon when all else is lost.[6]

Each of Frankl's meanings moves a person beyond a focus on self and pain. Through creativity or human connection, they can help those overwhelmed by multiple losses remain involved in life. This is particularly important, since Susan Folkman has found that among gay men affected by the epidemic, those who coped with stress by remaining involved in life became less depressed over time.[7] In addition, maintaining a positive attitude in the face of random suffering promotes coping by increasing self-esteem and maintaining a sense of purpose.

Interventions

Ultimately these theories are limited; an individual must forge his or her own meaning from loss. A synthesis of these theories, however, may provide therapists with a practical approach for dealing with multiple loss. Among the key interventions are:

1. Witness the pain. All bereaved people, particularly those struggling with multiple loss, have a tremendous need to tell their stories. Expressing the pain allows catharsis and healing.

2. Help clients stay involved. Anything that focuses a client outside of him or herself can promote involvement: work, social contact, education about HIV, activism, and protest.

3. Assist people in creating meaningful rituals. Ritual allows people to express feelings while connecting them to spirituality. Rituals also bind people together in a common expression of grief. The AIDS Memorial Quilt, funerals, and memorial marches are examples of rituals that bring people together.

4. Provide structure and support when emotional flooding overwhelms clients. Instruct clients in ways to divert attention from flooding by using activity and relaxation. Action, instead of immobility and fear, can promote a sense of mastery and control, and improves coping.

5. Refocus individual clients on the elevating emotions—joy and hope— by assisting with the development of an autobiography of joy. Encourage individuals to focus collective efforts to honor all that is good in a community overwhelmed by loss, perhaps by developing a community autobiography of joy.

The multiple losses that people experience as a result of HIV disease can be overwhelming and depressing. Therapists need to help individuals and communities maintain purpose while living with unending loss.

■

References

1. McKusick L, Hilliard R: Multiple loss accounts for worsening distress in a community hard hit by AIDS. Presentation from the VII International Conference on AIDS, Florence, Italy, June 1991.

2. Hays RB, Tobey LA: The social support networks of gay men with AIDS. Journal of Community Psychology 1990; 18: 374-385.

3. Worden W: Grief Counseling and Grief Therapy: a Handbook for the Mental Health Practitioner. New York: Springer Publishing, 1982.

4. Horowitz M: Stress Response Syndromes. Northvale, New Jersey: Jason Aronson Inc., 1986.
5. Kast V: Joy, Inspiration, and Hope. College Station: Texas A & M University Press, 1991.
6. Frankl V: Man's Search for Meaning. New York: Washington Square Press, 1959.
7. Folkman S, Chesney M, Pollack L, et al: Coping and changes in depression among gay men of San Francisco. Unpublished manuscript.

Behavioral Theories and Relapse

David Silven, PhD

At a recent discussion of health educators about relapse into unsafe sex among gay and bisexual men, a participant suggested that theory-based principles of behavior change be used as guides to develop relapse prevention interventions. Other participants responded with skepticism; the majority seemed to agree that theory should remain in the classroom.

What use, if any, does theory have in the critical area of sexual relapse prevention? To address this question, this article summarizes four basic behavior theories—The Health Belief Model, Social Cognitive Theory, Stages of Change, and Marlatt's Relapse Prevention Model—and examines the applicability of these theories in planning prevention interventions.

The Health Belief Model

The Health Belief Model grew out of research in the 1950s and 1960s—by Irving Rosenstock and colleagues at the United States Public Health Service—that investigated the widespread failure of people to take preventive health measures such as annual physical checkups, and screening tests for tuberculosis and dental disease. The model postulates that individuals will take preventive actions when they:

- believe that they are susceptible to a disease that would have at least moderately severe negative consequences;
- believe that taking such actions will be beneficial in reducing the threat of the disease and that this benefit will sufficiently outweigh the costs, such as the inconvenience and effort required, embarrassment, and financial expense;
- perceive a stimulus or "cue to action": either internal, for example, the perception of an uncomfortable bodily state; or external, for example, mass media campaigns, newspaper articles, or personal knowledge of someone affected by the disease.

The perception of threat and the occurrence of a cue to action, which raises awareness of feelings of threat, lead to the decision to act. The direction that action takes is influenced by beliefs about the relative availability and effectiveness of alternatives for reducing the threat, which, in turn, are influenced by social norms.

Social Cognitive Theory

Albert Bandura's Social Cognitive Theory suggests that in order to take a particular course of action, individuals must not only possess the required skills but must also believe that the action will lead to a desired outcome and that they are personally capable of performing the action. This belief in personal capability, known as "self-efficacy," is a pivotal concept in Bandura's theory: it influences how much effort a person invests in an action and how long he or she will persevere in the face of difficulties or disappointing results.

An individual develops self-efficacy by accumulating feedback from four primary sources: personal experience of successfully performing the behavior; vicarious experience through observing others perform the behavior ("modeling"); persuasion by others who convey that the individual is capable of performing the behavior; and physiological states.

Of these four sources of information, successful performance or "mastery" experiences are considered the most potent in raising levels of self-efficacy. Proficiency with new behaviors requires extensive practice. Ideally, this practice occurs with considerable external guidance, encouragement, and feedback; it progresses gradually to more challenging situations, the removal of external support, and increased opportunities for self-guided practice. Failure and difficulty during the learning process help build a resilient sense of self-efficacy by providing experience in overcoming setbacks.

Through modeling, people learn skills and judge their capabilities in comparison to others. It is crucial that individuals perceive themselves as similar to the models they observe, particularly in terms of the degree of hesitancy and fear they feel in challenging situations.

Persuasion by others provides encouragement that can lead people to believe they are capable of performing a desired behavior. The impact of persuasion varies according to the perceived credibility of the persuader.

Finally, individuals rely partly on their physiological state to judge their abilities to perform target behaviors. Self-efficacy is strengthened when people possess skills to reduce uncomfortable physiological reactions, such as agitation, and insight to interpret these reactions as normal rather than as a sign of inefficacy.

Stages of Change

In the early 1980s, James Prochaska and Carlo DiClemente outlined several fundamental stages through which individuals typically progress when making behavioral changes: precontemplation, contemplation, action, and maintenance of change. During the precontemplation stage, people are unaware—because they are uninformed or in denial—of having a problem in need of change, even though others may perceive the problem.

In the next stage, contemplators are seriously thinking about, but not committed to, changing their behavior. They tend to be relatively open to feedback and education about the problem behavior. The contemplation stage ends at the point that a commitment to change is made.

Progression through the stages is cyclical rather than linear. People will often revert to an earlier stage, which is then repeated. Relapse is seen as leading back to either the contemplation stage, from which the individual may again attempt to change, or to the precontemplation stage, during which the individual succeeds in avoiding, at least temporarily, having to think about the behavior as a problem.

People utilize different processes of change during the various stages. In the contemplation stage, for example, the processes include information-seeking and evaluation of one's behavior. In the action and maintenance stages, processes include changing the environment to build in supports for new behaviors and to minimize risk-associated stimuli, and developing new responses to these stimuli.

Marlatt's Relapse Prevention Model

Alan Marlatt and his colleagues developed in the mid-1980s a cognitive-behavioral model that focuses on coping during "high-risk situations," situations that pose a threat to the individual's sense of control and increase the risk of relapse. According to the theory, lapses—or single incidents of slipping into the avoided behavior—are considered important and expected components of the behavior change process. Through trial-and-error, new response patterns in high-risk situations are gradually acquired, corrected, and strengthened.

Whether lapses are followed by a total relapse, that is, a return to baseline levels of the behavior, is largely determined by how the individual reacts to the lapse: this is called the "Abstinence Violation Effect." If he or she perceives the slip as a response to a particularly difficult situation or as a sign that he or she needs more practice with the new behavior, the lapse is unlikely to lead to relapse. On the other hand, if the individual attributes the slip to personal weakness or failure, the risk of relapse is greatly increased.

Another aspect of the Abstinence Violation Effect is the experience of cognitive dissonance resulting from the contradiction between the individual's self-perception as an abstainer and the occurrence of the prohibited behavior. This dissonance creates conflict or guilt and motivates efforts to eliminate these unpleasant feelings. Thus, people may engage further in the prohibited behaviors in an attempt to produce positive feelings to replace these unpleasant ones. Alternately, there may be a change in self-image as lapsers begin to think of themselves as non-abstainers. In either of these cases, the stage is set for relapse.

Additional factors contributing to the risk of relapse include the use of denial to mask the potential negative consequences of slipping, and rationalization to justify the prohibited behavior based, for example, on the extreme demands of everyday life. Finally, relapse may be seen as the result of a chain of decisions leading to a high-risk situation.

Applying the Theories

These theories suggest several reasons why sexual relapse might occur and guidelines for how to minimize the risk of its occurrence. First, as suggested by the Health Belief Model, people may relapse because they no longer perceive unsafe sex as a significant problem. As suggested by the Stages of Change theory, behavior change may naturally involve back-and-forth movement among stages, including repeated reentry into the precontemplation stage of unawareness. Alternately, people may initially change behavior from unsafe to safer sex as a result of external pressure, and prior to a firm internal commitment to safer sex; once the external pressure diminishes, the behavior change breaks down. A third explanation, using Marlatt's model, is that people fail to perceive unsafe sex as a problem because of the psychological denial they employ to avoid anxiety.

HIV-infected people, in particular, may relapse because they question the legitimacy of warnings against the dangers of "re-infection" by HIV. Others may be unaware of the seriousness of the risk to their immune systems of other diseases that can be contracted through unsafe sex.

Successful prevention efforts should first establish whether the target audience is fully aware of the dangers of unsafe sex before proceeding with information about prevention strategies. For those who are not yet committed to avoiding unsafe sex, educators might direct efforts at mobilizing interest in exploring whether a problem really exists. For those who are misinformed or uninformed, providing information about risk is critical.

Second, as suggested by the Health Belief Model and Social Cognitive Theory, people may relapse because they are not convinced that safer sex adequately reduces the chances of infection. Specifically, they may question whether condoms are truly effective barriers against transmission. They may have heard stories about condoms breaking, or about people becoming infected presumably without having participated in unsafe sex or other high-risk activities. Again, supplying clear and credible information—in this case, about the effectiveness of condoms—would seem critical.

Third, people may relapse because, as the Health Belief Model further suggests, they do not feel convinced that the health benefits of safer sex outweigh the effort required to avoid unsafe sex. As Marlatt points out, those who experience day-to-day life as full of demands may reach a point where they no longer feel motivated to pursue long-term goals—in this case, health and longevity—that involve depriving themselves of short-term pleasure or relief. Or, they may not feel they have the internal strength and resources needed for prolonged efforts avoiding unsafe sex. This may be particularly true of many who are feeling the effects of loss and grief. Help in coping with extreme stress, depression, and loss may be necessary before these individuals can feel renewed commitment to safer sex.

Fourth, according to Social Cognitive Theory and Marlatt, people may relapse because they do not have, or do not feel they have, the necessary skills to avoid unsafe sex in all situations. This may result from insufficient trial-and-error learning. People may lack skill or confidence in using condoms or in having satisfying forms of safer sex that do not require condoms. They may also lack the skill or confidence required to effectively deal with various situations that can easily lead to unsafe sex. These include negotiating or talking about safer sex with partners; insisting on safer sex; coping with stress related to social anxiety; and responding to social or internal pressures to drink or use drugs in conjunction with sex.

Finally, according to Marlatt, people who relapse may lack the awareness or resolve to break the chain of events that tends to lead to high-risk situations. For example, a man may be unable to stop himself from going to a bar to find a sex partner, despite the fact that he knows that this will lead to the pressure to drink heavily, the likelihood that he will become intoxicated, and the heightened risk that he will engage in unsafe sex as a result. Furthermore, they may lack the ability to see failures or setbacks as normal parts of the learning process, leaving them unable to rebound when slips do occur.

Conclusion

These theories suggest that behavior change interventions must go beyond providing prevention information and limited practice with condoms. Educators must make efforts to identify additional areas in which target audiences lack skills, including negotiating safer sex and avoiding situations in which sex and mind-altering substances are mixed. They must help people acquire skills and achieve mastery, provide practice in coping with mistakes, and prepare individuals for the possibility that lapses may occur. Finally, for those not ready to commit to avoiding unsafe sex, supplying basic information may be ineffective without efforts to address the reluctance to change.

■

Further Reading

Bandura A: Self-efficacy: toward a unifying theory of behavior change. Psychological Review 1977; 84:191-215.

Bandura A: Social Foundations of Thought and Action: A Social Cognitive Theory. Englewood Cliffs, NJ: Prentice Hall, 1986.

Marlatt A, Gordon JR (eds.): Relapse Prevention: Maintenance Strategies in Addictive Behavior Change. New York: Guilford Press, 1985.

Prochaska JO, DiClemente CC: Transtheoretical therapy: Toward a more integrated model of change. Psychotherapy Theory, Research, and Practice 1982; 19(3): 276-288.

Prochaska JO, DiClemente CC: Stages and processes of self-change of smoking: toward an integrative model of change. Journal of Consulting and Clinical Psychology 1983; 51: 390-395.

Rosenstock IM: Historical origins of the health belief model. Health Education Monographs 1974; 2(4): 328-335.

■

Tom Grothe, RN, MA is Charge Nurse at Coming Home Hospice in San Francisco and a private mental health practitioner under supervision who focuses on chronically and terminally ill clients and multiple bereavement. Leon McKusick, PhD is a Research Psychologist at the Center for AIDS Prevention Studies of the University of California San Francisco (UCSF), and a therapist in private practice. He is a pioneer in AIDS behavioral and psychosocial research focusing on gay men.

David Silven, PhD is a clinical psychologist in private practice in San Francisco and Clinical Consultant to Community and Client Services at the UCSF AIDS Health Project.

Index

RELATED PUBLICATIONS

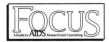

FOCUS: A Guide to AIDS Research and Counseling

This monthly newsletter reviews the counseling aspects of AIDS: how HIV-related counseling is affected by the medical, epidemiological, and social realities of AIDS, as well as the emotional response to the disease. Since 1985, FOCUS has been an indispensable reference for the 25,000 counselors, health providers, and scholars who read it.

**RISK
AND
RECOVERY**
AIDS, HIV
AND ALCOHOL

Risk and Recovery: AIDS, HIV and Alcohol

This book provides essential information about the connections between alcohol use and HIV disease—information that can save lives and protect sobriety; information that every counselor working in substance abuse treatment or HIV-related counseling should know. The book includes workshop guidelines on safer sex, deciding to take the HIV antibody test, and responding to HIV-related grief.

AIDS Law
for
Mental
Health
Professionals

AIDS Law for Mental Health Professionals

This book explores the legal and ethical issues confronting therapists when they treat people with concerns about HIV disease. Using clear, understandable, and jargon-free language, the book covers the variety of situations counselors are likely to encounter and makes them accessible and real by using case vignettes. While focusing on California law, the book discusses issues relevant to practitioners everywhere.

AIDS,
The Brain,
and Behavior
*A Practical Guide for
Mental Health Providers*

AIDS, The Brain, and Behavior:
A Practical Guide for Mental Health Providers

As people with HIV disease live longer, they are more likely to undergo neurological changes that alter thinking, movement, emotions, and personality. This 80-page guide provides practical diagnostic and treatment information about the range of neurological conditions that affect people with HIV disease including HIV-associated dementia, opportunistic conditions such as toxoplasmosis and lymphoma, and organic affective disorders such as mania and depression.

**THE EFFECTS
OF AIDS
ON THE BRAIN**

The Effects of AIDS on the Brain

Prepared for families, friends, and caregivers, this brochure examines the neurological symptoms of HIV infection and offers helpful information on the management of patients with these problems.

Order form on reverse

ORDER FORM   *See previous page for book descriptions*

NAME _____   DAY PHONE (___) _____

TITLE _____

ORGANIZATION _____

ADDRESS _____

CITY/STATE/ZIP _____

	Price x	Quantity =	Total
AIDS, The Brain, and Behavior: *A Practical Guide for Mental Health Providers*	$7.95 x	_____ =	_____
Face to Face: A Guide to AIDS Counseling	$16.95 x	_____ =	_____
Risk and Recovery: AIDS, HIV and Alcohol	$16.95 x	_____ =	_____
AIDS Law for Mental Health Professionals	$19.95 x	_____ =	_____
The Effects of AIDS on the Brain	$.65 x	_____ =	_____
$.45 *each for quantities of 25 - 249* x		_____ =	_____
$.40 *each for quantities of 250 - 499* x		_____ =	_____
$.35 *each for quantities of 500 or more* x		_____ =	_____
FOCUS/Individual Subscription	$36.00 x	_____ =	_____
foreign = $48.00 x		_____ =	_____
FOCUS/Institutional Subscription	$90.00 x	_____ =	_____
foreign = $110.00 x		_____ =	_____
Shipping	$4.00 *first item* x	_____ =	_____
$1.00 *additional items* x		_____ =	_____
does not apply to **FOCUS**			
Sales tax (add 8.5%)	*California residents only* x	_____ =	_____
does not apply to **FOCUS**			

Payment

❑ **Check enclosed** *Please make check payable to UCSF AIDS Health Project*

❑ **VISA**   ❑ **MasterCard**   *Account number* _____

Expiration date _____   *Signature* _____

❑ **Bill me** (*net 30 days*)   *Purchase order number* _____

Signature _____

Mail order to: UCSF AIDS Health Project, Box 0884, San Francisco, CA 94143-0884

To fax orders: 415/476-7996, **For further information call:** 415/476-6430